Handbook of Breast Cancer and Related Breast Disease

Handbook of Breast Cancer and Related Breast Disease

Editors

Katherine H. R. Tkaczuk, MD, FACP
Professor of Medicine
University of Maryland School of Medicine;
Director, Breast Evaluation and Treatment Program
University of Maryland Greenebaum Comprehensive Cancer Center
Baltimore, Maryland

Susan B. Kesmodel, MD
Assistant Professor of Surgery
University of Maryland School of Medicine;
Division of General and Oncologic Surgery, Department of Surgery
Director of Breast Surgery, University of Maryland Medical Center
Baltimore, Maryland

Steven J. Feigenberg, MD
Professor, Radiation Oncology
Department of Radiation Oncology
Director for Clinical Research
Director of Stereotactic Body Radiotherapy Program/Director of
    Emerging Technologies
University of Maryland School of Medicine
Baltimore, Maryland

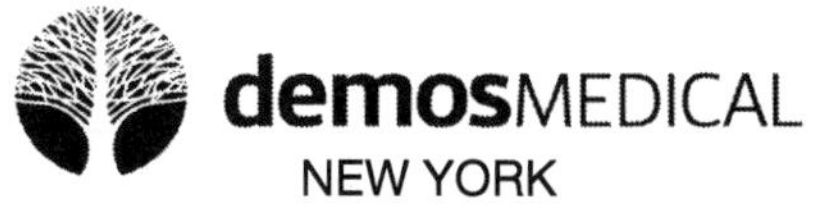

demosMEDICAL
NEW YORK

Visit our website at www.demosmedical.com

ISBN: 9781620700990
e-book ISBN: 9781617052767

Acquisitions Editor: David D'Addona
Compositor: Exeter Premedia Services Private Ltd.

Library of Congress Cataloging-in-Publication Data

Names: Tkaczuk, Katherine H. R., editor. | Kesmodel, Susan B., editor. |
    Feigenberg, Steven J., editor.
Title: Handbook of breast cancer and related breast disease/editors,
    Katherine H. R. Tkaczuk, Susan B. Kesmodel, Steven J. Feigenberg.
Description: New York: Demos Medical Publishing, [2017] | Includes
    bibliographical references and index.
Identifiers: LCCN 2016037911 | ISBN 9781620700990 | ISBN 9781617052767 (e-book)
Subjects: | MESH: Breast Neoplasms
Classification: LCC RC280.B8 | NLM WP 870 | DDC 616.99/449—dc23
LC record available at https://lccn.loc.gov/2016037911

Printed in the United States of America by McNaughton & Gunn.
16 17 18 19 20 / 5 4 3 2 1

*To all providers who take care of patients with
breast cancer and breast diseases and
to our patients and their families*

Contents

Contributors   *ix*
Preface   *xiii*

1. Breast Imaging: Breast Cancer Screening, Diagnosis, Staging, and Surveillance   *1*
   Cristina Campassi, Lyn Ho, Jessica Galandak, Sergio Dromi, Divya Awal, Daniel Maver, Jasleen Chopra, and Sonya Y. Khan

2. Management of High-Risk Breast Disease   *21*
   Arielle Cimeno, Stephanie Richards, Susan B. Kesmodel, Olga Ioffe, Katherine H. R. Tkaczuk, and Emily Bellavance

3. Phyllodes Tumor   *39*
   Jolinta Lin, Elizabeth Nichols, Susan B. Kesmodel, Dina Ioffe, Olga Ioffe, and Katherine H. R. Tkaczuk

4. Management of Ductal Carcinoma In Situ   *49*
   Susan B. Kesmodel, Natalie O'Neill, Steven J. Feigenberg, Alex Engelman, Katherine H. R. Tkaczuk, Susan Shyu, and Olga Ioffe

5. Early-Stage Invasive Breast Cancer   *73*
   Paula Rosenblatt, J. W. Snider III, Steven J. Feigenberg, Neha Bhooshan, Sally B. Cheston, Susan B. Kesmodel, Lindsay Hessler, Julia Terhune, Olga Ioffe, Rachel White, Yang Zhang, Ina Lee, Krista Chain, Chad Tarabolous, Rawand Faramand, Angela DeRidder, Jennifer Ding, and Katherine H. R. Tkaczuk

6. Metastatic Breast Cancer   *174*
   Katherine H. R. Tkaczuk, Paula Rosenblatt, Angela DeRidder, Syed S. Mahmood, Reshma L. Mahtani, Geetha Pukazhendhi, Susan B. Kesmodel, Jason Molitoris, and Randi Cohen

7. Breast Cancer in Pregnancy   *223*
   Ewa Mrozek, Susan B. Kesmodel, and Katherine H. R. Tkaczuk

8. Breast Cancer Reconstruction   *231*
   Rachel Bluebond-Langner, Erin M. Rada, and Sheri Slezak

9. Genetic Syndromes Associated With Increased Risk of
Breast Carcinoma   *251*
Jessica Scott and Carolyn Rogers

10. Integrative Approaches to Symptom Management in Breast
Cancer Patients   *264*
Ting Bao

11. Breast Cancer Survivorship   *286*
Paula Rosenblatt, Ikumi Suzuki, Angela DeRidder, and Nilam Patel

Index   *307*

Contributors

Divya Awal, MD, Clinical Fellow, Department of Radiology, University of Maryland Medical Center, Baltimore, Maryland

Ting Bao, MD, DABMA, MS, Integrative Medicine Specialist, Department of Integrative Medicine, Memorial Sloan Kettering Cancer Center, New York, New York

Emily Bellavance, MD, Assistant Professor, Department of Surgery, University of Maryland School of Medicine, Baltimore, Maryland

Neha Bhooshan, MD, PhD, Radiation Oncology Resident, Department of Radiation Oncology, University of Maryland Medical Center, Baltimore, Maryland

Rachel Bluebond-Langner, MD, Assistant Professor, Department of Surgery, University of Maryland School of Medicine, Baltimore, Maryland

Cristina Campassi, MD, Assistant Professor, Department of Radiology, University of Maryland School of Medicine, Baltimore, Maryland

Krista Chain, Medical Student, University of Maryland School of Medicine, Baltimore, Maryland

Sally B. Cheston, MD, Assistant Professor, University of Maryland School of Medicine, Baltimore; Medical Director, Central Maryland Radiation Oncology, Columbia, Maryland

Jasleen Chopra, MD, Radiology Resident, Department of Radiology, University of Maryland Medical Center, Baltimore, Maryland

Arielle Cimeno, MD, Surgical Resident, Department of Surgery, University of Maryland Medical Center, Baltimore, Maryland

Randi Cohen, MD, Assistant Professor, Department of Radiation Oncology, University of Maryland School of Medicine, Baltimore, Maryland

Angela DeRidder, MD, Hematology/Oncology Fellow, University of Maryland Greenebaum Comprehensive Cancer Center, Baltimore, Maryland

Jennifer Ding, MD, Resident, Department of Medicine, University of Maryland Medical Center, Baltimore, Maryland

Sergio Dromi, MD, Assistant Professor, Department of Radiology, University of Maryland School of Medicine, Baltimore, Maryland

Alex Engelman, MD, Radiation Oncology Resident, Department of Radiation Oncology, University of Maryland Medical Center, Baltimore, Maryland

Rawand Faramand, MD, Chief Resident, Department of Medicine, University of Maryland Medical Center, Baltimore, Maryland

Steven J. Feigenberg, MD, Professor, Radiation Oncology, Department of Radiation Oncology, Director for Clinical Research, Director of Stereotactic Body Radiotherapy Program/Director of Emerging Technologies, University of Maryland School of Medicine, Baltimore, Maryland

Jessica Galandak, MD, Assistant Professor, Department of Radiology, University of Maryland School of Medicine, Baltimore, Maryland

Lindsay Hessler, MD, General Surgery Resident, Department of Surgery, University of Maryland Medical Center, Baltimore, Maryland

Lyn Ho, MD, Assistant Professor, Department of Radiology, University of Maryland School of Medicine, Baltimore, Maryland

Dina Ioffe, Medical Student, University of Maryland School of Medicine, Baltimore, Maryland

Olga Ioffe, MD, Professor, Department of Pathology, Director, Anatomic Pathology, University of Maryland School of Medicine, Baltimore, Maryland

Susan B. Kesmodel, MD, Assistant Professor of Surgery, University of Maryland School of Medicine; Division of General and Oncologic Surgery, Department of Surgery, Director of Breast Surgery, University of Maryland Medical Center, Baltimore, Maryland

Sonya Y. Khan, MD, Diagnostic Radiology Resident, Department of Diagnostic Radiology & Nuclear Medicine, University of Maryland Medical Center, Baltimore, Maryland

Ina Lee, MD, Pathology Resident, Department of Pathology, University of Maryland Medical Center, Baltimore, Maryland

Jolinta Lin, MD, Radiation Oncology Resident, Department of Radiation Oncology, University of Maryland Medical Center, Baltimore, Maryland

Syed S. Mahmood, MD, Hematology/Oncology Fellow, University of Maryland Greenebaum Comprehensive Cancer Center, Baltimore, Maryland

Reshma L. Mahtani, DO, Assistant Professor, Division of Hematology/Oncology, Sylvester Comprehensive Cancer Center, University of Miami School of Medicine, Deerfield Beach, Florida

Daniel Maver, MD, Clinical Fellow, Department of Radiology, University of Maryland Medical Center, Baltimore, Maryland

Jason Molitoris, MD, Radiation Oncology Resident, Department of Radiation Oncology, University of Maryland Medical Center, Baltimore, Maryland

Ewa Mrozek, MD, Associate Professor, Division of Hematology/Oncology, Department of Medicine, Ohio State University, OSU James Cancer Hospital & Solove Research Institute, Columbus, Ohio

Elizabeth Nichols, MD, Assistant Professor, Department of Radiation Oncology, University of Maryland School of Medicine, Baltimore, Maryland

Natalie O'Neill, MD, General Surgery Resident, Department of Surgery, University of Maryland Medical Center, Baltimore, Maryland

Nilam Patel, MD, Resident, Department of Medicine, University of Maryland Medical Center, Baltimore, Maryland

Geetha Pukazhendhi, MD, Hematology/Oncology Fellow, Public Health Sciences, Division of Hematology/Oncology, Sylvester Comprehensive Cancer Center, University of Miami School of Medicine, Deerfield Beach, Florida

Erin M. Rada, MD, Plastic Surgery Resident, Department of Surgery, Johns Hopkins Hospital, Baltimore, Maryland

Stephanie Richards, MD, Pathology Resident, Department of Pathology, University of Maryland Medical Center, Baltimore, Maryland

Carolyn Rogers, Genetic Counseling Student, University of Maryland School of Medicine, Baltimore, Maryland

Paula Rosenblatt, MD, Assistant Professor, University of Maryland School of Medicine; Department of Medicine, University of Maryland Greenebaum Comprehensive Cancer Center, Baltimore, Maryland

Jessica Scott, MGC, CGC, Certified Genetic Counselor, University of Maryland Greenebaum Comprehensive Cancer Center, University of Maryland Medical Center, Baltimore, Maryland

Susan Shyu, MD, Pathology Resident, University of Maryland Medical Center, Baltimore, Maryland

Sheri Slezak, MD, Professor of Surgery, Division of Plastic Surgery, Department of Surgery, University of Maryland School of Medicine, Baltimore, Maryland

J. W. Snider III, MD, Radiation Oncology Resident, Department of Radiation Oncology, University of Maryland Medical Center, Baltimore, Maryland

Ikumi Suzuki, MD, Hematology/Oncology Fellow, University of Maryland Greenebaum Comprehensive Cancer Center, Baltimore, Maryland

Chad Tarabolous, MD, King's Daughters Medical Specialties, Ashland, Kentucky

Julia Terhune, MD, General Surgery Resident, Department of Surgery, University of Maryland Medical Center, Baltimore, Maryland

Katherine H. R. Tkaczuk, MD, FACP, Professor of Medicine, University of Maryland School of Medicine; Director, Breast Evaluation and Treatment Program, University of Maryland Greenebaum Comprehensive Cancer Center, Baltimore, Maryland

Rachel White, Medical Student, University of Maryland School of Medicine, Baltimore, Maryland

Yang Zhang, MD, Pathology Resident, Department of Pathology, University of Maryland Medical Center, Baltimore, Maryland

The breast oncology field is rapidly changing and smaller texts, which can be updated more often, are of clinical value to practitioners, especially those who do not have access to a multidisciplinary clinic. In this book, we have endeavored to provide enough current and clinically useful information for all subspecialists who routinely care for breast cancer and breast disease, and have included dedicated breast and plastic surgery, radiation, and medical approaches, recognizing the fact that the management should be multidisciplinary. We believe that this book structure will provide our readers with a balanced view of oncologic and non-oncologic approaches routinely utilized in the field in the management of patients. This handbook has been written especially for younger practitioners involved in the care of patients; in addition, we hope that experienced clinicians in all related fields will also find it a handy, 'on-the-go' resource and can use it in their busy clinics while they manage patients.

We do realize that given the smaller format of our handbook, we will not be able to completely satisfy all readers and some may still want to pursue the online search engines and larger textbooks when needed. We also recognize that not all management viewpoints may have been included; and some may disagree with us on certain, more controversial clinical issues; however, we have striven to point out these controversies and provide enough useful and up-to-date information that is relevant and clinically applicable, followed by the rationale behind the University of Maryland approach. We sincerely hope you will enjoy reading and using the *Handbook of Breast Cancer and Related Breast Disease* in your clinics, especially when you need a quick look or reminder on the clinical management approaches to the treatment of breast diseases. Finally, we would like to thank all the contributing authors for their time and effort, as well as Helen Spiker for her administrative help during production of this book.

Katherine H. R. Tkaczuk, MD, FACP
Susan B. Kesmodel, MD
Steven J. Feigenberg, MD

Handbook of Breast Cancer and Related
Breast Disease

Breast Imaging: Breast Cancer Screening, Diagnosis, Staging, and Surveillance

Cristina Campassi, Lyn Ho, Jessica Galandak, Sergio Dromi, Divya Awal, Daniel Maver, Jasleen Chopra, and Sonya Y. Khan

INTRODUCTION

Imaging is essential in detecting, diagnosing, staging, and providing surveillance of diseases of the breast. Breast imaging plays a fundamental role, as clinical examination of the breast and surrounding regional lymph nodes is extremely challenging and nonpalpable abnormalities in the breast are common.

Indications for Breast Imaging

Asymptomatic women undergo screening while women with clinical breast signs and symptoms undergo a diagnostic evaluation.

SCREENING EXAM

Mammography is the main screening modality. Breast MRI is a supplemental modality in women at increased risk for breast cancer. Periodic screening is recommended. The National Comprehensive Cancer Network (NCCN) recommends receiving an annual mammogram starting at age 40 for average-risk women and earlier screening mammography supplemented with breast MRI for high-risk women (1,2). Screening exams are performed by a technologist and interpreted by a radiologist at a later time. The Food and Drug Administration requires mammography providers to inform women of their screening mammogram results within 30 days of the exam date. At our institution we batch-read screenings that are usually interpreted within a few days unless prior mammograms performed at another facility are unavailable for comparison. In such cases, 2 weeks are allowed to receive the patients' prior mammograms before reading the current screening exam.

DIAGNOSTIC EXAM

Imaging evaluation is tailored to a specific clinical or imaging finding. The radiologist prescribes dedicated mammographic views and/or an ultrasound as needed and monitors the exam while it is in progress. The patient is informed of the results the same day.

Multimodality Breast Imaging

Breast imaging encompasses multiple modalities. Guidelines for the use of different modalities are outlined in the American College of Radiology (ACR) Appropriateness Criteria and Practice Guidelines (3–6).

MAMMOGRAPHY AND ULTRASOUND

Mammography and ultrasound are established conventional imaging modalities. In the screening setting, mammography is the only test proven to reduce mortality in randomized trials (7) and ultrasound has been shown to increase cancer detection in a subset of women with increased risk for breast cancer and dense breast tissue on mammography (8). In the setting of clinical symptoms, mammography and ultrasound are the first-line exam in women over and under the age of 30, respectively.

MRI

MRI is the best modality to detect silicone breast implant rupture. It is also the most sensitive imaging tool for detecting breast cancer and may identify cancer occult to clinical examination or conventional modalities such as mammography and ultrasound. MRI is used to supplement screening mammography in women with increased risk for breast cancer (2,9). In the setting of known breast cancer, MRI is used to assess the extent of disease in selected cases and response to systemic therapy in the neoadjuvant setting. In selected cases, it may be used for problem solving.

CONTRAST ENHANCED MAMMOGRAPHY (CEM)

Contrast enhanced mammography (CEM) is utilized in selected diagnostic cases, mostly as an alternative to breast MRI.

NUCLEAR MEDICINE MODALITIES

Nuclear medicine modalities such as positron emission mammography (PEM) and molecular breast imaging (MBI), also known as breast-specific gamma imaging (BSGI), are used for rare selected high-risk women in the diagnostic setting.

Breast Imaging Reporting and Data System (BI-RADS)

A standardized set of guidelines was developed by international experts in breast imaging with support from the ACR. The first edition, published in 1993, set guidelines for mammography. The most recent edition, published in 2013, provides guidelines for mammography, breast ultrasound, and breast MRI (10). The goal is to provide a common language for mammography and health care providers to facilitate communication and patient care. Standardization of finding description, assessment, recommendation, and reporting allows for easy communications, medical audit, and patient tracking.

BI-RADS PRINCIPLES

The guiding principle of BI-RADS is concordance. Finding descriptor, assessment, and recommendation need to be congruent (eg, a finding with a suspicious description cannot be classified as benign). Correlation of findings identified using different imaging modalities or at clinical breast examination (eg, a mass seen on mammogram correlated with ultrasound and clinical exam) is also required. Finally, desired benchmarks (eg, recall rate, sensitivity, specificity) are established and are reinforced through medical audit.

BI-RADS ASSESSMENT CATEGORIES AND RECOMMENDATION

At interpretation, findings are identified, analyzed, described, and then classified according to assessment categories. The assessment may be final or incomplete. A final assessment may apply to a screening or diagnostic exam. An incomplete assessment usually applies to a screening (eg, need comparison to prior mammograms or additional mammographic views). By convention, the assessment category is composed of a numeric code and a statement. Assessment category 0 is used for incomplete exams. The remaining six assessment categories, numbered from 1 to 6, are used for final assessment and span from negative exam to known malignancy (Table 1.1). The degree of abnormality and likelihood of malignancy are lowest with low BI-RADS assessment numeric code and highest for BI-RADS 5. The likelihood of malignancy for BI-RADS 3 is <2%, for BI-RADS 4 the likelihood ranges between >2% and 95%, and for BI-RADS 5 it is >95%. Notably, assessment category 4, used for suspicious findings, may be subdivided into three groups (ie, 4A, 4B, and 4C) based on level of suspicion (likelihood of malignancy is >2% to <10% for 4A, 10% to <50% for 4B, and >50% to 95% for 4C). The recommendation should be in keeping with the finding assessment category and clinical history. These guidelines ensure standardization across radiologists.

BREAST CANCER SCREENING

Breast cancer is the most common cancer in women of all races and ethnicities and a leading cause of premature mortality among U.S. women. Early detection is associated with reduced mortality. Mammogram is the primary test recommended to identify early breast cancer. Supplemental screening with other modalities, such as breast MRI and ultrasound, in selected subgroups of women has shown increased detection of breast cancer.

Table 1.1 BI-RADS Assessment Categories: Numeric Coding, Definition, and Pertinent Recommendation	
Assessment category	**Recommendation**
0. Incomplete	Need additional imaging evaluation (recall) and/or prior mammograms for comparison
1. Negative	Routine mammogram
2. Benign	Routine mammogram
3. Probably benign	Initial short-term (6 months) follow-up
4. Suspicious	Tissue diagnosis
5. Highly suggestive of malignancy	Tissue diagnosis
6. Known biopsy-proven malignancy	Appropriate action
BI-RADS, breast imaging reporting and data system.	

Mammography and Digital Breast Tomosynthesis

A meta-analysis of seven randomized controlled trials of screening mammography in women 39 to 74 years of age has demonstrated a 20% overall reduction in mortality from breast cancer with a 22% mortality reduction in women aged 50 to 74 and 15% reduction in women aged 39 to 49 (11). Despite the well-documented benefit of screening mammography, debate and uncertainty exist on the optimal screening strategy because exposure to screening generates false positives (ie, benign findings that require workup and biopsy to exclude cancer), identifies subclinical cancers that may not become clinically significant if undetected, and results in radiation exposure. As a result, recent screening strategies have deviated from the previously unanimous recommendation for annual screening mammography starting at age 40. The U.S. Preventive Services Task Force in 2009 and 2016 (12) and the American Cancer Society in late 2015 (13) have suggested more restrictive guidelines (Table 1.2). While recognizing the mortality reduction from screening mammography across all ages, both organizations encourage women to decide with their physician when to start and end, and how often to undergo screening mammography (12,13).

TECHNOLOGY

Mammography utilizes ionizing radiation, which is captured on a detector after passing through the breast. A major advancement in mammography technology over the past decade has been the development of digital technology, called full field digital mammography (FFDM) or 2D mammography. Compared to film screen, digital mammography uses a lower radiation dose, has a digital rather than film detector, and allows for separation of image acquisition, display, and archiving. The most recent improvement in mammography is digital breast tomosynthesis (DBT). While 2D mammography administers ionizing radiation through a stationary source perpendicular to the breast, DBT uses a moving x-ray source to image the breast at different angles. Thus, DBT obtains multiple digital images that can be reconstructed to obtain a quasi-tridimensional (3D) representation of the breast as opposed to FFDM, which obtains a bidimensional (2D) image. As a result,

Table 1.2 Summary of Screening Strategies and Relative Mortality Reduction According to the Guidelines of the American College of Radiology (ACR), National Comprehensive Cancer Network (NCCN), American Cancer Society (ACS), and U.S. Preventive Services Task Force (USPSTF)

Organization	Screening strategy			Mortality reduction
	When to start	When to stop	How often/when	
ACR and NCCN	40	Life expectancy <10 years	Annual	40%
ACS	45	Life expectancy <10 years	Annual 45–54, biennial >55	31%
USPSTF	50	74	Biennial	22%

while breast tissue is superimposed on a view obtained with FFDM, it is viewed separately with DBT. This improves lesion detection and characterization while decreasing superimposition of breast tissue and the rate of false positives.

TECHNIQUE

The same standard technique is used regardless of the technology utilized, film-screen mammography, FFDM, or DBT. A mammogram is performed with the patient standing or, if needed, sitting in a chair. The mammographic views are acquired with the breast under compression. A screening mammogram includes projections of each breast in two routine views: craniocaudal and mediolateral oblique (Figure 1.1). Therefore, typically a bilateral screening mammogram includes four views.

INTERPRETATION

The radiologist analyzes the mammographic views and classifies a screening mammogram as negative, benign, or incomplete, using the BI-RADS assessment categories 1, 2, and 0, respectively. Approximately 10% of screening mammograms are incomplete and require additional imaging with dedicated mammographic views and/or ultrasound in accordance with the ACR Practice Guidelines (4,5). Mammographic interpretation and detection of breast findings depend on breast composition (Figure 1.2). As the relative amount of fat decreases and glandular tissue increases, the breast becomes dense on a mammogram and cancer detection becomes more challenging (Figure 1.3). Additionally, dense breast tissue is considered an independent risk factor for breast cancer. Legislations to increase women's awareness of breast density and its effect on screening mammography in the setting of dense breast tissue has been passed in the majority of U.S. states since 2009. This state legislation requires mammography providers to share information about breast density and/or inform women

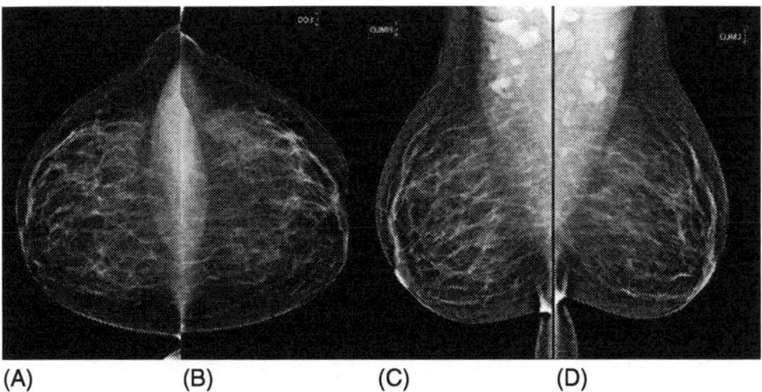

(A)   (B)   (C)   (D)

Figure 1.1 Digital mammogram with 2D technique. Screening mammogram includes two views of each breast: craniocaudal (CC) (A, B) and mediolateral oblique (MLO) (C, D). For viewing and interpretation, the mammographic views are displayed side by side to facilitate comparison of breast tissue and identification of findings that may represent breast cancer.

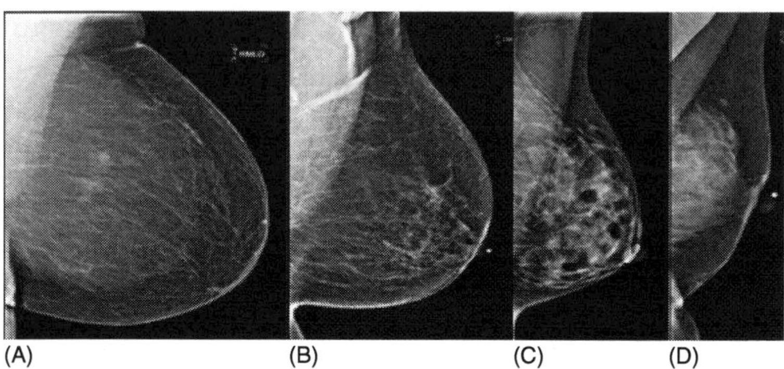

(A) (B) (C) (D)

Figure 1.2 Breast composition varies depending on the amount of fatty and glandular tissue. Classification of breast composition ranges from almost entirely fatty (A) to extremely dense (D). The majority of women have either scattered fibroglandular elements (B) or heterogeneously dense breast tissue (C) while less than 20% of the female population has either fatty (A) or extremely dense breast tissue (D).

of their own breast density. Federal legislation may follow as the Breast Density and Mammography Reporting Act introduced to the U.S. Congress in October 2013 and to the U.S. Senate in February 2015 is under consideration.

FULL FIELD DIGITAL MAMMOGRAPHY (FFDM) AND DIGITAL BREAST TOMOSYNTHESIS (DBT)

Compared to film screen, FFDM has shown improved cancer detection of 15% in women under the age of 50 years, women with radiographically dense breast tissue, and premenopausal or perimenopausal women (14). DBT has further increased breast cancer detection by 27% to 40% and decreased false-positive rates by 15% to 40% compared to FFDM (15).

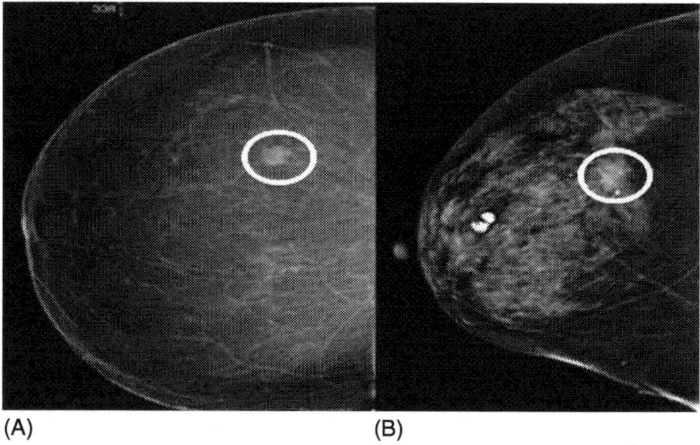

(A) (B)

Figure 1.3 Breast composition influences breast cancer detection. A breast cancer (circle) is easier to detect in a fatty breast (A) compared to a dense breast (B).

Breast MRI

Several trials performed throughout the United States, Canada, and Europe in the mid- to late 1990s assessed the benefit of adding screening MRI to annual mammography in women who were at increased risk of breast cancer. The consistent finding was a much higher sensitivity for MRI when compared to mammography with sensitivities between 71% and 100% with MRI and 16% and 40% with mammography. The specificity of mammography remained higher than MRI, ranging from 93% to 99% compared to 81% to 99% for MRI. While the combination of higher sensitivity and lower specificity with MRI results in higher callback and biopsy rates than mammography, it also results in a higher cancer detection rate (1.04% vs. 0.46% in the Netherlands trial and 1.44% vs. 0.69% in the UK trial).

TECHNOLOGY

MRI utilizes magnetic fields to create multiplanar cross-sectional images through the body. MRI does not utilize radiation and has extremely good soft tissue contrast resolution, making it an excellent imaging modality for evaluating the breast. An intravenous gadolinium-based contrast agent is needed to reliably detect cancers, cancer extension, and other lesions.

TECHNIQUE

Patients are positioned prone. Both breasts are accommodated within an open padded platform (coil) that allows imaging without compression. The patient is placed into the bore of the MRI machine. Claustrophobic patients may need open magnets or premedication with anxiolytic. Multiple sequences are performed including precontrast and postcontrast. The overall scan time is usually 15 to 25 minutes. Although the scan requires that the patient be able to hold still during the entire examination, sedation is not required. Contraindications to MRI include a prior allergic reaction to contrast or severe renal insufficiency. The use of gadolinium is not recommended if the glomerular filtration rate (GFR) is below 30 mL/min due to the risk of nephrogenic systemic fibrosis (16). The use of gadolinium-based agents for elective exams such as breast MRI is contraindicated during pregnancy and is not needed if the examination is performed to evaluate for silicone breast implant rupture only.

RECOMMENDATIONS

The American Cancer Society guidelines for screening breast MRI as an adjunct to mammography (9), the NCCN (2), and the practice guidelines of the ACR (6) are used as a reference across specialties in the medical community. In our practice, screening breast MRI is used for all groups of high-risk women listed in the American Cancer Society guidelines (see Table 1.3). In particular, our experience on breast cancer survivors has shown that when breast MRI is used in adjunct to mammography, cancer detection rate increases compared to mammography alone; see Figure 1.4.

Breast Ultrasound

Historically ultrasound has been used as a diagnostic problem-solving tool in patients who present with either a physical finding (nipple discharge, palpable

<table>
<tr><td colspan="1">Table 1.3 American Cancer Society Guidelines for Supplemental Screening Breast MRI</td></tr>
<tr><td>

Evidence-based recommendation for annual screening MRI
    BRCA mutation carrier
    First degree relative of BRCA carrier, but untested
    Lifetime risk for breast cancer >20% when evaluated with a model
       dependent on family history

</td></tr>
<tr><td>

Consensus expert opinion recommendation for annual screening MRI
    Radiation to the chest between age 10–30 years
    Patients with Li–Fraumeni, Cowden, or Bannayan–Riley–Ruvalcaba
       syndromes and their first degree relatives

</td></tr>
<tr><td>

Insufficient evidence for or against annual screening MRI
    Lifetime risk for breast cancer of 15%–20% when evaluated with a model
       dependent on family history
    Lobular carcinoma in situ or atypical lobular hyperplasia
    Atypical ductal hyperplasia
    Heterogeneously or extremely dense breast on mammography
    Women with a personal history of breast cancer, including ductal carcinoma
       in situ

</td></tr>
<tr><td>

Consensus expert opinion recommendation against annual MRI screening
    Lifetime risk for breast cancer <15%

</td></tr>
</table>

lump), a mammographic finding (asymmetry, mass), or, less commonly, an MRI finding (second look ultrasound for enhancing mass) (see "Imaging Assessment After Breast Cancer Diagnosis"). It is also the main modality for image-guided procedures (see "Image-Guided Breast Biopsies"). In addition, breast ultrasound has been investigated as a modality for breast cancer screening (see this section).

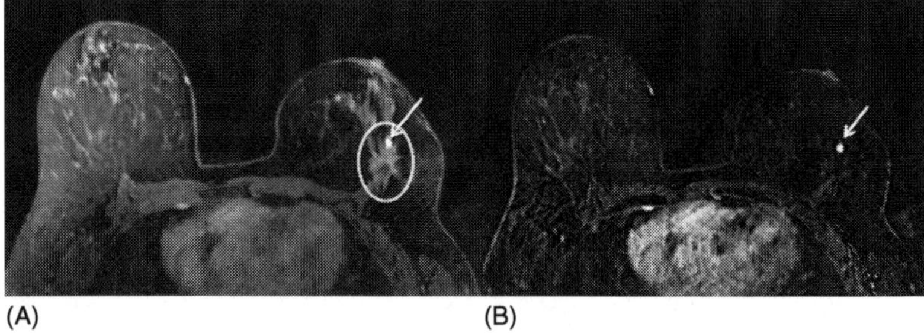

(A)   (B)

Figure 1.4 MRI detected, mammographically occult, local recurrence in a high-risk woman with personal history of breast cancer treated 5 years earlier with partial mastectomy and radiation therapy. (A) Postcontrast MR image shows a 5-mm circumscribed homogeneously enhancing round mass (arrow) along the anterior aspect of the operative bed (circle). Asymmetric size, contour, and skin thickening of the left breast are due to prior treatment for breast cancer. (B) Subtracted postcontrast MR image better shows the focal nature of the enhancing mass (arrow). MR-guided breast biopsy shows ductal carcinoma in situ (DCIS).

TECHNOLOGY

Ultrasound is an imaging modality that uses sound waves to create cross-sectional images through the body. Ultrasound does not use radiation, is portable and inexpensive, and produces excellent imaging of the breast.

a. **Grayscale ultrasound** shows the tissue in different shades of gray and is best for anatomic evaluation and characterization of lesion morphology (Figure 1.5).
b. **Color Doppler ultrasound** is best for evaluating the presence of blood flow and distinguishing venous and arterial flow.
c. **Power Doppler ultrasound** is best for detecting a subtle amount of blood flow without the capability of differentiating between arterial and venous flow.
d. **Ultrasound elastography** allows quantitative and qualitative evaluation of tissue deformation in response to an applied force. This is a simple and rapid method that can improve the sensitivity and specificity of grayscale images.

TECHNIQUE

Patients are positioned supine with the ipsilateral arm raised above their head. The ultrasound probe is placed on the breast with interposed conductive gel. Conventionally, the exam is performed with a handheld transducer operated by an ultrasound technologist or a physician. Whole breast ultrasound may also be performed with automated equipment positioned by a technologist. During handheld ultrasound, representative static images are saved for interpretation. During automated breast ultrasound the entire breast is imaged, allowing for improved consistency and reproducibility of images as well as decreased operator dependence.

SCREENING BREAST ULTRASOUND

The ACRIN 6666 trial (NCT00072501) was performed to compare screening mammography alone to combined screening mammography and physician-performed handheld screening breast ultrasound. The study was targeted at women

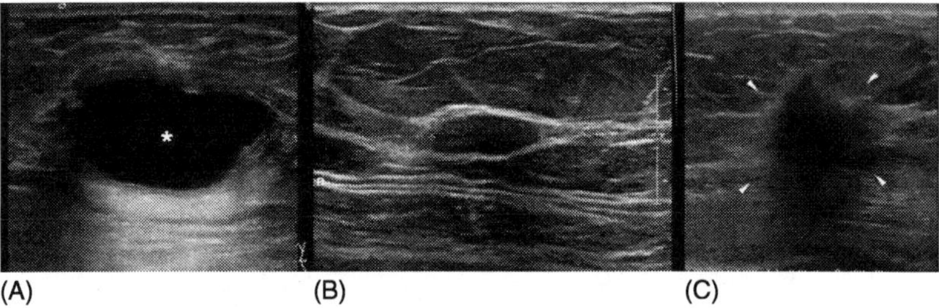

(A) (B) (C)

Figure 1.5 Ultrasound of three breast masses. (A) Anechoic mass (asterisk) with imperceptible wall and posterior through transmission pathognomonic for simple cyst. (B) Benign appearing solid mass (calipers) with circumscribed margins, homogenous hypoechoic echotexture, orientation parallel to the chest wall, and no posterior shadowing. Pathology: fibroadenoma. (C) Highly suspicious solid mass (arrowheads) with irregular margins and shape, hypoechoic echotexture, orientation not parallel to the chest wall, and with marked posterior shadowing. Pathology: invasive ductal carcinoma.

with dense breasts and increased risk of breast cancer. The addition of screening breast ultrasound to screening mammography resulted in an increased cancer detection rate (4.2 additional cancers/1,000 patients screened). However, the combination of screening breast ultrasound and mammography resulted in a 250% increase in biopsy rate and a low positive predictive value for biopsied findings (17).

SCREENING BREAST ULTRASOUND CONCEPTS FOR GUIDELINES

Although guidelines for screening breast ultrasound are currently not standardized, there is agreement that screening breast ultrasound may be performed as an adjunct to and in conjunction with screening mammography when indicated. Given the superior sensitivity of screening breast MRI, this is the preferred supplemental screening modality in women at high risk for breast cancer. There may be some role for the use of screening breast ultrasound in women with >20% lifetime risk for developing breast cancer who have a contraindication to breast MRI, or women with 15% to 20% lifetime risk for developing breast cancer (18).

DIAGNOSIS OF BREAST DISEASES BY IMAGING

In contrast to screening mammography, diagnostic breast imaging is a tailored exam for evaluation of a specific clinical finding or an abnormality detected at screening. Appropriate diagnostic imaging tests for common indications are outlined in the following text.

Palpable Breast Lump

Mammography and ultrasound are primarily utilized. Breast MRI is typically not indicated as a first-line diagnostic exam due to cost, necessity of intravenous contrast, and likely higher rate of incidental false-positive findings unrelated to the palpable abnormality (19), although it may occasionally be used for problem solving.

FEMALE PATIENTS 30 YEARS OF AGE OR OLDER

Diagnostic mammogram (including spot compression views) with a skin marker placed at the site of palpable concern is the first-line modality. Following mammography, targeted ultrasound of the palpable area of concern is typically performed for further evaluation (19).

FEMALE PATIENTS YOUNGER THAN 30 YEARS OLD

Evaluation should begin with an ultrasound, targeting the region of palpable concern. Mammography is generally not performed due to density of breast tissue in young patients limiting sensitivity and in order to avoid unnecessary exposure to radiation (20). If no sonographic finding is detected at the site of palpable concern, mammography may or may not be recommended, depending on the level of clinical suspicion (20). Mammography may also be utilized to further characterize an indeterminate sonographic finding (eg, fat necrosis, which is typically better evaluated mammographically).

MALE ADULT PATIENT

Evaluation should begin with diagnostic mammogram. If the mammographic findings are indeterminate or suspicious, ultrasound should follow (21).

MALE CHILDREN/ADOLESCENTS

Palpable breast masses are rare in the pediatric male population (22). Male children and adolescents with physical exam and clinical history consistent with gynecomastia require no imaging evaluation (23). If there is suspicion for etiology other than gynecomastia (ie, male breast cancer) ultrasound is the primary imaging modality (22). Breast cancer comprises less than 1% of pediatric cancers, and is exceedingly rare in pediatric males. Malignant lesions are almost always metastatic or primary tumors of nonbreast tissue origin (22).

PREGNANT AND LACTATING PATIENTS

Ultrasound is the initial imaging modality of choice recommended for a palpable breast mass in a pregnant or lactating patient. However, mammography is not contraindicated in pregnancy and should be performed if malignancy is suspected. With proper abdominal shielding, mammography poses little risk of radiation exposure to the fetus, estimated at less than 0.01 Gy (24).

In the absence of any mammographic or sonographic findings corresponding to a palpable mass, clinical follow-up is indicated. A highly suspicious physical exam should prompt biopsy by palpation in the absence of the imaging findings.

Breast Pain

Pain can be cyclical or noncyclical, depending on its temporal relation to the menstrual cycle, unilateral or bilateral, and the distribution can be diffuse or focal (involving less than 25% of the breast tissue) (25).

CYCLICAL, BILATERAL, OR NONFOCAL BREAST PAIN

Imaging is not indicated due to the low yield of finding a specific cause; results vary in regard to whether imaging provides reassurance in this group of patients (25).

NONCYCLICAL, UNILATERAL, FOCAL BREAST PAIN

Evaluation may begin with ultrasound or mammography depending on whether the patient's age is under or above 40. Imaging may identify a treatable cause of the pain, provide reassurance, and usually exclude malignancy (26).

Nipple Discharge

Clinically concerning features of nipple discharge in a nonlactating patient include: bloody, clear, or serosanguinous discharge; unilateral symptoms; and spontaneous (as opposed to expressed) discharge.

PATIENT LESS THAN 30 YEARS OF AGE

Evaluation should begin with ultrasound, followed by mammogram if findings are equivocal or suspicious.

PATIENT OLDER THAN 30 YEARS OF AGE

Evaluation should include mammogram and ultrasound.

If no etiology is identified with initial imaging studies and discharge is clinically concerning, breast MRI should be considered. At the surgeon's request, a ductogram may be performed. A ductogram is a radiologic exam performed by cannulating and injecting contrast through the discharging duct. This test may identify and localize intraductal disease.

Implant Abnormalities

Most silicone breast implant ruptures are clinically silent or asymptomatic, making diagnosis difficult. Physical exam alone is unreliable with an approximate sensitivity of 30% for rupture detection. MRI is the test of choice to evaluate implant integrity or rupture. Sensitivity of mammography for implant rupture is 68%, of ultrasound is 77%, and of MRI is 93% (27). Ultrasound may be considered if MRI is unavailable as it is more specific than mammography and does not expose the patient to radiation.

IMAGE-GUIDED BREAST BIOPSIES

The mainstay of establishing pathological diagnosis of suspicious lesions is image-guided percutaneous biopsy. This has been shown to have excellent accuracy and is now the standard of care (28). Surgical biopsy is reserved for those lesions that are not amenable to image-guided biopsy. The advantages of minimally invasive image-guided breast biopsy over surgical biopsy are numerous and include shorter recovery time, lower cost, higher safety, and minimal scarring (28,29). Image-guided biopsies are utilized for nonpalpable, image-detected findings and palpable findings to direct the needle to the most suspicious portion of a lesion.

Type of Image-Guided Biopsy

The choice of modality used for biopsy depends on optimal lesion visualization, efficiency, and safety.

ULTRASOUND-GUIDED BIOPSY

Ultrasound-guided biopsy is the most commonly used image-guided biopsy that is performed with the patient lying comfortably supine. Advantages of ultrasound guidance include lack of ionizing radiation, accessibility to all areas of the breast, real-time visualization of the needle and lesion, readily available equipment, and greater patient comfort since it does not require breast compression. For these reasons, it is the preferred method for lesions that are visualized by ultrasound. Either spring-loaded or vacuum-assisted biopsy devices can be utilized.

STEREOTACTIC BIOPSY

Stereotactic biopsy is typically utilized for lesions that are only seen mammographically. The patient is positioned either prone, upright in a chair, or in lateral decubitus and the breast is placed in compression. The lesion is centered in an aperture within the compression plate and images are obtained from multiple angles to determine the depth of the lesion. After the biopsy needle is advanced to the calculated location and needle position is verified, tissue samples are taken using a vacuum-assisted biopsy device (29). A specimen radiograph is performed to evaluate for the presence of the lesion (typically calcifications) within the sample and a clip is placed to mark the biopsy site for future reference.

MRI-GUIDED BIOPSY

MRI-guided biopsy is utilized for lesions seen with MRI only. The patient is placed inside the scanner for imaging and outside of the scanner for the biopsy. The breast is immobilized and biopsied using a compression grid system designed to fit the breast coil. After contrast administration and imaging, the grid provides landmarks for calculation of lesion position (29). A needle sheath is placed at the lesion site and an obturator is used for confirmation of position with additional MR images. When appropriate position is confirmed, an MR-compatible vacuum-assisted biopsy device is placed through the sheath and used to sample the lesion.

Type of Needle Biopsy

The type of needle utilized for a breast biopsy depends on the lesion characteristics, level of suspicion, and modality used for biopsy. Large (12G, 14G) core needles and (8G, 9G, 10G) vacuum-assisted biopsy devices are the preferred sampling method yielding the highest diagnostic accuracy. Fine (23G or 25G) needle aspiration of the breast is limited to selected cases (eg, benign solid masses in teenagers) due to the high rate of inadequate sampling.

For all image-guided breast biopsies, metallic markers are placed at the biopsy sites following sampling to facilitate follow-up or excision. The radiologist should review pathology results in conjunction with imaging features of each lesion to determine concordance of results and ensure appropriate patient management recommendations (28).

IMAGE-GUIDED NEEDLE LOCALIZATIONS

Image-guided needle localization and subsequent surgical excision is indicated if percutaneous biopsy cannot be performed or is inconclusive, for high-risk lesions, if there is discordance between imaging and pathology results from percutaneous biopsy, or for treatment purposes after percutaneous biopsy yields a malignant diagnosis. Localizations are typically performed using a needle–wire system. There are several available needle–wire systems, all of which allow placement of a wire through an introducing needle that has been positioned in the breast at the lesion. Mammographic, ultrasound, or MRI guidance can be utilized (Figure 1.6). Bracketed localization using multiple wires can be performed for multiple lesions or for extensive microcalcifications, in coordination with the surgeon (29).

RADIOLOGIC–PATHOLOGIC CORRELATION

Image-guided percutaneous breast biopsies have become an integral part of the diagnosis of breast diseases. Prior to performing an image-guided biopsy, the radiologist should predetermine the likelihood of malignancy based on imaging characteristics. Following biopsy, the radiologist needs to correlate radiologic and pathologic findings to validate their concordance and to recognize discordant or false-negative or false-positive biopsy results. Assessment of concordance can be performed via case review at a multidisciplinary conference or independent review

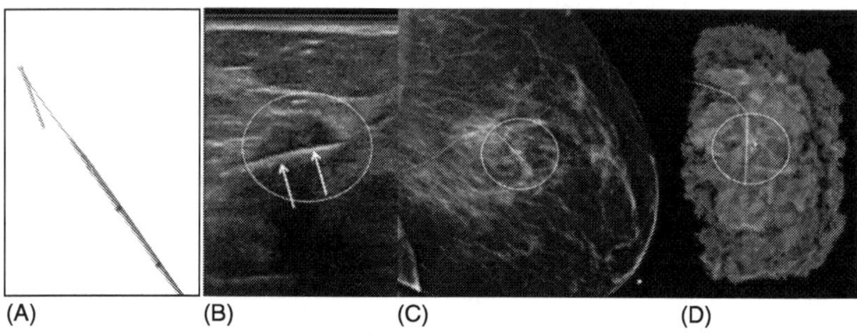

Figure 1.6 Ultrasound-guided needle localization biopsy-proven breast cancer. (A) Needle–wire device utilized for preoperative localization. The needle is used to introduce the thin wire within the lesion to be excised. This type of wire has a hook shape. (B) Ultrasound guidance utilized for needle–wire localization placement shows the wire (arrows) as a bright line through the solid mass (circle). (C) Post-procedure mammogram confirms successful localization of the mass and metallic clip placed at the time of biopsy (circle). (D) Magnification radiograph of the surgical specimen shows the wire, the spiculated mass, and the clip (circle) within the excised tissue.

of imaging and pathology findings concurrently. With knowledge of the pathology results, images from the procedure should be scrutinized to determine if the lesion was appropriately targeted and sampled. Specimen radiographs from the biopsy and postbiopsy mammogram after clip placement should also be re-evaluated. Particular attention to radiologic–pathologic correlation is required for those few selected cases of fine needle aspiration, as the diagnostic accuracy of fine needle aspiration is lower than core needle or a vacuum-assisted biopsy, in particular if a cytologist is not on site to assess the specimen for adequacy. In cases of discordant or high-risk lesions, the breast surgeon, radiologist, and pathologist must review the case and reach a consensus of the best management plan to avoid delay in diagnosis. The possible clinical scenarios are outlined in the following list:

1. **Concordant benign lesions.** Imaging favors a benign etiology, and pathology results are benign. The patient should return for follow-up imaging in 6 months or 1 year and continue clinical follow-up if the lesion was palpable. Overall, the false-negative rate from image-guided core needle biopsy is reported to be approximately 2% (30).
2. **Concordant malignant lesions.** Imaging favors suspicious etiology, and pathology results are malignant. The patient should be promptly referred to a multidisciplinary team for discussion of treatment.
3. **Discordant benign lesions.** Imaging favors suspicious etiology, but pathology results are benign. Image-guided needle biopsies can yield false-negative results secondary to sampling error, mostly at fine needle aspiration. It is prudent to repeat the image-guided needle biopsy with a larger needle or refer the patient to a surgeon for excisional biopsy to ensure adequate tissue sampling.

4. **Discordant malignant lesions.** Imaging favors benign etiology, but pathology results are malignant. False-positive results may occur, mostly at fine needle aspiration, and require sampling with a larger biopsy device, either a core needle or vacuum-assisted biopsy device. In view of malignant pathology, the patient should be ultimately referred for surgical consultation.
5. **High-risk lesions.** Histopathology yields a high-risk lesion with associated increased risk for developing breast cancer (see Chapter 2). Patients should be referred for surgical consultation.

IMAGING ASSESSMENT AFTER BREAST CANCER DIAGNOSIS

After a patient is diagnosed with breast cancer, a staging evaluation is pursued to determine the extent of disease, guide management decisions, and estimate prognosis.

DIAGNOSTIC MAMMOGRAPHY

Diagnostic mammography and targeted diagnostic ultrasound are the first-line imaging evaluation during initial workup and staging. The ipsilateral breast should be evaluated for multifocal or multicentric disease. The contralateral breast should also be evaluated for synchronous cancer. Additional suspicious lesions detected on MRI that may change the treatment plan should undergo image-guided biopsy (stereotactic or ultrasound-guided) prior to surgery. For lesions not amenable to percutaneous needle biopsy, needle localization and excisional biopsy should be performed to aid in staging.

AXILLARY ULTRASOUND AND AXILLARY NODE SAMPLING

Axillary ultrasound and axillary node sampling may be performed to assess ipsilateral and contralateral lymph nodes as indicated and agreed upon with the oncologists (31).

BREAST MRI

Breast MRI can define the anatomic extent of the cancer more accurately than mammography and ultrasound (32). MRI identifies additional ipsilateral disease in up to 30% of patients (33) and contralateral synchronous malignancy in approximately 5% of patients with known breast cancer (34), which may impact surgical management (Figure 1.7). In addition, breast MRI is recommended for invasive lobular carcinoma and inflammatory breast cancer to assess tumor involvement of the nipple or chest wall (35,36). Other indications for breast MRI following a cancer diagnosis include determining response to neoadjuvant chemotherapy and evaluating patients with metastatic axillary adenopathy of unknown primary.

PET–CT

PET–CT is indicated in the initial staging of a selected group of breast cancer patients. Currently, PET/CT is used to evaluate nodal involvement and distant disease in patients with stage 2B or higher in which PET/CT may identify clinically occult internal mammary, supraclavicular, and infraclavicular lymph nodes (37). NCCN guidelines recommend PET/CT in patients with clinical stage IIIA (T3, N1, M0) or higher breast cancer (category 2B recommendation). At our institution

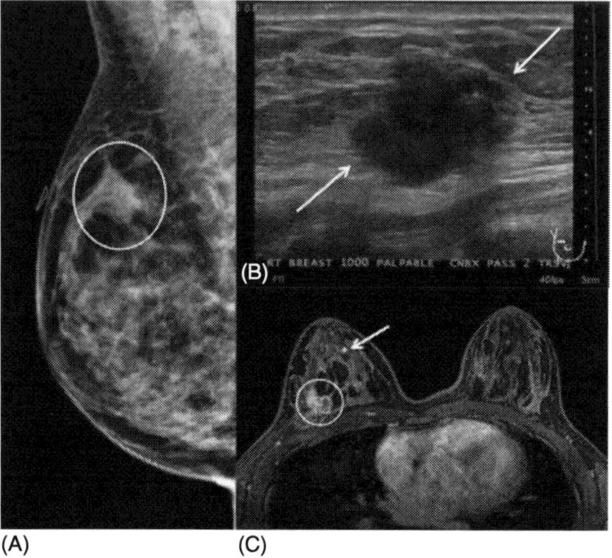

(A)   (C)

Figure 1.7 MRI-detected multicentric disease in a 52-year-old postmenopausal patient with newly diagnosed right breast cancer manifested as a palpable lump. (A) Diagnostic mammogram demonstrates an irregular mass (circle) at the palpable lump (triangular marker on skin) in the upper outer right breast. (B) Ultrasound shows a suspicious irregular solid mass (arrows), proven to represent an invasive ductal carcinoma at ultrasound-guided biopsy. (C) Preoperative breast MRI shows the biopsy-proven cancer in the posterior upper outer quadrant (circle) and an additional 6-mm enhancing mass in the anterior upper inner quadrant (arrow). MRI-guided breast biopsy of the 6-mm mass reveals invasive ductal carcinoma confirming multicentric disease.

we recommend PET/CT for patients with lesser disease burden if they have an aggressive phenotype such as triple negative or Her2+ disease. PET/CT may also be useful when CT or MRI is equivocal, when evaluating response to systemic chemotherapy in the setting of distant metastases, and when evaluating clinically asymptomatic treated breast cancer survivors with rising levels of tumor markers (38).

CT

CT is recommended by the NCCN in patients with symptoms or laboratory values suspicious for pulmonary or abdominal metastases.

IMAGING SURVEILLANCE OF BREAST CANCER SURVIVORS

Currently, there are over 3 million breast cancer survivors in the United States (2,39,40). These patients are monitored both on clinical and imaging bases. A meta-analysis of 13 studies with 2,263 breast cancer survivors demonstrated better survival in asymptomatic patients with imaging-detected local–regional and contralateral recurrence compared to symptomatic patients with clinically detected recurrence (41). Imaging surveillance of breast cancer survivors may entail multiple imaging modalities.

MAMMOGRAPHY

Mammography is considered the main surveillance-imaging modality for patients following curative primary breast conservation treatment. Studies have shown improved survival for early detection of recurrence in posttreatment patients (42). Current guidelines from the American Society of Clinical Oncology (ASCO) and NCCN suggest annual mammogram based on expert opinion (41). Mammography alone detects 8% to 50% of recurrent cancer in the ipsilateral breast and 18% to 80% of contralateral metachronous cancers (43). Postoperative and postradiation changes can decrease sensitivity and specificity of mammography (41). Therefore, additional adjunct surveillance-imaging modality may be considered. In our practice we perform annual screening mammography, preferably with DBT, and often add screening breast MRI in women aged 65 and under.

BREAST ULTRASOUND

ASCO and NCCN do not recommend routine surveillance ultrasound in women with a personal history of breast cancer. The ACR suggests that screening ultrasound is an option for women with intermediate risk (eg, personal history of breast cancer) and women with high risk for breast cancer who are unable to undergo breast MRI (18,41).

BREAST MRI

Breast MRI is a resource-intensive modality and can be more difficult for patients to tolerate compared to ultrasound or mammography. However, breast MRI has been shown to be superior in differentiating postoperative and posttreatment changes from recurrent tumor (41). In addition, a large retrospective study by Brennan et al demonstrated a benefit to MRI surveillance in patients with a personal history of breast cancer, detecting malignancy in 12% of patients (44). At our institution, we compared cancer detection with screening mammography and breast MRI on 249 asymptomatic breast cancer survivors treated with breast conserving therapy or mastectomy. Supplemental screening breast MRI identified the vast majority of cancers: of the 11 diagnosed cancers, 8 were detected by MRI alone, 3 by MRI and mammography, and none by mammography alone (45). Respectively, sensitivity and specificity were 84.6% and 95.3% for breast MRI and 23.1% and 96.4% for mammography. Therefore, breast MRI should be considered an important adjunct surveillance-imaging tool for breast cancer survivors.

F-18 FLUORO-DEOXYGLUCOSE (FDG) POSITRON EMISSION TOMOGRAPHY (PET)

Once recurrent disease is suspected based on clinical or other imaging findings, F-18 FDG PET is considered appropriate to evaluate the extent of disease and distant metastasis, as its sensitivity and specificity have been reported up to 97% and 82%, respectively, compared to conventional imaging (46). Otherwise, given the radiation exposure, high cost, and low sensitivity for primary tumor detection of only 68% for tumors <2 cm (47), PET–CT is not routinely recommended for initial surveillance of patients with a personal history of breast cancer.

➤ MANAGEMENT PEARLS

1. Screening mammogram is performed in asymptomatic women to detect breast cancer before it is clinically evident.
2. Women with clinical symptoms or signs of breast cancer should undergo diagnostic imaging evaluation. Women under 30 should start with ultrasound and have a diagnostic mammogram only if deemed necessary by the interpreting radiologist. Women aged 30 and above should start with a diagnostic mammogram immediately followed by ultrasound.
3. Screening breast MRI is considered supplemental to screening mammogram in women with high risk for breast cancer.
4. Breast MRI may be indicated to evaluate diagnostic patients such as patients with newly diagnosed breast cancer, history of breast cancer, suspected breast silicone implant rupture, free silicone injections, and inconclusive conventional imaging.
5. Image-guided needle breast biopsies are accurate and minimally invasive. They usually allow a definitive benign diagnosis, identification of high-risk lesions, and preoperative diagnosis of malignancy. Therefore using image-guided needle breast biopsy avoids unnecessary surgery for benign lesions and allows a single step surgery for malignancies.

REFERENCES

1. Bevers TB, Anderson BO, Bonaccio E, et al. NCCN clinical practice guidelines in oncology: breast cancer screening and diagnosis. *J Natl Compr Canc Netw*. 2009;7(10): 1060–1096.
2. Bevers EB, Helvie M, Bonaccio E, et al. NCCN clinical practice guidelines in oncology version 1.2015. Breast cancer screening and diagnosis. https://www.nccn.org/professionals/physician_gls/f_guidelines.asp
3. Mainero MB, Lourenco A, Mahoney MC, et al. ACR Appropriateness Criteria breast cancer screening. https://acsearch.acr.org/list
4. Patel SB, Mahoney MC, Newell MA, et al. ACR practice parameters for the performance of screening and diagnostic mammogram. http://www.acr.org/Quality-Safety/Standards-Guidelines/Practice-Guidelines-by-Modality/Breast-Imaging
5. Mendelson EB, Mahoney MC, Bassett LW, et al. ACR practice parameters for the performance of a breast ultrasound examination. http://www.acr.org/Quality-Safety/Standards-Guidelines/Practice-Guidelines-by-Modality/Breast-Imaging
6. Mahoney MC, Newell MS, Bailey L, et al. ACR practice parameters for the performance of contrast enhanced magnetic resonance imaging (MRI) of the breast. http://www.acr.org/quality-safety/standards-guidelines/practice-guidelines-by-modality/breast-imaging
7. Tabár L, Vitak B, Chen TH, et al. Swedish two-county trial: impact of mammographic screening on breast cancer mortality during 3 decades. *Radiology*. 2011;260(3):658–663.
8. Brem RF, Tabár L, Duffy SW, et al. Assessing improvement in detection of breast cancer with three-dimensional automated breast ultrasound in women with dense breast tissue: the SomoInsight study. *Radiology*. 2015;274(3):663–673.

9. Saslow D, Boetes C, Burke W, et al. American Cancer Society guidelines for breast screening with MRI in adjunct to mammography. *CA Cancer J Clin.* 2007;57:75–89.

10. D'Orsi CJ, Sickles EA, Mendelson EB, et al. *ACR BI-RADS® Atlas, Breast Imaging Reporting and Data System.* 5th ed. Reston, MD: American College of Radiology; 2013:147–163.

11. Smith RA, Duffy SW, Gabe R, et al. The randomized trials of breast cancer screening: what have we learned? *Radiol Clin North Am.* 2004;42:793–806.

12. U.S. Preventive Services Task Force 2016. http://www.uspreventiveservicestaskforce.org/Page/Document/UpdateSummaryFinal/breast-cancer-screening1

13. Oeffinger KC, Fontham TH, Etzioni R, et al. Breast cancer screening for women at average risk: 2015 guideline update from the American Cancer Society. *JAMA.* 2015;314(15):1599–1614.

14. Pisano ED, Gatsonis C, Hendrick E, et al. Diagnostic performance of digital versus film mammography for breast-cancer screening. *N Engl J Med.* 2005;353:1773–1783.

15. Skaane P, Bandos AI, Gullien R, et al. Comparison of digital mammography alone and digital mammography plus tomosynthesis in a population based screening program. *Radiology.* 2013;267:47–56.

16. Ellis J, Davenport M, Dillman J, et al. ACR manual on contrast media version 10.1. http://docplayer.net/7062512-Acr-committee-on-drugs-and-contrast-media-acr-manual-on-contrast-media-version-10-1-2015.html

17. Berg WA, Blume JD, Cormack JB, et al. Combined screening with ultrasound and mammography vs mammography alone in women at elevated risk of breast cancer. *JAMA.* 2008;299(18):2151–2163.

18. Lee C, Dershaw D, Kopans D, et al. Breast cancer screening with imaging: recommendations from the Society of Breast Imaging and the ACR on the use of mammography, breast MRI, breast ultrasound, and other technologies for the detection of clinically occult breast cancer. *J Am Coll Radiol.* 2010;7:18–27.

19. Harvey JA, Mahoney MC, Newell MS, et al. ACR Appropriateness Criteria palpable breast masses. https://acsearch.acr.org/docs/69495/Narrative

20. Lehman CD, Lee AY, Lee CI. Imaging management of palpable breast abnormalities. *AJR Am J Roentgenol.* 2014;203:1142–1153.

21. Mainiero MB, Lourenco AP, Barke LD, et al. ACR Appropriateness Criteria evaluation of the symptomatic male breast. https://acsearch.acr.org/docs/3091547/Narrative

22. Welch ST, Babcock DS, Ballard ET. Sonography of pediatric male breast masses: gynecomastia and beyond. *Pediatr Radiol.* 2004;34:952–957.

23. West KW, Rescoria FJ, Scherer LR, et al. Diagnosis and treatment of symptomatic breast masses in the pediatric population. *J Pediatr Surg.* 1995;30:182–187.

24. Yang WT, Dryden MJ, Gwyn K, et al. Imaging and diagnosis of breast cancer diagnosed and treated with chemotherapy during pregnancy. *Radiology.* 2006;239:52–60.

25. Jokich PM, Newell MS, Bailey L, et al. ACR Appropriateness Criteria breast pain. https://acsearch.acr.org/docs/3091546/Narrative

26. Howard MF, Battaglia T, Prout M, et al. The effect of imaging on the clinical management of breast pain. *J Gen Inter Med.* 2012;27:817–824.

27. Margolis NE, Morley C, Lofti P, et al. Update on imaging of the post-surgical breast. *Radiographics.* 2014;32:642–660.

28. Ho CP, Gillis GE, Atkins KA, et al. Interactive case review of radiology and pathologic findings from breast biopsy: are they concordant? How do I manage the results? *Radiographics.* 2013;33:E149–E152.

29. Brant WE, Helms CA. *Fundamentals of Diagnostic Radiology.* 3rd ed. Philadelphia, PA: Lippincott Williams and Wilkins; 2007:565–599.

30. Lee CH, Philpotts LE, Horvath LJ, et al. Follow-up of breast lesions diagnosed as benign with stereotactic core needle biopsy: frequency of mammographic change and false-negative rate. *Radiology.* 1999;212:189–194.

31. Humphrey K, Saksena MA, Freer PE, et al. To do or not to do: axillary nodal evaluation after ACOSOG Z0011 trial. *Radiographics.* 2014;34:1807–1816.

32. Boetes C, Mus RD, Holland R, et al. Breast tumors: comparative accuracy of MR imaging relative to mammography and US for demonstrating extent. *Radiology.* 1995;197:743–747.

33. Gundry KR. The application of breast MRI in staging and screening for breast cancer. Oncology (Willston Park). 2005;19:159–169.

34. Liberman L, Morris EA, Kim CM, et al. MR imaging findings in the contralateral breast of women with recently diagnosed breast cancer. *AJR Am J Roentgenol.* 2003;180:333–341.

35. Mann RM. The effectiveness of MR imaging in the assessment of invasive lobular carcinoma of the breast. *Magn Reson Imaging Clin N Am.* 2010;18:259–276.

36. Le-Petross CH, Bidaut L, Yang WT. Evolving role of imaging modalities in inflammatory breast cancer. *Semin Oncol.* 2008;35:53–61.

37. Groheux D, Hindié E, Delord M, et al. Prognostic impact of [18]FDG-PET-CT findings in clinical stage III and IIB breast cancer. *J Natl Cancer Inst.* 2012;104:1879–1887.

38. Rosen EL, William BE, Mankoff DA. FDG PET, PET/CT, and breast cancer imaging. *Radiographics.* 2007;27:S215–S229.

39. Cancer Among Women. Cancer Prevention and Control. Centers for Disease Control and Prevention. http://www.cdc.gov/cancer/dcpc/data/women.htm

40. American Cancer Society. *Cancer Treatment and Survivorship Facts & Figures 2014–2015.* Atlanta, GA: American Cancer Society, Inc; 2015.

41. Schneble EJ, Graham LJ, Shupe MP, et al. Current approaches and challenges in early detection of breast cancer recurrence. *J Cancer.* 2014;5:281–290.

42. Lu WL, Jansen L, Post WJ, et al. Impact on survival of early detection of isolated breast recurrences after the primary treatment for breast cancer: a meta-analysis. *Breast Cancer Res Treat.* 2009;114:403–412.

43. Arasu VA, Joe BN, Lvoff NM, et al. Benefit of semiannual ipsilateral mammographic surveillance following breast conservation therapy. *Radiology.* 2012;264:371–377.

44. Brennan S, Liberman L, Dershaw DD, et al. Breast MRI screening of women with a personal history of breast cancer. *AJR Am J Roentgenol.* 2010;195:510–516.

45. Weinstock H, Campassi C, Goloubeva O, et al. Breast magnetic resonance imaging (MRI) surveillance in breast cancer survivors. *SpringerPlus.* 2015;4:459.

46. Gallowitsch HJ, Kresnik E, Gasser J, et al. F-18 fluorodeoxyglucose positron-emission tomography in the diagnosis of tumor recurrence and metastases in the follow-up of patients with breast carcinoma: a comparison to conventional imaging. *Invest Radiol.* 2003;38:250–256.

47. Almuhaideb A, Papathanasiou, N, Bomanji J. ^{18}F-FDG PET/CT imaging in oncology. *Ann Saudi Med.* 2011;31:3–13.

Arielle Cimeno, Stephanie Richards, Susan B. Kesmodel, Olga Ioffe,
Katherine H. R. Tkaczuk, and Emily Bellavance

INTRODUCTION

General Characteristics

High-risk breast lesions represent a category of disease that, while "benign," confers an increased risk of future malignancy. These lesions may require surgical excision to exclude the presence of an invasive breast cancer or ductal carcinoma in situ (DCIS). Included in this category are atypical ductal hyperplasia (ADH), atypical lobular hyperplasia (ALH), lobular carcinoma in situ (LCIS), flat epithelial atypia (FEA), and intraductal papillomas (IPs). These lesions are typically asymptomatic. The actual incidence of high-risk breast lesions is unknown, primarily because they are often clinically silent. Up to 4% of core needle biopsies (CNBs) and 23% of excisional biopsies are reported to contain a high-risk lesion (1,2). Atypical hyperplasia is found in 10% to 17% of biopsies (3–5). LCIS is an incidental finding in up to 3.8% of benign breast biopsies (3), FEA is a rare lesion found in 1.2% of CNB (6), and 5% of lesions on CNB are identified as IPs (7).

Workup

A. Improvements in breast imaging have resulted in more abnormalities detected on screening mammography, leading to an increased number of breast biopsies.
B. Image-guided CNB is the first modality utilized to obtain tissue for diagnosis.
C. Studies of CNB techniques show that larger gauge needles, higher number of cores obtained, and the use of vacuum-assisted devices result in a lower rate of upgrading of the pathology upon excision, need for rebiopsy, and radiologic–pathologic discordance (8,9,10).

Management

A. A high-risk lesion found on CNB is considered for surgical excision based on the likelihood of malignancy (risk of upgrading) on final pathology. Discordance or concern that the intended lesion was not sampled is also an indication for surgical excision (11).
B. Depending on the results of surgical excision and lifetime risk of breast cancer, patients may be eligible for chemoprevention.
C. Select patients may be candidates for prophylactic mastectomy.

ATYPICAL DUCTAL HYPERPLASIA

Histology

ADH is a proliferative intraductal lesion that fulfills some, but not all, of the criteria for DCIS (Figure 2.1). Like DCIS, it carries an increased risk for the development of invasive breast cancer (12,13). Clinically, ADH is a lesion that does not present as a palpable mass; it is usually identified on screening mammography by the presence of microcalcifications. ADH identified on core biopsy may signify the presence of a higher grade adjacent lesion; cases of ADH on biopsy are not infrequently upgraded to DCIS or invasive carcinoma on excision (1). ADH confers a mildly increased risk of breast cancer—4–5× relative risk (RR).

There are no universally accepted criteria to reliably distinguish between ADH and DCIS (14). Generally, though, a diagnosis of DCIS requires the presence of at least two duct cross-sections that are fully involved by the atypical proliferative lesion (14). Anything less than two fully involved ductal cross-sections is more appropriately characterized as ADH.

ADH may also have significant microscopic overlap with usual ductal hyperplasia (UDH) or benign intraductal hyperplasia. Unlike DCIS, UDH is characterized by cells of nonuniform shape with nuclei oriented parallel to their long axes (streaming cells) and indistinct cell borders. However, atypical features need to be present in order to diagnose a lesion as ADH. ADH is a proliferation of atypical epithelial cells that involve individual ductal spaces. The distinction between ADH and DCIS is the extent of proliferation, with ductal involvement of <2mm and less than two ductal spaces in ADH (3).

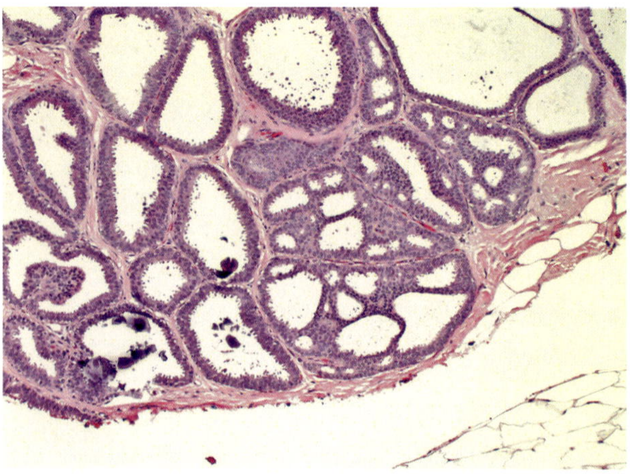

Figure 2.1 Atypical ductal hyperplasia (ADH). The ductal profiles in this field exhibit focal cribriforming and monotonous cellular proliferation; however, this process does not fulfill criteria for ductal carcinoma in situ (does not involve two profiles completely) and is therefore classified as ADH.

Upgrade Rate

A. Surgical excision of ADH found on biopsy has variable published upgrade rates in the range of 18% to 31% (1,8). In a study that assessed upgrade rates in 685 women with ADH, 123 (18%) were found to have more significant pathology in the breast at surgical excision (1). The majority of these cases showed DCIS (82%), with invasive cancer identified in the remaining 18%. In a smaller study that examined pathology in 70 patients with ADH undergoing surgical excision, malignancy was identified in 31% of the patients (8). Again, the majority of patients had DCIS (74%) on final pathology.

Treatment

A. Based on the reported upgrade rates, ADH found on biopsy is considered an indication for surgical excision.

> ➤ We currently recommend excision in women with ADH on image-guided biopsy who are surgical candidates.

B. There is interest in elucidating a set of criteria that would determine which patients can forgo surgical excision for imaging surveillance; however, currently there is no consensus and individualized treatment approaches are recommended.

C. Based on cumulative risk factors for breast cancer, patients with a diagnosis of ADH may be eligible for chemoprevention, which is covered later in this chapter.

Risk of Future Malignancy

The cumulative risk of in situ or invasive cancer in patients with ADH is approximately 20% at 20 years (11), an RR of 4 (15). In a study conducted by the Mayo Clinic that examined the risk of subsequent breast cancer in women with atypical hyperplasia, 698 women were identified from pathology review (16). This study included patients with ADH and ALH. With a mean follow-up of 12.5 years, breast cancer was detected in 143 patients (20.4%), with similar rates in patients with ADH and ALH. The majority of cancers developed in the ipsilateral breast and most patients with ADH were diagnosed with invasive breast cancer.

Factors associated with an increased risk of developing breast cancer after a diagnosis of atypical hyperplasia include multifocal disease, less age-related lobular involution in the breast, and younger age at diagnosis.

ATYPICAL LOBULAR HYPERPLASIA

Histology

Like ADH, ALH is an atypical proliferative lesion that is not sufficiently developed to meet the criteria for LCIS. Histologically, ALH—like LCIS—is composed of bland cells that lack E-cadherin expression and fill preexisting lobular structures. However, unlike in LCIS, these cells do not expand the lobules (17). ALH confers a mildly increased bilateral breast cancer risk of the same magnitude as ADH (4–5× RR). ALH and LCIS are distinguished by the degree of lobular involvement, with distortion of <50% of involved lobular acinar spaces categorized as ALH and >50% as LCIS (3).

Upgrade Rate

Published pathology upgrade rates for excision of ALH vary widely, from 0% to 43% (8,10,11), because ALH is commonly found with other lesions on biopsy. In a pooled analysis of studies that examined the results of surgical excision in patients with high-risk breast lesions and included 280 patients with ALH, breast cancer was identified in 53 cases (19%) on surgical excision with 74% of these showing DCIS.

Treatment

A. Because of variable upgrade rates and the high frequency of incidental ALH and concomitant lesions, surgical excision of ALH is controversial. Surgical biopsy should be offered in patients with ALH diagnosed on CNB for definitive diagnosis. Patients should also be offered the option of clinical and imaging follow-up in 6 to 12 months after careful consideration of the risks and benefits of surgical excision.
B. Based on cumulative risk factors for breast cancer, patients with a diagnosis of ALH may be eligible for chemoprevention, which is covered later in this chapter.

Risk of Future Malignancy

A. The RR of developing cancer with ALH is similar to ADH (RR of 4) (15). Cumulative incidence of developing a malignancy in either breast approaches 20% at 20 years, 30% at 25 years, and 35% at 30 years (4,11,18). Breast cancers that develop in women with ALH are more commonly invasive ductal carcinomas than other histologies and, similar to ADH, occur more frequently in the ipsilateral breast (16).
B. The same factors that increase the risk of breast cancer in patients with ADH, including multifocal disease and younger age at diagnosis, apply for ALH (16,18).

LOBULAR CARCINOMA IN SITU

Histology

LCIS is a proliferative intralobular lesion that is often incidentally detected on biopsy of an unrelated lesion (Figure 2.2). It is often multifocal and bilateral, and as such, it is considered to be a marker of increased bilateral risk (8–10 × RR) (19) for invasive breast cancer rather than a true precursor lesion (20,21). LCIS rarely forms a discrete mass; occasionally, a palpable region of firmness will be present due to surrounding tissue reaction (17). LCIS is characterized by lobules that are filled and expanded by discohesive neoplastic bland round cells with eccentric nuclei and occasional signet ring forms. On immunohistochemistry, LCIS cells exhibit loss of E-cadherin, a cellular adhesion protein. Pagetoid spread of LCIS cells into the ducts underneath the normal ductal epithelium is relatively common.

Upgrade Rate

A. The rate of upgrade at surgical excision ranges widely from 0% to 60% in published studies, as many have small sample sizes and include LCIS found with other lesions (8,10,22). In a pooled analysis that reported results of surgical excision in 241 patients with LCIS, upgrade to DCIS or invasive cancer was observed in 32% of cases. The majority of these cases were invasive cancer (64%). Upgrade rates are higher when other high-risk lesions (ADH) are identified in combination with LCIS (22).

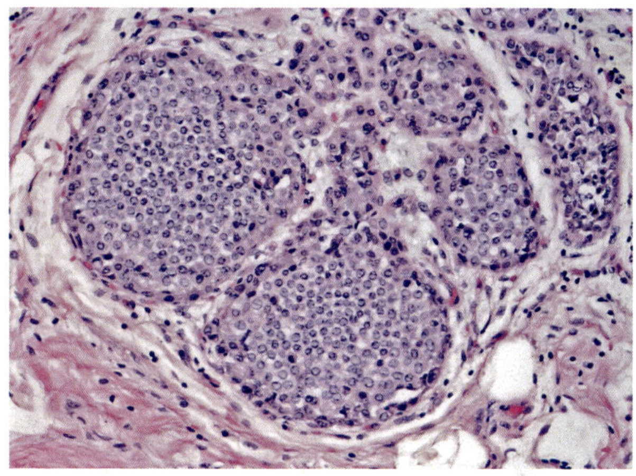

Figure 2.2 Lobular carcinoma in situ (LCIS). Small monotonous discohesive cells fill acini in this lobule.

B. One subtype, pleomorphic LCIS, is a more aggressive lesion with a higher risk of concurrent malignancy.

Treatment

A. Surgical excision for LCIS is controversial and should depend on institutional upgrade rates. Similar to ALH, surgical biopsy should be offered in patients for definitive diagnosis. Patients should also be offered the option of clinical and imaging follow-up in 6 to 12 months after careful consideration of the risks and benefits of surgical excision. Since surgical excision is performed for sampling, negative margins are not necessary.

> ➤ Patients should be offered the option of surgical excision as well as the alternative of close follow-up with imaging.

B. Pleomorphic LCIS is a more aggressive subtype and may represent a precursor lesion to invasive cancer.

> ➤ We currently recommend treating this entity with surgical excision. The importance of obtaining microscopically negative margins in the excision of pleomorphic LCIS is controversial. Invasive cancer is identified more frequently on excision of pleomorphic LCIS than standard LCIS (10).

C. Based on cumulative risk factors for breast cancer, patients with a diagnosis of LCIS may be eligible for chemoprevention (see the following).
D. Patients with a diagnosis of LCIS may be considered for more aggressive screening strategies including more frequent clinical breast exams and breast MRI. This should be considered in the context of the patients' other risk factors for breast cancer.

Risk of Future Malignancy

A. LCIS confers an RR of lifetime malignancy of 10 (19). The risk of developing an invasive cancer is about 0.7% to 1% per year (11).
B. LCIS confers a greater risk for both ductal and lobular cancers, which can occur in either breast (10,11).

ATYPICAL COLUMNAR CELL CHANGE (FLAT EPITHELIAL ATYPIA)

Histology

Columnar cell change is a ubiquitous alteration of benign breast epithelium characterized by tall cuboidal to columnar epithelial cells replacing the normal low cuboidal ductal cells. Features that signify atypical columnar cell change (FEA) are similar to those of ADH: a uniformly sized cell population with basally oriented, hyperchromatic monotonous nuclei. Similar to ADH, though, FEA does not meet the criteria to diagnose DCIS (14). FEA is currently considered to represent a non-obligate precursor to estrogen receptor (ER)/progesterone receptor (PR) positive, low-grade DCIS and invasive carcinoma; as such, it imparts a slightly increased risk of future breast cancer—between that of ADH and florid proliferative breast disease.

Upgrade Rate

A. Published upgrade rates vary from 0% to 25% in small series (2,23).
B. Rates are higher when found with ADH or DCIS. A study that examined upgrade rates in patients with FEA and included 95 patients with pure FEA who underwent surgical excision showed an upgrade rate of only 3.2%, with 1 patient having DCIS and 2 patients having invasive cancer and DCIS. In those patients with concomitant FEA and ADH who underwent surgical excision (43 patients), the upgrade rate was 18.6%, with 4 patients having DCIS alone and 4 patients having an invasive component (2).
C. Upgrade rates with pure FEA may be lower. In a study that assessed upgrade rates to DCIS or invasive cancer in 104 patients with pure FEA who underwent surgical excision, an upgrade rate of 9.6% was observed, with 5 patients having invasive cancer and 5 patients having DCIS. Other histopathology that was identified on surgical excision included LCIS, ADH, ALH, and FEA (6).

Treatment

A. FEA found with other lesions warranting excision should be excised given the higher upgrade rates when found in combination with ADH, ALH, or LCIS (24).
B. The need for excision of pure FEA is unclear. The decision to excise FEA should take into account imaging studies, the findings on pathology, and the overall health of the patient. If there is concern that the finding on imaging has not been adequately sampled or that the imaging and pathology are discordant, then surgical excision is warranted. In general, we consider excision for all patients with FEA given that even in pure FEA, the upgrade rates can be as high as 10%.

Risk of Future Malignancy

A. FEA is a relatively new diagnosis, and long-term studies on the risk of malignancy associated with FEA have not been reported (11).

INTRADUCTAL PAPILLOMAS

Histology

IP is a lesion consisting of a fibrovascular stalk and surrounding epithelial proliferation (7).

Upgrade Rate

A. Upgrade rates for IP vary from 2% to 35% and depend on whether atypia is present in the biopsy (Table 2.1) (1,11).
B. In a study that looked at upgrade rates at surgical excision for 99 papillary lesions without atypia, the upgrade rate was only 2% and both patients had DCIS.
C. Upgrade rates are higher when atypia is present and are closer to rates seen with ADH, ALH, and LCIS. A comparison of upgrade rates in patients with IP without atypia to those with atypia showed an upgrade rate of 6% in patients with IP without atypia and a rate of 21% in patients with IP with atypia (27).

Table 2.1 Upgrade Rates of High-Risk Lesions

Lesion	Study	N	Upgrade rate (%)
ADH	Margenthaler et al (8)	61	31
	Menes et al (1)	685	18
ALH	Margenthaler et al (8)	19	16
	Hussain, Cunnick (10)	280	19
	Rendi et al (22)	53	4.1
	Shah-Khan et al (25)	81	1.2
	Murray et al (26)	34	11
LCIS	Margenthaler et al (8)	16	25
	Hussain, Cunnick (10)	241	32
	Rendi et al (22)	23	5
	Shah-Khan et al (25)	20	5
	Murray et al (26)	46	4.3
Pleomorphic LCIS	Hussain, Cunnick (10)	22	41
FEA	Lavoue et al (2)	60	13
	Uzoaru et al (24)	95	3.2
	Khoumais et al (6)	104	9.6
IP	Menes et al (1)	99	2
	Nakhlis et al (27)	97	10

ADH, atypical ductal hyperplasia; ALH, atypical lobular hyperplasia; FEA, flat epithelial atypia; IP, intraductal papilloma; LCIS, lobular carcinoma in situ.

Treatment

IP with or without atypia should be excised if the presenting symptom is a mass or pathologic nipple discharge, there is radiologic–pathologic discordance, or if the CNB was not obtained with a vacuum-assisted device (7). Patients with IP with atypia should always be considered for surgical excision given the similar upgrade rates to other proliferative breast lesions with atypia.

Risk of Future Malignancy

A. The long-term risk of malignancy is linked to the presence of atypia with an RR of 4 with atypia and 2 without atypia (Table 2.2) (11).

CHEMOPREVENTION

Risk Reduction

The use of hormonal (endocrine) therapy has been shown to reduce the incidence of breast cancer in women with increased risk. Only a very small proportion of women who might benefit from chemoprevention are prescribed and/or take these medications, largely due to fear of adverse side effects (4). In a meta-analysis of endocrine prevention of breast cancer with selective estrogen receptor modulators (SERMs), incidence of invasive ER-positive breast cancer was reduced both during treatment and for at least 5 years after completion. Careful consideration of risks and benefits is needed to identify women who are most likely to benefit from prevention (28).

Selective Estrogen Receptor Modulators

A. Agents
1. Tamoxifen—in 1999 the U.S. Food and Drug Administration (FDA) approved tamoxifen for primary prevention of breast cancer.
2. Raloxifene—in 2007 the FDA approved raloxifene for reducing the risk of invasive breast cancer in postmenopausal women with osteoporosis and in postmenopausal women at high risk for invasive breast cancer.
B. Mechanism of action: competitive inhibitor of ERs on breast tissue

Table 2.2 Long-Term Risk of Breast Cancer With High-Risk Lesions	
Lesion	**Relative risk of breast cancer**
ADH	4
ALH	4
LCIS	10
FEA	1.5
Papillary lesions	2
ADH, atypical ductal hyperplasia; ALH, atypical lobular hyperplasia; FEA, flat epithelial atypia; LCIS, lobular carcinoma in situ.	

C. Indications: premenopausal women at increased risk of breast cancer (tamoxifen only); postmenopausal (tamoxifen and raloxifene) women at increased risk of breast cancer

D. Side effects: vasomotor symptoms, venous thromboembolic (VTE) events, tamoxifen (not raloxifene) increases the risk of endometrial cancer; contraindications: pregnancy, history of VTE, history of stroke

Aromatase Inhibitors

A. Agents
   1. Exemestane—irreversible steroidal aromatase inactivator
   2. Anastrozole—nonsteroidal aromatase inhibitor (AI)
B. Mechanism of action-block conversion of androgens to estrogens in peripheral tissues. AIs are contraindicated in premenopausal women or pregnant women.
C. Indications: Neither anastrozole nor exemestane is FDA approved for prevention of breast cancer. However, based on available data from several prevention studies discussed in the following, these agents can be considered for prevention in women with increased risk of developing breast cancer such as Gail risk of ≥1.6% in 5 years.
D. **Most common side effects:** Side-effect profiles for anastrozole and exemestane are expected to be similar. In the Anastrozole, Tamoxifen, Alone or in Combination (ATAC) study, a randomized, placebo-controlled study of tamoxifen versus anastrozole versus the combination, the most common side effects observed in >10% of women taking anastrozole compared to tamoxifen included: hot flashes, asthenia, arthritis, pain, arthralgia, pharyngitis, hypertension, depression, nausea and vomiting, rash, osteoporosis, fractures, back pain, insomnia, headache, peripheral edema, and lymphedema, regardless of causality. In women with preexisting ischemic heart disease, an increased incidence of ischemic cerebrovascular stroke (CVS) events occurred with anastrozole (17%) compared to tamoxifen (10%). Increases in total cholesterol and decreased bone mineral density may occur and should be monitored.
E. **Contraindications:** pregnancy, osteoporosis

KEY PREVENTION TRIALS (Table 2.3)

International Breast Cancer Intervention Study I (IBIS-I)

DESIGN

A randomized, placebo-controlled double-blind trial of premenopausal and postmenopausal women aged 35 to 70 at increased risk of breast cancer who received tamoxifen or placebo for 5 years. Increased risk was defined as at least a twofold increased risk for breast cancer based on risk factors for breast cancer in patients aged 45 to 70 and greater than a twofold increased risk in women younger than 45.

RESULTS

There was a reduction in breast cancer incidence including DCIS with a hazard ratio (HR) of 0.71 ($P < .0001$) at a median follow-up of 16 years. The greatest risk reduction was seen for ER-positive breast cancer and DCIS. There was no impact on the development of ER-negative breast cancer. Reduction continued for invasive cancer after the treatment period with an absolute risk reduction of 4.5% at

Table 2.3 Prevention Trials

Trial	Design	Participants	Intervention	Results
IBIS-I	Randomized (8) placebo-controlled double-blind	Pre- and postmenopausal women aged 35–70 with increased risk of breast cancer (>2× risk)	Tamoxifen vs. placebo for 5 years	29% reduction in BC incidence including DCIS ($P < .0001$) at a median follow-up of 16 years Increased rates of VTE and endometrial cancer
NSABP (P-1)	Randomized placebo-controlled double-blind	Women at increased risk of breast cancer (age >60, age 35–59 with risk >1.66%, or history of LCIS)	Tamoxifen vs. placebo for 5 years	49% risk reduction of invasive breast cancer, 50% risk reduction of noninvasive cancer Increased risk of endometrial cancer, PE, and DVT
Royal Marsden	Randomized placebo-controlled double-blind	Women aged 30–70 with a family history of breast cancer	Tamoxifen vs. placebo for 8 years	Lower risk of ER-positive breast cancer in the post treatment period
MORE	Randomized placebo-controlled double-blind	Postmenopausal women younger than 81 with osteoporosis	Raloxifene vs. placebo for 3 years	76% decreased risk of invasive cancer

(continued)

Table 2.3 Prevention Trials (*continued*)

Trial	Design	Participants	Intervention	Results
STAR P-2	Randomized blinded	Women with >1.66% 5-year risk based on Gail model	Tamoxifen vs. Raloxifene for 5 years	Raloxifene 76% as effective as tamoxifen at reducing invasive BC and Raloxifene reduced risk 39% vs. placebo Raloxifene had lower risk of VTE and endometrial cancer
MAP3	Randomized placebo-controlled double-blind	Postmenopausal women >60 or women >35 with 5-year risk >1.66% based on Gail model, ADH, ALH, LCIS, or DCIS	Exemestane vs. placebo	65% relative risk reduction in annual incidence of invasive cancer
IBIS-II	Randomized placebo-controlled double-blind	Postmenopausal women 40–70 with increased risk of breast cancer	Anastrozole vs. placebo for 5 years	Significantly less cancers in the anastrozole group with hazard ratio of 0.47

ADH, atypical ductal hyperplasia; ALH, atypical lobular hyperplasia; DCIS, ductal carcinoma in situ; DVT, deep venous thrombosis; ER, estrogen receptor; IBIS-I, International Breast Cancer Intervention Study I; IBIS-II, International Breast Cancer Intervention Study II; LCIS, lobular carcinoma in situ; MAP3, Mammary Prevention 3; MORE, Multiple Outcomes of Raloxifene Evaluation; NSABP, National Surgical Adjuvant Breast and Bowel Project; PE, pulmonary embolism; STAR, Study of Tamoxifen and Raloxifene;
VTE, venous thromboembolic.

20 years. The number of patients needed to treat for 5 years to prevent 1 incidence of cancer at 20 years is 22 patients.

SIDE EFFECTS

Tamoxifen was shown to cause increased rates of VTE mainly in the first 10 years of follow-up, 1.4% in patients receiving tamoxifen versus 0.8% in patients receiving placebo, and endometrial cancer mainly in the first 5 years of follow-up, 15 patients (0.4%) receiving tamoxifen versus 4 patients (0.1%) receiving placebo in the first 5 years, and 29 patients (0.8%) receiving tamoxifen versus 20 patients (0.6%) receiving placebo overall (28).

National Surgical Adjuvant Breast and Bowel Project, Prevention-1 (NSABP P-1)

DESIGN

Randomized, placebo-controlled double-blind trial of women who received tamoxifen for 5 years. 8.9% of participants had a history of atypical hyperplasia and 6.2% has a history of LCIS. Women (N = 13,388) at increased risk for breast cancer because they (a) were 60 years of age or older, (b) were 35 to 59 years of age with a 5-year predicted risk for breast cancer of at least 1.66%, or (c) had a history of LCIS were randomly assigned to receive placebo (N = 6,707) or 20 mg/day tamoxifen (N = 6,681) for 5 years.

RESULTS

Tamoxifen reduced the risk of invasive breast cancer by 49% (two-sided $P < .00001$), with cumulative incidence through 69 months of follow-up of 43.4 versus 22.0 per 1,000 women in the placebo and tamoxifen groups, respectively. The decreased risk occurred in women aged 49 years or younger (44%), 50 to 59 years (51%), and 60 years or older (55%); risk was also reduced in women with a history of LCIS (56%) or atypical hyperplasia (86%) and in those with any category of predicted 5-year risk. Tamoxifen reduced the risk of noninvasive breast cancer by 50% (two-sided $P < .002$) and reduced the occurrence of ER-positive tumors by 69%, but there was no difference in the occurrence of ER-negative tumors.

SIDE EFFECTS

Endometrial cancer was increased in the tamoxifen group (risk ratio = 2.53), predominantly in women aged 50 years or older. Increased risk of pulmonary embolus was also seen again primarily in women aged 50 years or older and deep venous thrombosis (DVT) (RR—1.60; 95% CIs [0.91, 2.86]) (29).

Royal Marsden Trial

DESIGN

Randomized, placebo-controlled double-blind trial of women (N = 2,494) aged 30 to 70 with a family history of breast cancer who received tamoxifen or placebo for 8 years. The primary outcome was occurrence of invasive breast cancer. A secondary planned analysis of ER-positive invasive breast cancer was also done.

RESULTS

A statistically significant reduction in the incidence of ER-positive breast cancer was observed in the tamoxifen arm that occurred predominantly during the posttreatment follow-up, indicating long-term prevention of estrogen-dependent breast cancer by tamoxifen. The risk of ER-positive breast cancer was not statistically significantly lower in the tamoxifen arm than in the placebo arm during the 8-year treatment period (HR = 0.77, 95% CIs [0.48, 1.23]; P = .3) but was statistically significantly lower in the posttreatment period (HR = 0.48, 95% CIs [0.29, 0.79]; P = .004), suggesting a carryover effect of prevention with tamoxifen (30).

Multiple Outcomes of Raloxifene Evaluation (MORE)

DESIGN

Randomized, placebo-controlled double-blind trial of postmenopausal women less than 81 years old with osteoporosis who received raloxifene or placebo for 3 years.

RESULTS

Raloxifene was shown to decrease the risk of invasive cancer by 76%. The risk of all ER-positive cancers decreased by 90% but there was no effect on ER-negative cancers. The number needed to treat to prevent one incidence of breast cancer was 126.

SIDE EFFECTS

Raloxifene did confer an increased risk of VTE events with an RR of 3 (0.6%) (1). Raloxifene did not significantly increase the risk of endometrial cancer (31).

National Surgical Adjuvant Breast and Bowel Project, Study of Tamoxifen and Raloxifene (STAR) P-2 (NCT00003906)

DESIGN

Randomized blinded trial of postmenopausal women at increased risk of breast cancer defined as 5-year risk at least 1.66% based on the Gail model, who received tamoxifen 20 mg daily or raloxifene 60 mg daily for 5 years. 23% of participants had a history of atypical hyperplasia and 9.2% had a history of LCIS.

RESULTS

Initial results showed that raloxifene was as effective as tamoxifen at reducing the incidence of invasive breast cancer but worse in terms of prevention of noninvasive disease. There were an equal number of cases of invasive breast cancer in women assigned to tamoxifen and raloxifene. There were fewer cases of noninvasive breast cancer in the tamoxifen group than in the raloxifene group (risk ratio: 1.40; 95% CIs [0.98, 2.02]). Longer follow-up of 81 months showed that this benefit did not persist past the treatment period. Raloxifene was 76% as effective as tamoxifen at reducing invasive breast cancer risk and grew closer to tamoxifen over time in preventing noninvasive disease; it also reduced risk by 39% compared to placebo.

SIDE EFFECTS

Raloxifene had a significantly lower risk of VTE events and endometrial cancer (32). Toxicity risk ratios (raloxifene:tamoxifen) were 0.55 (95% CI; P = .003) for endometrial cancer; this difference was not significant in the initial results, 0.19

(95% CIs [0.12, 0.29]) for uterine hyperplasia and 0.75 (95% CIs [0.60, 0.93]) for thromboembolic events, and there were fewer cataracts and cataract surgeries in the women taking raloxifene (risk ratio: 0.79; 95% CIs [0.68, 0.92]).

Mammary Prevention 3 (MAP3) (NCT00083174) Trial
DESIGN

Randomized placebo-controlled double-blind trial of postmenopausal women aged 60 and over or aged 35 and over with a Gail 5-year risk >1.66%, ADH, ALH, LCIS, or DCIS treated with mastectomy, who were treated with exemestane for a median follow-up of 3 years. Eleven percent of the participants had a history of ADH, ALH, LCIS, or DCIS.

RESULTS

A 65% relative reduction in the annual incidence of invasive cancer was seen in the exemestane group.

SIDE EFFECTS

There was no difference in the number of fractures between the exemestane and placebo groups (33).

International Breast Cancer Intervention Study II (IBIS-II) (NCT00072462)
DESIGN

Randomized, placebo-controlled double-blind trial of postmenopausal women aged 40 to 70 with an increased risk of breast cancer who received anastrozole for 5 years. Nine percent of participants had a high-risk breast lesion.

RESULTS

At 5-year follow-up there were significantly fewer cancers in the anastrozole group with an HR of 0.47. Women taking anastrozole were also found to have a lower frequency of high-grade cancers.

SIDE EFFECTS

Anastrozole did not increase the risk of VTE events but did increase musculoskeletal and vasomotor side effects (28).

SERM Clinical Trials Meta-Analysis
DESIGN

A meta-analysis with individual participant data from nine prevention trials comparing four SERMs (tamoxifen, raloxifene, arzoxifene, and lasofoxifene) with placebo, or in one study with tamoxifen. Primary endpoint was incidence of all breast cancer (including DCIS) during a 10-year follow-up period. Analysis of outcomes data for 83,399 healthy women was done by intention to treat; median follow-up was 65 months (range 54–93 months).

RESULTS

Treatment resulted in a 38% reduction (HR 0.62, 95% CIs [0.56, 0.69]) in breast cancer incidence; 42 women would need to be treated to prevent one breast cancer event in the first 10 years of follow-up. The reduction was larger in the first 5 years of follow-up than in years 5 to 10 (42%, HR 0.58, $P < .0001$ vs. 25%, 0.75; $P = .007$), but no heterogeneity between time periods was observed.

SIDE EFFECTS

Thromboembolic events were significantly increased with all SERMs (odds ratio 1.73, 95%; $P < .0001$) while there was a significant reduction of 34% in vertebral fractures (0.66, 0.59–0.73), but only a small effect for nonvertebral fractures (0.93, 0.87–0.99).

In Figure 2.3 we show possible breast cancer prevention strategies based on menopausal status, as well as presence or absence of bone loss or uterus.

PROPHYLACTIC MASTECTOMY

Surgical prophylaxis in the form of bilateral mastectomy is an option for a select group of patients. Prophylactic mastectomy should be considered individually based on cumulative risk factors (rather than the presence of a high-risk breast lesion alone). Consultation with a genetics counselor to assess breast cancer risk and with a medical oncologist to discuss chemoprophylaxis can aid patient decision making. Prophylactic mastectomy can decrease the risk of developing breast cancer in a high-risk population by >90% (34).

SURVEILLANCE

In addition to annual screening mammography, MRI has been considered in patients with an increased risk of breast cancer. The American Cancer Society recommends annual breast MRI in addition to mammography for women with a cumulative lifetime risk of breast cancer greater than 20% to 25%, but there is insufficient evidence to recommend it for women with LCIS or atypical hyperplasia alone (35). Recommendations for surveillance in patients with high-risk lesions should be based on the calculated lifetime risk.

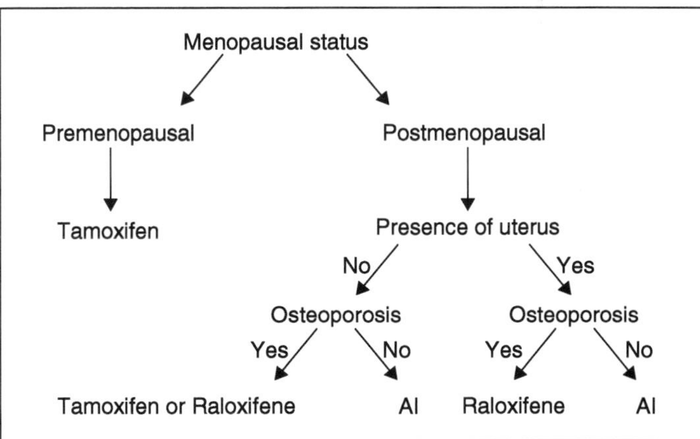

Figure 2.3 Suggested prevention strategies for selection of systemic treatments for 5 years.

AI, aromatase inhibitor.

➤ MANAGEMENT PEARLS

1. Image-guided CNB is the preferred method to obtain a tissue diagnosis of a suspicious breast lesion.
2. Recommendations for surgical excision of high-risk breast lesions are based on the risk of finding an invasive breast cancer or DCIS in the excised specimen.
3. Chemoprophylaxis with SERMs or AIs should be offered to eligible candidates for breast cancer risk reduction.

REFERENCES

1. Menes TS, Rosenberg R, Balch S, et al. Upgrade of high-risk breast lesions detected on mammography in the Breast Cancer Surveillance Consortium. *Am J Surg.* 2014;207(1):24–31.
2. Lavoue V, Roger CM, Poilblanc M, et al. Pure flat epithelial atypia (DIN 1a) on core needle biopsy: study of 60 biopsies with follow-up surgical excision. *Breast Cancer Res Treat.* 2011;125(1):121–126.
3. Morrow M, Schnitt SJ, Norton L. Current management of lesions associated with an increased risk of breast cancer. *Nat Rev Clin Oncol.* 2015;12(4):227–238.
4. Hartmann LC, Degnim AC, Santen RJ, et al. Atypical hyperplasia of the breast—risk assessment and management options. *N Engl J Med.* 2015;372(1):78–89.
5. Caplain A, Drouet Y, Peyron M, et al. Management of patients diagnosed with atypical ductal hyperplasia by vacuum-assisted core biopsy: a prospective assessment of the guidelines used at our institution. *Am J Surg.* 2014;208(2):260–267.
6. Khoumais NA, Scaranelo AM, Moshonov H, et al. Incidence of breast cancer in patients with pure flat epithelial atypia diagnosed at core-needle biopsy of the breast. *Ann Surg Oncol.* 2013;20(1):133–138.
7. Krishnamurthy S, Bevers T, Kuerer H, Yang WT. Multidisciplinary considerations in the management of high-risk breast lesions. *AJR Am J Roentgenol.* 2012;198(2):W132–W140.
8. Margenthaler JA, Duke D, Monsees BS, et al. Correlation between core biopsy and excisional biopsy in breast high-risk lesions. *Am J Surg.* 2006;192(4):534–537.
9. Brem RF, Lechner MC, Jackman RJ, et al. Lobular neoplasia at percutaneous breast biopsy: variables associated with carcinoma at surgical excision. *AJR Am J Roentgenol.* 2008;190(3):637–641.
10. Hussain M, Cunnick GH. Management of lobular carcinoma in-situ and atypical lobular hyperplasia of the breast—a review. *Eur J Surg Oncol.* 2011;37(4):279–289.
11. Degnim AC, King TA. Surgical management of high-risk breast lesions. *Surg Clin North Am.* 2013;93(2):329–340.
12. Collins LC, Tamimi RM, Baer HJ, et al. Outcome of patients with ductal carcinoma in situ untreated after diagnostic biopsy: results from the Nurses' Health Study. *Cancer.* 2005;103(9):1778–1784.
13. Coopey SB, Mazzola E, Buckley JM, et al. The role of chemoprevention in modifying the risk of breast cancer in women with atypical breast lesions. *Breast Cancer Res Treat.* 2012;136(3):627–633.

14. Hoda SA. Ductal hyperplasia: usual and atypical. In: Hoda SA, Brogi E, Koerner FC, Rosen PP, eds. *Rosen's Breast Pathology*. 4th ed. Philadelphia, PA: Lippincott Williams & Wilkins; 2014:230–263.

15. Dupont WD, Page DL. Risk factors for breast cancer in women with proliferative breast disease. *N Engl J Med*. 1985;312(3):146–151.

16. Hartmann LC, Radisky DC, Frost MH, et al. Understanding the premalignant potential of atypical hyperplasia through its natural history: a longitudinal cohort study. *Cancer Prev Res (Phila)*. 2014;7(2):211–217.

17. Hoda SA. Lobular carcinoma in situ and atypical lobular hyperplasia. In: Hoda SA, Brogi E, Koerner FC, Rosen PP, eds. *Rosen's Breast Pathology*. 4th ed. Philadelphia, PA: Lippincott Williams & Wilkins; 2014:637–789.

18. Degnim AC, Visscher DW, Berman HK, et al. Stratification of breast cancer risk in women with atypia: a Mayo cohort study. *J Clin Oncol*. 2007;25(19):2671–2677.

19. Page DL, Kidd TE, Jr, Dupont WD, et al. Lobular neoplasia of the breast: higher risk for subsequent invasive cancer predicted by more extensive disease. *Hum Pathol*. 1991; 22(12):1232–1239.

20. Oppong BA, King TA. Recommendations for women with lobular carcinoma in situ (LCIS). *Oncology (Williston Park)*. 2011;25(11):1051–1056, 1058.

21. King TA, Pilewskie M, Muhsen S, et al. Lobular carcinoma in situ: a 29-year longitudinal experience evaluating clinicopathologic features and breast cancer risk. *J Clin Oncol*. 2015;33(33):3945–3952.

22. Rendi MH, Dintzis SM, Lehman CD, et al. Lobular in-situ neoplasia on breast core needle biopsy: imaging indication and pathologic extent can identify which patients require excisional biopsy. *Ann Surg Oncol*. 2012;19(3):914–921.

23. Sohn V, Porta R, Brown T. Flat epithelial atypia of the breast on core needle biopsy: an indication for surgical excision. *Mil Med*. 2011;176(11):1347–1350.

24. Uzoaru I, Morgan BR, Liu ZG, et al. Flat epithelial atypia with and without atypical ductal hyperplasia: to re-excise or not. Results of a 5-year prospective study. *Virchows Arch*. 2012;461(4):419–423.

25. Shah-Khan MG, Geiger XJ, Reynolds C, et al. Long-term follow-up of lobular neoplasia (atypical lobular hyperplasia/lobular carcinoma in situ) diagnosed on core needle biopsy. *Ann Surg Oncol*. 2012;19(10):3131–3138.

26. Murray MP, Luedtke C, Liberman L, et al. Classic lobular carcinoma in situ and atypical lobular hyperplasia at percutaneous breast core biopsy: outcomes of prospective excision. *Cancer*. 2013;119(5):1073–1079.

27. Nakhlis F, Ahmadiyeh N, Lester S, et al. Papilloma on core biopsy: excision vs. observation. *Ann Surg Oncol*. 2015;22(5):1479–1482.

28. Cuzick J, Sestak I, Forbes JF, et al. Anastrozole for prevention of breast cancer in high-risk postmenopausal women (IBIS-II): an international, double-blind, randomised placebo-controlled trial. *Lancet*. 2014;383(9922):1041–1048.

29. Fisher B, Costantino JP, Wickerham DL, et al. Tamoxifen for prevention of breast cancer: report of the National Surgical Adjuvant Breast and Bowel Project P-1 Study. *J Natl Cancer Inst*. 1998;90:1371–1388.

30. Powles TJ, Ashley S, Tidy A, et al. Twenty-year follow-up of the Royal Marsden randomized, double-blinded tamoxifen breast cancer prevention trial. *J Natl Cancer Inst*. 2007;99(4):283–290.

31. Cummings SR, Eckert S, Krueger KA, et al. The effect of raloxifene on risk of breast cancer in postmenopausal women: results from the MORE randomized trial. Multiple Outcomes of Raloxifene Evaluation. *JAMA*. 1999;281(23):2189–2197.

32. Vogel VG, Costantino JP, Wickerham DL, et al. Update of the National Surgical Adjuvant Breast and Bowel Project Study of Tamoxifen and Raloxifene (STAR) P-2 Trial: Preventing breast cancer. *Cancer Prev Res (Phila)*. 2010;3(6):696–706.

33. Goss PE, Ingle JN, Ales-Martinez JE, et al. Exemestane for breast-cancer prevention in postmenopausal women. *N Engl J Med*. 2011;364(25):2381–2391.

34. Hartmann LC, Schaid DJ, Woods JE, et al. Efficacy of bilateral prophylactic mastectomy in women with a family history of breast cancer. *N Engl J Med*. 1999;340(2):77–84.

35. Saslow D, Boetes C, Burke W, et al. American Cancer Society guidelines for breast screening with MRI as an adjunct to mammography. *CA Cancer J Clin*. 2007;57:75–89.

Jolinta Lin, Elizabeth Nichols, Susan B. Kesmodel, Dina Ioffe, Olga Ioffe, and Katherine H. R. Tkaczuk

EPIDEMIOLOGY

Phyllodes tumors (PTs) are uncommon, biphasic, fibroepithelial neoplasms of the breast that were originally named "cystosarcoma phyllodes" for their leaf-like papillary projections seen on histology. PTs account for approximately 0.5% of primary breast neoplasms (1,2). Population studies have estimated an incidence of 2.1 per 1 million women. Most PTs are benign, but some have malignant potential (18%–25%) (3–5). Thus, the broader term "phyllodes tumor" is used as opposed to the previous term of "cystosarcoma phyllodes."

CLINICAL PRESENTATION

Although they can occur at any age, the majority of PTs present in women in their fourth decade of life and are most commonly detected as rapidly enlarging, painless, palpable breast masses. They tend to be larger and present 10 to 20 years later than the peak age for fibroadenomas. On imaging, these appear as round, sharply defined masses with cysts or clefts, and occasionally coarse calcifications (6,7).

PATHOLOGY

Like fibroadenomas, PTs arise from intralobular stroma, which distorts lobules and ducts and incorporates them within the mass; while the tumor contains epithelial elements, only the stromal component is neoplastic (3). Compared to fibroadenomas, PTs have increased cellularity of the stroma, a higher mitotic rate, and a leaf-like architecture with periepithelial stromal condensation, also known as cuffing. Histologically, PTs are characterized by elongated, branching epithelial cleft-like spaces within leaf-like hypercellular epithelial-lined stromal fronds that protrude into cystically dilated spaces, creating a staghorn appearance. Increased stromal cellularity is a characteristic feature of PT; this feature helps differentiate PTs from fibroadenomas and helps to histologically grade PTs.

PATHOLOGIC CLASSIFICATION OF PHYLLODES TUMORS

While many classification systems have been proposed for these neoplasms, none is universally honored. In 1951, Treves and Sunderland classified PTs as benign, borderline, or malignant based on histological parameters (8), a classification system that is still most widely used to date. In 2003, the World Health Organization (WHO) proposed a classification system based on Treves and Sutherland's three categories, only with better defined criteria, which were amended in 2012 (9). The histological parameters in this classification system include the degree of stromal cellularity and atypia, mitotic count, stromal overgrowth (defined as presence of stroma without epithelium in at least one low-power field), and invasion into the surrounding breast tissue (10).

BENIGN PHYLLODES TUMORS

Benign PTs comprise 60% to 75% of all PTs and are characterized by mildly increased stromal cellularity, minimal stromal atypia, well-defined pushing borders, <5 mitoses/10 high power field (HPF), and no stromal overgrowth. Although they are not likely to metastasize, they have the potential for local recurrence (LR), making it important to distinguish them from fibroadenomas. Many of these histologic features overlap with fibroadenomas (pushing/circumscribed borders and modest stromal cellularity), making it particularly difficult to distinguish the two on core needle biopsy, largely due to limited sample size. The key features distinguishing PTs from fibroadenomas are the characteristic leaf-like structures and increased stromal cellularity around the epithelial clefts—stromal cuffing (Figure 3.1).

MALIGNANT PHYLLODES TUMOR

On the other end of the spectrum are malignant PTs, which account for 10% to 20% of all PTs. They have marked cellular atypia (coarse chromatin, significant variation in nuclear size, and irregular membranes with discernible nucleoli), moderate to marked stromal atypia, >10 mitoses/10 HPF, infiltrative borders, and stromal overgrowth. All of these features must be present to be graded as a malignant PT; otherwise, it is considered a borderline PT (Figure 3.2). Alternatively, a PT is graded as malignant if a heterologous element is present (eg, liposarcoma, chondrosarcoma, osteosarcoma), regardless of the other parameters.

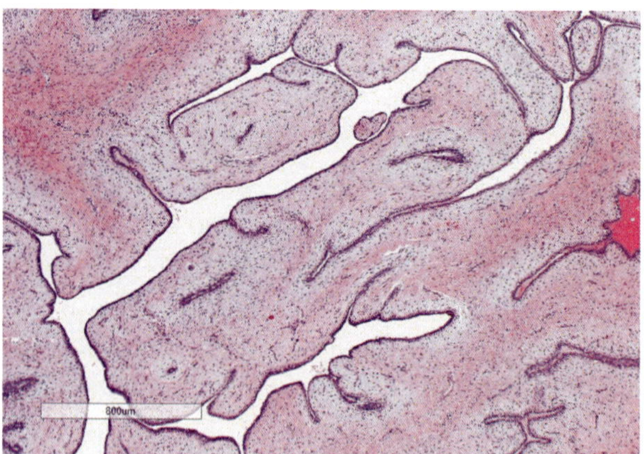

Figure 3.1 Benign phyllodes tumor. Note the leaf-like architecture and stromal condensation under the epithelial lining of the spaces.

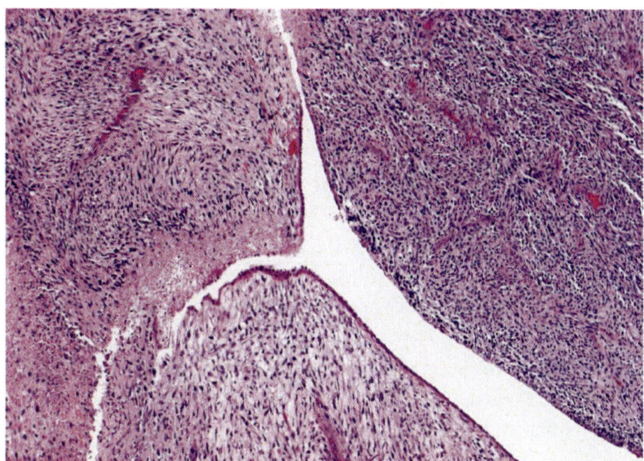

Figure 3.2 Malignant phyllodes tumor. The leaf-like architecture is still present but stroma is very hypercellular, highly pleomorphic, with necrosis and frequent mitotic figures.

BORDERLINE PHYLLODES TUMOR

As their name implies, borderline PTs fall in between these two extremes, making precise definitions difficult. They comprise 15% to 20% of all PTs and generally have intermediate features or do not fully meet malignant criteria. They have moderate stromal cellularity, mild to moderate stromal atypia, 5 to 9 mitoses/10 HPF, and may have focal infiltrative borders. Predicting tumor behavior based on these histologic parameters alone has proved futile, as benign PTs have been known to metastasize while malignant ones may neither recur nor metastasize after wide local excision. However, stromal overgrowth is consistently associated with aggressive behavior and metastatic potential. There have been efforts to identify tumor markers as predictors of clinical course and outcome, including Ki-67, p53, CD117, and CD34, but all have failed to consistently and reliably predict outcomes. The major clinical concern is LR, which can be seen with all types of PTs, and is best mitigated with adequate wide local excision (3,6,11,12).

DIAGNOSIS

Core needle biopsy is the preferred method of evaluating breast lesions; however, the limited specimen from a core biopsy can make it difficult to accurately distinguish a benign PT from a fibroadenoma (3,13).

TREATMENT

Wide local excision of the mass with a margin of normal breast tissue remains the standard of care for PT (6); total mastectomy is generally reserved for large tumors where breast conserving surgery (BCS) would not lead to an acceptable cosmetic outcome or for cases of LR when a reexcision is not possible (5,14). Routine axillary staging or lymph node dissection is not recommended for PT since the incidence of axillary lymph node metastasis is low (6,14). Negative margins, wide excision (microscopic margins ≥1 cm), and mastectomy can have high rates of local control (80%–100%) (6,14,15). Some groups report better local control with total mastectomy for patients with borderline or malignant PT (5,16).

PROGNOSIS

Given the rarity of PT in general, most studies that have examined local control and survival rates have been either retrospective single-institution studies or population-based studies. Population-based studies have noted high rates of cancer-specific survival even for malignant PTs, with 15-year cancer-specific survival of 89% (1). Other groups have combined borderline and malignant PTs together and estimated 10-year disease-free survival (DFS) and overall survival (OS) rates to be 68% and 88%, respectively (5). Histopathologic factors associated with disease recurrence include the degree of stromal hypercellularity (17), stromal atypia, and permeative margins (11), although this is not consistent in all reported studies (6). While few patients develop metastatic disease, some groups have noted that patients with infiltrating tumor margin, severe stromal overgrowth (14), atypia, and cellularity are at higher risk for metastasis (6). Belkacémi et al collected data from 443 women in the Rare Cancer Network with PT and reported LR of 19% and incidence of distant metastases of 3.4% at a median follow-up of 106 months (5). Patients with borderline or malignant PT were more likely to develop LR than patients with benign PT, with 10-year local control rates of 64% and 87%, respectively (P < .0001). Adjuvant radiation therapy (RT) in patients with borderline or malignant PT also significantly increased local control rates compared to BCS alone.

Benign PT carries a good prognosis even when treated with surgery alone; most LRs are salvaged by secondary surgery, likely contributing to the excellent survival rates. Belkacémi et al observed LR rates of 13% at 10 years in women with benign PT (5). Kim et al reported even fewer LR (3.4%) among 143 women with benign PT regardless of surgical margins or adjuvant radiation (RT) (16). Our approach for the management of benign PT is wide local excision to obtain negative pathologic margins with no adjuvant therapy.

RADIATION THERAPY FOR BORDERLINE AND MALIGNANT PHYLLODES TUMOR

Patients with borderline and malignant tumors have higher rates of LR after surgery than benign PT, 18% to 26% and 36% to 47%, respectively (5,16). In women with borderline and malignant PT who opt for BCS, improvement in local control rates may be observed with adjuvant RT (5,18). Given the rarity of borderline and malignant PT, the role of adjuvant RT has not been well established. Prior to 2009, most studies reported surgery as the primary treatment, with approximately 9% of PTs treated with adjuvant RT (1,5,19). A Surveillance, Epidemiology, and End Results (SEER) analysis of patients with malignant PT suggested that patients who received adjuvant RT had worse cause-specific survival compared to those who had surgery alone; however, the authors note that only a small percentage of patients (9%) received adjuvant RT, which would suggest selection bias that the worst tumors likely received adjuvant RT (1). The authors recognize that important clinical and pathologic data such as presence of stromal overgrowth, tumor necrosis, tumor grade, margin status, lymph node status, histologic subtype, hormone receptor status, specifics of the surgical and radiotherapy procedures, and clinical reasoning for mastectomy versus wide excision were not available or were incomplete within the SEER record (1).

A recent meta-analysis focusing on borderline and malignant PT showed a lower relative risk of LR with adjuvant RT with an absolute risk difference of 10.1% (20). Despite a clear reduction in LR in the patients who had BCS, no statistically significant differences were seen in OS or DFS between patients who received adjuvant RT and those who had surgery alone (20).

A population study using data collected from the National Cancer Data Base from 1998 to 2009 revealed that the use of adjuvant RT for PT has been increasing over recent years. Use of RT doubled over the study period from 9.5% (1998–1999) to 19.5% (2008–2009). Among the 3,120 women with malignant PT, women were significantly more likely to receive RT if they were diagnosed later in the study, were age 50 to 59 years old, had tumors >10 cm, or had lymph nodes removed. While recurrence data was only available for 1,774 patients, the overall recurrence rate was 14.1%, and LR was 5.9%. The multivariate model demonstrated that adjuvant RT significantly reduced LR (hazard ratio 0.43, 95% CIs [0.19, –0.95]) (19).

Pezner et al from the City of Hope published local control rates for 478 patients with malignant PT undergoing surgery alone with the important finding that tumor size was associated with tumor recurrence. With a median follow-up of just over 5 years, the recurrence rate following a lumpectomy was 9% for tumors <2 cm, 15% for tumors between 2 and 5 cm, and 41% for tumors >5 cm. Based on this data, we recommend whole breast radiation to 50 Gy at 1.8 to 2 Gy per fraction followed by a boost to the tumor cavity for an additional 10 Gy for tumors >5 cm following a BCS with negative margins (15).

Adjuvant RT to the chest wall after mastectomy may also be performed in patients with malignant PT, especially when the tumor is large; however, the benefit is not completely clear given the limited data (4,15). In Table 3.1 we summarize studies including adjuvant RT for borderline or malignant PT.

CHEMOTHERAPY

A role for adjuvant chemotherapy in patients with borderline or malignant PT has not been established and remains controversial. Since most retrospective analyses report excellent OS and low rates of systemic recurrence, it is unlikely that the use of systemic chemotherapy for management of adequately resected PT is beneficial. Due to the low incidence of this malignancy, it is also unlikely that prospective clinical trials will be conducted to address the role of adjuvant chemotherapy in management of PT. Genetic tumor analysis will supplement classical histologic examination and may potentially identify targetable mutations in order to improve our management of these rare tumors.

A small prospective observational study in 28 patients with malignant PT reported outcomes in patients who were assigned to chemotherapy or observation. Seventeen patients received adjuvant chemotherapy consisting of four cycles of 65 mg/m^2 doxorubicin infusion over 48 hours and 960 mg/m^2 dacarbazine infusion over 48 hours. Eleven patients were in the observation group. All patients had

Table 3.1 Studies Including Adjuvant Radiation Therapy for Borderline or Malignant Phyllodes Tumor

Study	No.	Time period	Surgery type (TM/BCS/ unknown)	Negative margins? (yes/no/ unknown)	Mean tumor size (cm)	Tumor grade, malignant/ borderline	Adjuvant RT/no RT	Dose range (Gy)	Conclusions
Pandey et al (21)	36	1982–1998	26/6/4	17/6/13	10.8	All malignant	25/11	45–50	Adjuvant RT decreases LR and increases survival
Soumarová et al (4)	25	1970–1995	21/4/0	Unknown	10	All malignant	17/8	46–70	Adjuvant RT decreases LR in malignant PT
Macdonald et al (1)	821	1983–2002	428/393/0	Unknown	Unknown	All malignant	76/745	Unknown	Role of adjuvant RT is uncertain
Belkacémi et al (5)	159	1971–2003	50/109/0	Unknown	4.6	79/80	36/123	36–60	Consider adjuvant RT according to histologic criteria if patient had BCS, with no effect on survival
Barth et al (18)	46	1999–2006	0/46/0	43/3/0	3.7	30/16	46/0	All received 60.4	Margin negative BCS with adjuvant RT has lower LR rate com-pared to observed LR rate in patients treated with negative margins–BCS alone

(continued)

Table 3.1 Studies Including Adjuvant Radiation Therapy for Borderline or Malignant Phyllodes Tumor (*continued*)

Study	No.	Time period	Surgery type (TM/BCS/ Unknown)	Negative margins? (yes/no/ unknown)	Mean tumor size (cm)	Tumor grade, malignant/ borderline	Adjuvant RT/no RT	Dose range (Gy)	Conclusions
Haberer et al (22)	25	1969–2006	20/5/0	20/0/2	6.5	All malignant	7/18	45–55	More studies investigating the role of adjuvant RT are needed
Badar et al (23)	32	1995–2012	Unknown	Unknown	9.2	All malignant	21/11	Unknown	Role of adjuvant RT is uncertain
Kim et al (16)	48	2000–2010	6/42/0	41/7/0	4.2 cm borderline; 6.2 cm malignant	15/33	6/42	Unknown	Additional information needed
Gnerlich et al (19)	3120	1998–2009	1,363/ 1838/9	2,787/275/ 148	4.2 (median)	All malignant	458/ 2,752	Unknown	Adjuvant RT significantly reduced LR but had no effect on DFS or OS

BCS, breast conserving surgery; DFS, disease-free survival; LR, local recurrence; OS, overall survival; PT, phyllodes tumor; RT, radiation therapy; TM, total mastectomy.

surgical resection, 38% had an axillary lymph node dissection, and 25% received adjuvant RT. The median age was 42 years (range, 23–76 years) and median tumor size was 13 cm (range, 3–30 cm). With median follow-up of 15 months (range, 2–81 months), 7 recurrences and 5 deaths were observed. The 5-year recurrence-free survival rate was 58% (95% CI = 36% and 92%) for the patients who received adjuvant therapy and 86% (95% CI = 63% and 100%) for the patients who did not (P = .17). The median survival after recurrence was 6.5 months. The authors concluded that adjuvant chemotherapy with doxorubicin and dacarbazine did not affect recurrence-free and OS, although there was a clear selection bias for which patients received chemotherapy in this study. In addition, the choice of dacarbazine instead of ifosfamide is considered less standard since ifosfamide plus doxorubicin is superior to dacarbazine plus doxorubicin in treatment of other soft tissue sarcomas (24).

Another unresolved management issue is whether systemic chemotherapy may have clinical benefit in those patients who develop LR after initial adequate surgical resection or local or systemic recurrence after surgical resection followed by local RT. Again we found no conclusive evidence that systemic chemotherapy is of benefit and management should be considered on a case-by-case basis as the majority of available information is from case reports of clinical response after systemic chemotherapy for recurrent or metastatic disease; agents used in this setting include cisplatin, etoposide, or ifosfamide (25–28).

➤ MANAGEMENT PEARLS

1. PT is a rare breast tumor that is more common in young women. **Surgery:** The majority of PTs are benign tumors that can be treated by wide local excision with negative margins followed by observation. Mastectomy is typically reserved for larger tumors or in cases of LR when reexcision is not possible. Lymph node assessment is usually not necessary for PT, given the low likelihood of lymph node involvement.
2. **Radiation therapy:** For patients with borderline and malignant PT, adjuvant RT may improve local control rates, and we typically recommend this in patients with larger tumors (≥5 cm) or when margins are close due to anatomical considerations.
3. **Adjuvant chemotherapy:** This is not recommended for patients with borderline or malignant PTs that have been adequately resected. Patients with large (>5 cm), high-risk, or recurrent malignant PT can be assessed for chemotherapy using soft tissue sarcoma protocols and after detailed discussion with the patient about the risks and benefits of such approach as it is unproven.
4. **Follow-up:** Since these women are often young, we extrapolate follow-up schedules from invasive breast cancer guidelines with clinical follow-up every 3 to 6 months for 5 years with annual mammography, prior to switching to yearly clinical exams with mammography (29).

REFERENCES

1. Macdonald OK, Lee CM, Tward JD, et al. Malignant phyllodes tumor of the female breast: association of primary therapy with cause-specific survival from the Surveillance, Epidemiology, and End Results (SEER) program. *Cancer.* 2006;107(9):2127–2133.
2. Reinfuss M, Mitus J, Duda K, et al. The treatment and prognosis of patients with phyllodes tumor of the breast: an analysis of 170 cases. *Cancer.* 1996;77(5):910–916.
3. Giri D. Recurrent challenges in the evaluation of fibroepithelial lesions. *Arch Pathol Lab Med.* 2009;133(5):713–721.
4. Soumarová R, Seneklova Z, Horova H, et al. Retrospective analysis of 25 women with malignant cystosarcoma phyllodes—treatment results. *Arch Gynecol Obstet.* 2004;269(4):278–281.
5. Belkacémi Y, Bousquet G, Marsiglia H, et al. Phyllodes tumor of the breast. *Int J Radiat Oncol Biol Phys.* 2008;70(2):492–500.
6. Chen WH, Cheng SP, Tzen CY, et al. Surgical treatment of phyllodes tumors of the breast: retrospective review of 172 cases. *J Surg Oncol.* 2005;91(3):185–194.
7. Plaza MJ, Swintelski C, Yaziji H, et al. Phyllodes tumor: review of key imaging characteristics. *Breast Dis.* 2015;35(2):79–86.
8. Treves N, Sunderland DA. Cystosarcoma phyllodes of the breast: a malignant and a benign tumor; a clinicopathological study of seventy-seven cases. *Cancer.* 1951;4(6):1286–1332.
9. Lakhani S, Ellis IO, Schnitt SJ, et al, eds. *WHO Classification of Tumours of the Breast.* Lyons, France: International Agency for Research on Cancer; 2012.
10. Tan BY, Acs G, Apple SK, et al. Phyllodes tumours of the breast: a consensus review. *Histopathology.* 2016;68(1):5–21.
11. Tan PH, Jayabaskar T, Chuah KL, et al. Phyllodes tumors of the breast: the role of pathologic parameters. *Am J Clin Pathol.* 2005;123(4):529–540.
12. Pietruszka M, Barnes L. Cystosarcoma phyllodes: a clinicopathologic analysis of 42 cases. *Cancer.* 1978;41(5):1974–1983.
13. Jara-Lazaro AR, Akhilesh M, Thike AA, et al. Predictors of phyllodes tumours on core biopsy specimens of fibroepithelial neoplasms. *Histopathology.* 2010;57(2):220–232.
14. Chaney AW, Pollack A, Mcneese MD, et al. Primary treatment of cystosarcoma phyllodes of the breast. *Cancer.* 2000;89:1502–1511.
15. Pezner RD, Schultheiss TE, Paz IB. Malignant phyllodes tumor of the breast: local control rates with surgery alone. *Int J Radiat Oncol Biol Phys.* 2008;71(3):710–713.
16. Kim S, Kim JY, Kim do H, et al. Analysis of phyllodes tumor recurrence according to the histologic grade. *Breast Cancer Res Treat.* 2013;141(3):353–363.
17. Onkendi EO, Jimenez RE, Spears GM, et al. Surgical treatment of borderline and malignant phyllodes tumors: the effect of the extent of resection and tumor characteristics on patient outcome. *Ann Surg Oncol.* 2014;21(10):3304–3309.
18. Barth RJ, Jr, Wells WA, Mitchell SE, Cole BF. A prospective, multi-institutional study of adjuvant radiotherapy after resection of malignant phyllodes tumors. *Ann Surg Oncol.* 2009;16(8):2288–2294.
19. Gnerlich JL, Williams RT, Yao K, et al. Utilization of radiotherapy for malignant phyllodes tumors: analysis of the National Cancer Data Base, 1998–2009. *Ann Surg Oncol.* 2014;21(4):1222–1230.
20. Zeng S, Zhang X, Yang D, et al. Effects of adjuvant radiotherapy on borderline and malignant phyllodes tumors: a systematic review and meta-analysis. *Mol Clin Oncol.* 2015;3(3):663–671.

21. Pandey M, Mathew A, Kattoor J, et al. Malignant phyllodes tumor. *Breast J.* 2001;7(6): 411–416.
22. Haberer S, Lae M, Seegers V, et al. Management of malignant phyllodes tumors of the breast: the experience of the Institut Curie. *Cancer Radiother.* 2009;13(4):305–312.
23. Badar F, Mahmood S, Syed AA, Siddiqui N. Malignant phyllodes tumour of the breast. *J Ayub Med Coll Abbottabad.* 2012;24(3–4):47–49.
24. Morales-Vasquez F, Gonzalez-Angulo AM, Broglio K, et al. Adjuvant chemotherapy with doxorubicin and dacarbazine has no effect in recurrence-free survival of malignant phyllodes tumors of the breast. *Breast J.* 2007;13(6):551–556.
25. Allen R, Nixon D, York M, Coleman J. Successful chemotherapy for cystosarcoma phyllodes in a young woman. *Arch Intern Med.* 1985;145(6):1127–1128.
26. Burton GV, Hart LL, Leight GS, Jr, et al. Cystosarcoma phyllodes. Effective therapy with cisplatin and etoposide chemotherapy. *Cancer.* 1989;63(11):2088–2092.
27. Hawkins RE, Schofield JB, Fisher C, et al. The clinical and histologic criteria that predict metastases from cystosarcoma phyllodes. *Cancer.* 1992;69(1):141–147.
28. Hawkins RE, Schofield JB, Wiltshaw E, et al. Ifosfamide is an active drug for chemotherapy of metastatic cystosarcoma phyllodes. *Cancer.* 1992;69(9):2271–2275.
29. Khatcheressian JL, Hurley P, Bantug E, et al. Breast cancer follow-up and management after primary treatment: American Society of Clinical Oncology clinical practice guideline update. *J Clin Oncol.* 2013;31(7):961–965.

Susan B. Kesmodel, Natalie O'Neill, Steven J. Feigenberg, Alex Engelman, Katherine H. R. Tkaczuk, Susan Shyu, and Olga Ioffe

INTRODUCTION

Ductal carcinoma in situ (DCIS) of the breast is a neoplastic lesion confined to the breast ducts and lobules without evidence of invasion into the surrounding stroma by light microscopic examination. Pure DCIS is considered a localized disease and is not associated with metastases to nodal basins (axillary, internal mammary, or supraclavicular lymph nodes) or distant metastases. The risk of metastases or death in a patient with pure DCIS is extremely low (less than 1%).

Epidemiology

The incidence of DCIS has significantly increased in the United States, from 1.87 per 100,000 women in 1973–1975 to 32.5 per 100,000 women in 2004. The incidence increased in all age groups but in particular for women older than 50 years (1). About 25% of breast cancers in the United States are DCIS and approximately 65,000 new cases of DCIS will be diagnosed in the United States alone in 2016 (Surveillance, Epidemiology, and End Results [SEER]).

Risk Factors

Similar to invasive breast cancer, risks for developing DCIS include older age, increased breast density, nulliparity or late age at first live birth, obesity, and family history.

Clinical Presentation

The majority of patients with DCIS have no clinical symptoms and are diagnosed via screening mammography. However, abnormal nipple discharge, a palpable mass, or Paget disease of the nipple can be associated with DCIS. **Microcalcifications** (Figure 4.1) seen on mammogram are very commonly associated with DCIS (90%). Certain mammographic patterns are highly suggestive of DCIS, such as linear branching or segmental types of pleomorphic microcalcifications (Chapter 1).

Diagnostic Evaluation

An abnormal lesion detected by mammogram or breast MRI should be assessed by core tissue sampling to obtain tissue confirmation of pathologic diagnosis. Excisional or incisional biopsy is rarely needed for diagnosis of DCIS and we typically do not recommend it unless the patient cannot have an image-guided biopsy. Fine needle aspiration (FNA) is not recommended because it may not provide enough tissue to confirm the diagnosis of noninvasive versus invasive breast carcinoma.

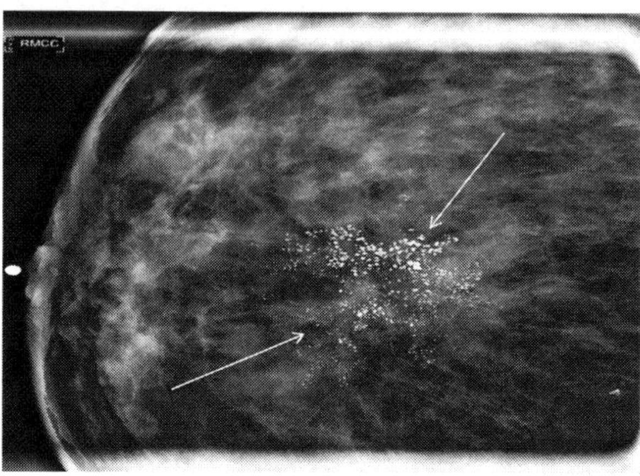

Figure 4.1 Mammographic magnification view of calcifications detected on screening mammogram; suspicious calcifications with pleomorphic morphology and grouped distribution (arrows) are noted; pathology: ductal carcinoma in situ (DCIS).

Pathology

DCIS is a neoplastic intraductal lesion characterized by the clonal proliferation of malignant epithelial cells, which, unlike invasive carcinoma, remain limited to the basement membrane of the ducts. DCIS is considered a direct precursor to invasive breast cancer and patients with DCIS have a risk 8 to 11 times greater than that of the general population for developing invasive carcinoma.

Grading

There is currently no universal agreement on a grading system for DCIS. Recently, there has been a shift toward nuclear grade and the presence of necrosis, as these factors are predictive of clinical outcome. The grade of DCIS is divided into three tiers: low, intermediate, and high. The characteristics of DCIS documented in the surgical pathology report are: (a) nuclear grade (based on nuclear atypia), (b) necrosis, and (c) architectural pattern.

Other key associated features noted on the pathology report include margin status, size of the lesion, and the presence of microcalcifications.

It is important to note that the tiered grading system does not necessarily imply a pathophysiologic progression from low- to high-grade DCIS. The current proposed sequence for the development of breast cancer involves two distinct pathways. Low/intermediate-grade DCIS is part of the low-grade/estrogen receptor-(ER) positive pathway thought to arise from the ER-expressing luminal cells and proliferative precursor lesions such as atypical ductal hyperplasia (ADH) before progressing to low-grade invasive carcinoma. In contrast, high-grade DCIS is considered part of the high-grade/ER-negative pathway with an unknown precursor that progresses to high-grade invasive breast cancer.

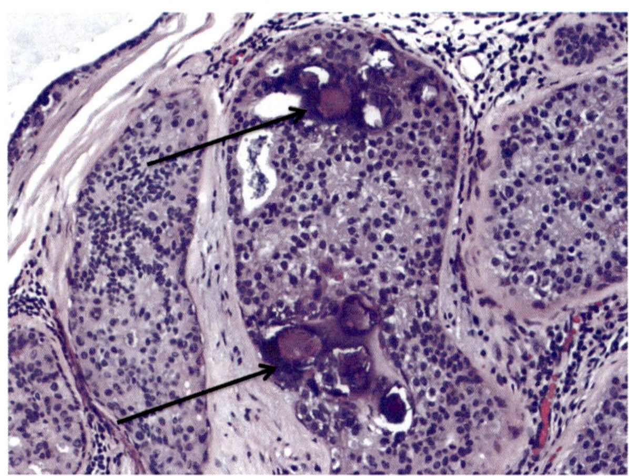

Figure 4.2 Low-grade ductal carcinoma in situ (DCIS), cribriform type, with calcifications (arrows).

Low-grade DCIS consists of small, round, monotonous cells, typically growing in a cribriform, micropapillary, or solid pattern (Figure 4.2). In the cribriform pattern, the cells are polarized around punched out ("cookie cutter") luminal spaces evenly distributed throughout the lesion. The cells within the intervening strands or bridges are arranged regularly or lie at a right angle ("Roman arches"). In the micropapillary pattern, cells protrude into the lumens as club-like fronds or pseudopapillae lacking fibrovascular cores. True papillary growth pattern with fibrovascular cores may occur, as well as free floating clusters of polarized cells detached from the papillae. In the solid pattern, the involved duct is distended by solid growth of the proliferating neoplastic cells. Calcifications are frequent. Limited areas of central necrosis may be present.

Intermediate DCIS consists of cells with features intermediate between those of low-grade and high-grade DCIS. Calcifications are often present. Necrosis may or may not be seen. Of the three grades, intermediate DCIS has been shown to have the least interobserver reproducibility.

High-grade DCIS consists of cells with overt morphologic features of malignancy (Figure 4.3). There is marked nuclear pleomorphism and high nuclear grade with prominent nucleoli. Polarization is lost and mitotic figures are numerous. Extensive necrosis is common; comedo-type necrosis—necrotic debris in a duct lumen surrounded by solid growth of viable tumor cells—is considered a defining feature of comedo DCIS, a subtype of high-grade DCIS commonly associated with a mass and most likely to have an associated invasive carcinoma.

Paget disease of the nipple is caused by high-grade DCIS involving the underlying subareolar ducts; these malignant cells creep up into the nipple skin and undermine it, causing ulceration. The malignant cells in the epidermis, known as Paget cells, are large with abundant pale cytoplasm often containing mucin, pleomorphic nuclei, and prominent nucleoli.

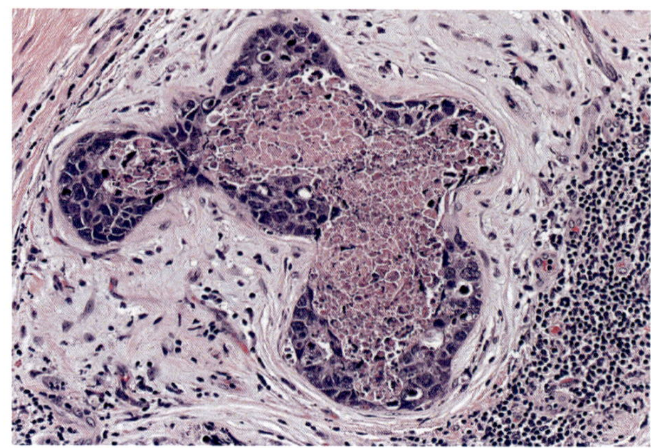

Figure 4.3 High-grade solid DCIS with central comedo-type necrosis (comedocarcinoma). The neoplastic cells are highly atypical, with frequent mitoses. Note stromal reaction and inflammatory infiltrate around DCIS.

Unusual variants include apocrine, neuroendocrine, mucinous and signet ring cell DCIS, and DCIS with basal-like phenotype (ER/PR/HER2-neu "triple negative"). The same assessment of nuclear grade and necrosis as that of the more usual DCIS applies to these variants.

Hormone receptor expression: The majority of DCIS, particularly low or intermediate grade, express receptors for estrogen (ER) and progesterone (progesterone receptor [PR]). The American Society of Clinical Oncology (ASCO)/College of American Pathologists (CAP) guidelines recommend classifying all cases with <1% positive cells as receptor negative. For DCIS with >1% positive cells, the percentage of positive cells is reported along with the intensity of staining.

SURGICAL MANAGEMENT OF DUCTAL CARCINOMA IN SITU

The surgical management of DCIS is similar to that of early-stage invasive breast cancer.

Management of the Breast

Although there are no randomized controlled trials (RCTs) that have compared mastectomy to breast conserving surgery (BCS) in patients with DCIS, based on the results of clinical trials for early-stage, invasive breast cancer, both of these surgical approaches are accepted for DCIS (see Surgery, Early-Stage Invasive Breast Cancer, Chapter 5).

Breast Conserving Surgery

The use of BCS for DCIS has increased steadily. A review of patients treated from 1992 to 1999 demonstrated an increase in the use of BCS over time, and overall during this time period 64% of patients were treated with BCS (2). A more recent analysis that examined patients treated at different time points from 1991 to 2005 also demonstrated an increase in the use of BCS for DCIS in more recent years (3).

Patients with biopsy-proven DCIS are considered candidates for BCS if the area of involvement can be removed with negative margins and results in acceptable cosmesis. BCS is not recommended for patients with DCIS who have diffuse malignant appearing or indeterminate calcifications in the breast.

PROCEDURE

BCS refers to removal of the area of malignancy in the breast with a margin of normal surrounding breast tissue.

Since DCIS is usually a nonpalpable lesion, preoperative wire-guided localization via either ultrasound or stereotactic guidance is generally utilized to localize the area of abnormality in the breast. Larger areas of calcifications in the breast may be bracketed with two or more wires. The area can then be targeted by the surgeon for removal. A specimen radiograph is typically obtained in the operating room to confirm that the appropriate tissue has been removed with a margin.

Shave margins are additional margins that may be taken after a lumpectomy is performed. These margins may encompass the entire surgical cavity in all directions or may be selectively taken in certain directions based on gross examination of the lumpectomy specimen or review of the specimen radiograph. These margins provide pathologists with additional tissue for examination and have been shown to decrease the rate of positive margins.

OUTCOMES

> ➤ Long-term survival for patients with DCIS is excellent whether BCS or mastectomy is utilized for treatment.

Adjuvant radiation therapy (RT) and endocrine therapy after BCS for DCIS have both been shown to decrease the risk of ipsilateral (invasive and noninvasive) breast tumor recurrence (IBTR).

The National Surgical Adjuvant Breast and Bowel Project (NSABP) B-17 trial randomized patients with localized DCIS to lumpectomy alone versus lumpectomy with adjuvant RT. Eight-year follow-up data from this trial showed that for those patients who received adjuvant external radiation therapy (XRT), the incidence of noninvasive IBTR was reduced from 13.4% to 8.2% ($P = .007$), and invasive IBTR was reduced from 13.4% to 3.9% ($P < .0001$) (4). A 15-year follow-up evaluation of results from the NSABP B-17 trial and a second trial, NSABP B-24, which randomized patients with localized DCIS to lumpectomy and adjuvant XRT with or without adjuvant tamoxifen, showed that invasive IBTR was lowest in patients who received adjuvant XRT and tamoxifen after lumpectomy. The overall prognosis was excellent for patients with DCIS regardless of treatment, with breast-cancer-related deaths of <5% at 15 years for all treatment groups (5).

MARGINS FOR BCS IN PATIENTS WITH DCIS

> ➤ Studies are inconsistent in their definition of negative margins following BCS for patients with DCIS; however, based on recent studies, a margin of at least 2 mm is recommended.

A retrospective, single-institution analysis of 469 patients treated for DCIS with BCS with or without radiation demonstrated that the likelihood of local recurrence (LR) was significantly greater for patients with a margin of <1 mm and that these patients benefitted the most from adjuvant RT. In patients with margins of <1 mm who did not receive adjuvant RT, the relative risk (RR) of recurrence was 2.54 compared to patients who received adjuvant RT (6). Similar results were reported from an analysis of patients treated on the European Organisation for Research and Treatment of Cancer (EORTC) 10853 trial, which found a hazard ratio (HR) of 2.07 for recurrence in patients with involved or close margins <1 mm compared to negative margins (7).

A recent meta-analysis of 22 trials that examined risk of recurrence in patients with DCIS treated with BCS and adjuvant RT showed that risk of recurrence was lower with negative margins compared to close/positive margins. When specific margin widths were compared, there was a significant difference in risk of recurrence when comparing margins of at least 5 mm to no tumor on ink or <1-mm margins. However, when margins of at least 5 mm were compared to 2-mm margins, there was no significant difference in LR rates (OR = 1.51; 95% CIs [0.51, 5.04]; P > .05). In addition, when a specific threshold margin was examined, a 2-mm margin was found to be superior to a margin <2 mm (OR = 0.53; 95% CIs [0.26, 0.96]; P < .05) (8).

> ➤ Based on these studies, we typically recommend obtaining a margin of at least 2 mm in patients with pure DCIS.

Mastectomy

Mastectomy may be considered in all patients with a diagnosis of DCIS. However, it is usually recommended for patients with a large area of involvement of the breast that does not appear to be amenable to BCS. This includes patients with diffuse malignant-appearing or indeterminate calcifications in the breast, a large area of involvement in the breast relative to breast size, and persistently positive margins after multiple excisions. It may also be recommended in patients who are not candidates for adjuvant RT.

Outcomes

A large meta-analysis of long-term outcomes for treatment of DCIS with mastectomy estimated an LR rate of 2.6% and breast-cancer-related death rate of 2% at 10 years (9).

SKIN-SPARING MASTECTOMY

Skin-sparing mastectomy (SSM) is a procedure that removes all breast tissue including the nipple–areolar complex (NAC) while preserving the skin envelope of the breast. This improves the cosmetic results from reconstruction. SSM is generally performed in patients with early-stage breast cancer including DCIS.

Outcomes

A retrospective, single-institution review of 223 patients with DCIS treated with SSM and immediate reconstruction with a median follow-up of 82.3 months showed an LR rate of 3.3% (10). In another study that included patients with invasive and noninvasive breast cancer undergoing SSM, 54 patients with DCIS were evaluated. The median follow-up time for all patients in the study was 119 months, with an LR rate of 2% in those patients with DCIS (11). **Therefore, SSM is an oncologically safe procedure in appropriately, selected patients with DCIS.** This approach may not be possible in patients with diffuse involvement of the breast tissue due to difficulty obtaining adequate margins.

NIPPLE-SPARING MASTECTOMY

Nipple-sparing mastectomy (NSM) removes all breast tissue and preserves the entire skin envelope of the breast including the NAC. This procedure may be considered in patients with DCIS when the DCIS does not involve the NAC. Typically, it is recommended that the tumor be at least 1 to 2 cm away from the NAC.

Outcomes

In a small review that examined NSM in 51 patients with DCIS in which 19 patients were followed for recurrence, an LR rate of 5.3%, 1/19 patients, was observed (12). A similar study that examined LR rates in patients undergoing NSM who were treated at the University of California San Francisco and Duke University and included 111 patients with DCIS showed an LR rate alone of 1.8%, 2/111 patients, and simultaneous local and distant recurrence in 1 patient (0.9%). The median follow-up in this study was only 28 months (13).

LYMPH NODE EVALUATION

In patients with DCIS, lymph node evaluation using sentinel lymph node biopsy (SLNB) is utilized in select cases. This includes patients who are undergoing mastectomy, since this precludes subsequent SLNB at a second operation, and physical exam or imaging findings that are concerning for invasive cancer, especially the presence of a mass lesion, DCIS that encompasses a large area on imaging (≥ 5 cm), and multicentric disease. We also perform SLNB for DCIS in cases where the location of the surgery may prevent a successful SLNB from being performed at a second surgery if invasive disease is identified.

BREAST CONSERVATION FOLLOWED BY RADIATION THERAPY FOR DCIS

The role of radiotherapy for patients with DCIS was established with the publication of four large prospective trials designed to address the effectiveness of BCS and RT for women with DCIS compared to BCS alone (5,14–16). The results of all four showed similar findings: the addition of RT resulted in an RR reduction of ipsilateral breast events (local failure) by 50%. With median follow-up intervals now of 13 to 17 years, omission of RT was associated with local failure rates of 23% to 35% compared to 10% to 20% in the irradiated arms. Of the local failures, approximately half were DCIS and half were invasive breast cancer. Despite higher local failure rates in surgery alone arms, survival is excellent and breast-cancer-related mortality is not different between arms. These findings are summarized in Table 4.1.

The Early Breast Cancer Trialists' Collaborative Group (EBCTCG) performed a meta-analysis of the randomized trials and found that radiotherapy reduced the

Table 4.1 Randomized Trials Comparing Lumpectomy With and Without Radiation Therapy for DCIS

Trial	Patients (n)	Median follow-up (y)	Resection margins	IBE (%)		DFS (%)		Breast cancer mortality (%)	
				No RT	RT	No RT	RT	No RT	RT
NSABP B-17	813	17.25	21% C/I/NS	35	20	–	–	3	5
SweDCIS	1,046	17	10% + / 9% NS	32	20	3	4	4	4
EORTC 10853	1,010	15.8	21% C/I/NS	31	18	9	10	4	5
UKCCCR	1,030	12.7	NTOI	23	9	–	–	3	2
EBCTCG Meta-Analysis	3,729	8.9		28	13	–	–	4	4

C, close; DFS, disease-free survival; I, involved; IBE, ipsilateral breast event; NS, not stated; NTOI, nontumor on ink, RT, radiation therapy.

absolute 10-year risk of any ipsilateral breast event (IBE) by 15.2%, an effect regardless of age at diagnosis, extent of BCS, use of tamoxifen, method of DCIS detection, margin status, focality, grade, the presence of comedonecrosis, architecture, or tumor size (17). They noted that the proportional reduction in ipsilateral breast events was greater in older than in younger women but did not significantly differ according to other available factors. However, after 10 years of follow-up, there was no significant effect on breast cancer mortality, mortality from causes other than breast cancer, or all-cause mortality, suggesting the effectiveness of salvage therapy or the long natural history of the disease.

FACTORS PROGNOSTIC FOR RECURRENCE

With the advent of breast screening and the trend for identification of smaller lesions, as well as the greater attention paid to surgical margin status (both factors associated with lower rates of IBE), there was general sentiment that the historic outcomes of BCS alone may not reflect current standards. Prognostic factors for recurrence were thus identified in an effort to characterize a population of women at sufficiently low risk such that radiotherapy could be safely omitted. These factors include: age, size, mode of detection, grade, architecture, focality, and margin status (5–7,18,19). In the Van Nuys Predictive Index, these factors were consolidated into a score, which predicted the risk of relapse after lumpectomy with or without RT. In unirradiated patients with scores of 4 to 6 there was a 10-year IBE rate of only 6% (20). These findings were confirmed with median follow-up of nearly 11 years showing a 5% event rate in "low-score" patients (21). The relative impact of these factors is depicted in Table 4.2.

Additionally, analysis of tumor genetics and molecular phenotype may further improve patient selection over classic pathologic and clinical factors. A 12-gene DCIS score (Genomic Health, Inc. Redwoods, California) was created from tissue samples of 327 patients treated with BCS alone in the ECOG 5194 trial. Patients with a low score (≤38) had a 10-year IBE rate of 12% compared to 25% and 27% in patients with intermediate (39–54) or high scores (≥55) (22). A study from Milan of over 1,100 women treated for DCIS with 10-year follow-up found Ki-67 labeling index and molecular phenotype to be significantly associated with recurrence risk. Five-year IBE rates were 9.4% for tumors with Ki-67 <14%, as compared to 10.3% for Ki-67 14% to 20% and 13% for Ki-67 >20% (23). The same study found 5-year IBE rates of 9.1%, 10.3%, and 15.3% for luminal A, luminal B/HER2-negative, and luminal B/HER2-positive subtypes, respectively. Notably, the use of clinical and pathologic factors seems to predict subgroups that have a low recurrence rate at a much lower cost.

BREAST CONSERVATION WITHOUT RADIOTHERAPY FOR SELECTED PATIENTS

Despite low local failure rates in individuals with favorable prognostic features, the EBCTCG meta-analysis still demonstrated an absolute reduction in the 10-year risk of IBE of 18.0% (12.1% vs. 30.1%) for women with negative margins and small low-grade tumors.

In a more recent SEER analysis of over 108,000 women, among patients who underwent BCS, radiotherapy was associated with a 2.4% absolute reduction in the

Table 4.2 Prospective Trials Omitting Radiotherapy in Selected Patients With "Low-Risk" DCIS

Trial	n	Inclusion criteria	HT	Median age	Median tumor size (mm)	Follow-up (y)		IBE	DCIS recurrence	Invasive recurrence
ECOG 5194	561	I: Low–intermediate grade, ≤2.5 cm, margin ≥3 mm	31%	60	6	12.3		14.4%	6.9%	7.5%
	104	II: High grade, ≤1 cm, margin ≥3 mm	24%	58	7			24.6%	11.2%	13.4%
Dana-Farber	158	Low–intermediate grade, ≤2.5 cm, margin ≥1 cm	None	51	8	11		16.1%	9.8%	6.3%
RTOG 9804	636	Mammographically detected, ECOG cohort 1	62%	58	5	7.17	No RT	6.7%	3.9%	2.8%
							RT	0.9%	0.45%	0.45%

DCIS, ductal carcinoma in situ; HT, hormonal therapy; IBE, ipsilateral breast event; RT, radiation therapy.

risk of ipsilateral invasive recurrence at 10 years (2.5% vs. 4.9%) (24). Interestingly, the risk of dying of breast cancer increased after experiencing an ipsilateral invasive breast cancer (HR 18.1). However, receipt of radiotherapy after BCS was not associated with a change in breast-cancer-specific mortality at 10 years (0.8% vs. 0.9%).

To answer the question of the clinical implications of BCS alone for patients with low-risk DCIS, several prospective trials were designed, which now have recently reported long-term follow-up (Table 4.1) (25–27). Paralleling the previous evidence, survival and breast-cancer-related mortality were excellent. In these well-selected women, BCS alone resulted in a 1% to 2% per year rate of IBEs. The local control rates of these trials are outlined in Table 4.3.

Within the ECOG-ACRIN 5194 trial, additional prognostic factors emerged: study cohort (HR 1.84 for cohort 2) and tumor size were both significantly associated with developing an IBE. Compared to tumors sized 5 mm or less, tumors 6 to 10 mm were associated with an HR of 1.42 and tumors greater than 10 mm with an HR of 2.11 for IBE. Variables not statistically significant were age, menopausal status, minimum negative margin width, method of detection, and tamoxifen use.

DECIDING WHEN IT IS SAFE TO WITHHOLD RADIOTHERAPY

In the previously discussed studies of patients with DCIS selected for favorable clinical and pathologic characteristics and treated with surgical excision without radiation, the risks of developing an IBE and an invasive IBE increased over time without plateau through 12 years of follow-up, confirming the known risk of late LRs. At the same time, RT substantially reduces local failures, but it does not impact the risk of metastases or breast cancer mortality.

The decision to accept a 1% to 2% per year risk of LR must be individualized and weighed against comorbidities, comfort level, and life expectancy (Table 4.2). Potential clinical criteria necessary to quote this low event rate include the presence of all of the following: age older than 40 years; highest nuclear grade 1 or 2; maximum extent 2.5 cm or less; and margins greater than 2 mm or no tumor on reexcision (Table 4.3) (28).

RADIOTHERAPY OPTIONS

Adjuvant radiotherapy has consisted of tangential irradiation of the whole breast delivered over 5 weeks to a total dose of 50 Gy in once-daily fractions of 2 Gy. Several alternatives to standard whole breast irradiation (WBI) exist to reduce the duration of adjuvant RT, including hypofractionation and accelerated partial breast irradiation (APBI). A full discussion of all technical details is beyond the scope of this text; however, certain areas of interest are highlighted.

USE OF A BOOST

The use of a tumor bed boost (in addition to WBI) as a part of adjuvant radiotherapy for patients with invasive breast cancer has been found to improve local control; however, the role of a boost after BCS in patients with DCIS has not been addressed in prospective trials.

A meta-analysis of 12 studies including nearly 7,000 patients showed no difference in the risk of LR between the patients who received boost and no boost in the general cohort (29). A reduced risk for LR, however, was found for the use of a

Table 4.3 Factors Associated With Increased Risk of Local Recurrence in Prospective Series of BCS Alone

Factor	HR	Factor	HR	Factor	HR	Factor	HR	Factor	HR
Age ≤45	2.14	Nonmammographically detected	1.37	Grade	NS	Comedonecrosis	2.21	Margins C/I/NS	2.61
Age ≤40	1.94	Nonmammographically detected	1.48	High grade	1.4	Cribriform/Comedo	2	Margins C/I/NS	1.69
Multifocality	1.8	–	–	High grade	1.65	–	–	Margins <4 mm	1.74
USC/Van Nuys Prognostic Index									
Age 40–60	2.3	Size 16–40 mm	2.2	Grade II	1.2	Necrosis	1.6	Margin 1–9 mm	6.4
Age <40	3.2	Size >40 mm	3.3	Grade III	2.2			Margin <1 mm	12.1

BCS, breast conserving surgery; C, close; HR, hazard ratio; I, involved; NS, not stated.

boost in patients with positive margins compared to no boost (OR 0.56). In a multi-institutional study included in the meta-analysis, 166 women received radiotherapy without a boost (median dose 50 Gy [range 40–60 Gy]) and 150 received radiotherapy with a boost (60 Gy [53–76 Gy]) (30). Local relapse-free survival at 10 years was 72% in those given radiotherapy without boost and 86% in those given radiotherapy with boost, despite more patients having positive or uncertain margins in the boost arm. Compared to radiotherapy without boost, radiotherapy with boost had an HR for local failure of 0.45 but no difference in overall survival. The use of a boost did not alter the proportion of invasive to in situ local recurrences (which was ~50:50, similar to the proportion in the randomized trials of BCS).

HYPOFRACTIONATION

Hypofractionation is an alternative form of WBI where treatment duration is reduced, typically to 3 weeks. A commonly used schedule is 40 to 42.5 Gy delivered in 15 to 16 treatments, respectively. With over 10 years follow-up in the setting of invasive disease, no differences in outcomes or toxicity profiles have been noted when compared to standard fractionation in trials from the UK and Canada (31,32).

Hypofractionation for DCIS has also been the subject of meta-analysis (29). No difference was observed in LR rates between patients who received hypofractionated versus standard radiotherapy, paralleling the long-term data for treatment of invasive disease. Similar results have been noted in several studies, and there has been increased utilization of hypofractionation for DCIS in the United States (33). Reflecting this change, hypofractionation (42.5 Gy in 16 daily fractions) was allowed in the RTOG 9804 randomized study. The schedules and results for studies of hypofractionation in DCIS are depicted in Table 4.4.

Table 4.4 Evidence for Hypofractionation as Part of Adjuvant Radiotherapy for DCIS

Trial	n	% HF	Follow-up (y)	HF schedule	Local failure SF	Local control HF
Ontario (34)	1,609	40%	9.2	40–44 Gy in 16 Fx	14%*	11%*
British Columbia (35)	478	77%	9.3	42.5 Gy in 16 Fx	–	HR 0.5
Princess Margaret (36)	266	61%	3.76	42.4 Gy in 16 Fx	6%	7%
McGill (37)	220	100%	3.75	45 Gy in 20 Fx/42.5 Gy in 16 Fx	–	HR 0.15 (0.02–1.36)

*statistically not significant

DCIS, ductal carcinoma in situ; HF, hypofractionation; HR, hazard ratio; SF, standard fractionation.

ACCELERATED PARTIAL BREAST IRRADIATION

Another alternative to standard WBI is APBI, treating only the area surrounding the lumpectomy cavity, typically in 1 week or less. There are many ways to accomplish partial breast irradiation, including interstitial, intraoperative, intracavitary balloon-based, and external beam techniques. Randomized trials comparing APBI with WBI demonstrate equivalent clinical outcomes for selected patients with early-stage invasive disease (38).

Pure DCIS had been a "cautionary" criterion for the use of APBI as recommended by the American Society for Radiation Oncology (ASTRO) consensus statement (39); however, the American Brachytherapy Society APBI consensus statement now includes DCIS in the acceptable treatment category (40). In the setting of invasive disease, the presence of extensive intraductal component increases local failure rates (41). Data are emerging on patients with DCIS treated with APBI. With early follow-up, control rates appear acceptable. Results of several retrospective series are detailed in Table 4.5.

SYSTEMIC THERAPY FOR DCIS

DCIS is considered a localized disease with a very low risk of developing nodal or distant metastases and prognosis is excellent. Estrogen and/or progesterone receptor expression is high in DCIS (50%–70%) (46). Studies have shown that the significantly elevated risk of development of invasive carcinoma after diagnosis of DCIS persists for up to 25 years (47). After diagnosis of DCIS approximately 50% of breast cancer recurrences are invasive rather than noninvasive (48).

Chemotherapy has no role in management of patients with DCIS given the low likelihood of metastatic disease. Endocrine therapy is the mainstay of systemic treatment for DCIS following completion of surgery and as long as the patient has residual breast tissue.

SYSTEMIC ENDOCRINE THERAPY

Definition of ER expression in DCIS: The 2010 ASCO/CAP guidelines recommend classifying all cases with <1% positive cells by immunohistochemistry (IHC)

Table 4.5 The Evidence for APBI as Adjuvant Radiotherapy for DCIS

Trial	n	Follow-up (y)	Median patient characteristics	Local failure
MammoSite Registry (42)	194	4.5	Age 62, size 8 mm, negative margins 88%	3.39%
ASTRO Cautionary (43)	46	3	17% age 50–59, 30% close margins	none
Georgia (44)	126	2	Age 59, 52% high grade, size 6 mm	2.4%
Promis (45)	240	6.9	HR (IDC vs. DCIS) 0.57 [0.3–1.09, $P = .09$]	

APBI, accelerated partial breast irradiation; DCIS, ductal carcinoma in situ; HR, hazard ratio; IDC, invasive ductal carcinoma.

as receptor negative. For DCIS with >1% positive cells, the percentage of positive cells is reported along with the intensity of staining.

ER-positive DCIS: That is completely excised, but where the patient has not had bilateral mastectomy and has residual breast tissue. We recommend chemoprevention with tamoxifen 20 mg daily for 5 years for premenopausal women and either tamoxifen 20 mg daily or anastrozole 1 mg daily for 5 years for postmenopausal women.

ER-negative DCIS: We do not routinely recommend chemoprevention with tamoxifen or an aromatase inhibitor such as anastrozole, although some women may still choose to take either of these agents to prevent subsequent ER-positive invasive or noninvasive breast cancers.

DCIS and BRCA1 or 2 mutation: The role and benefit of tamoxifen or aromatase inhibitors for chemoprevention for women with BRCA1 and 2 mutations and DCIS is largely unknown but it is likely similar to women without these mutations as long as other criteria for endocrine treatment are met as discussed previously. When these situations arise and the patient is not interested in prophylactic mastectomy surgery, we recommend chemoprevention with tamoxifen or anastrozole as long as other criteria for treatment are met (ER-positivity).

SYSTEMIC CHEMOPREVENTION TRIALS

RCTs have been conducted to investigate the benefit of tamoxifen or anastrozole after local treatments for DCIS.

Tamoxifen, a selective estrogen receptor modulator (SERM), is a nonsteroidal agent that has demonstrated potent antiestrogenic properties in animal test systems. The antiestrogenic effect is thought to be related to its ability to compete with estrogen for binding sites in target tissues such as the breast. Tamoxifen is Food and Drug Administration (FDA) approved at a dose of 20 mg daily for 5 years for prevention of invasive breast cancer recurrences in women with DCIS (FDA package insert).

Anastrozole is a triazole and type 2 nonsteroidal inhibitor of the aromatase enzyme; it binds reversibly to the enzyme substrate binding site and prevents the azole nitrogen's interaction with the heme prosthetic group, allowing for exquisite potency for the binding site and specificity against the aromatase enzyme (49). Dr. Angela Brodie and collaborators established a tumor model in nude mice to simulate several aspects of the postmenopausal breast cancer patient (50). These studies showed that aromatase inhibitors are more effective than tamoxifen at reducing tumor volume and that the combination of an aromatase inhibitor plus tamoxifen did not improve the antiproliferative results obtained with the aromatase inhibitor alone. This was later substantiated clinically in the Arimidex, Tamoxifen, Alone or in Combination (ATAC) adjuvant clinical trial.

DCIS CHEMOPREVENTION TRIALS

National Surgical Adjuvant Breast and Bowel Project *B-24*

This was a double-blind, randomized trial of tamoxifen versus placebo in women with DCIS following treatment with lumpectomy and RT. The primary objective was to determine if 5 years of tamoxifen (20 mg/day) would reduce the incidence of invasive breast cancer in the ipsilateral or contralateral breast; 1,804 women were randomized to either tamoxifen 10 mg twice daily (N = 902) or placebo (N = 902) treatment for 5 years.

RESULTS

At 5-year follow-up, 83.3% (95% CIs [80.8, 85.8]) of patients who received placebo were event-free compared to 87.4% (85.1–89.6) of tamoxifen-treated patients and there was no difference in survival (51); with a median follow-up of 74 months, the incidence of invasive breast cancer was reduced by 43% among women assigned to tamoxifen versus placebo (44 cases vs. 74 cases); $P = .004$; RR = 0.57, 95% CIs [0.39, 0.84]). The risk of developing ipsilateral or contralateral DCIS was also reduced with 5 years of tamoxifen prevention.

ADVERSE EVENTS

The overall frequency of side effects was similar between the groups and 62.8% of placebo and 57.1% of tamoxifen patients reported no adverse events. Grade 4 toxic effects not usually associated with tamoxifen occurred with similar rates in the two groups. There was an increase in the rate of endometrial cancer in tamoxifen-treated patients (1.53 vs. 0.45 per 1,000 patients per year in the placebo group). No deaths from endometrial cancer occurred in the tamoxifen group. The rates of phlebitis/thromboembolism were low overall; deep venous thrombosis (DVT) 0.2% in placebo versus 1% in tamoxifen group and nonfatal pulmonary embolism, 1 case in placebo versus 2 in tamoxifen. No strokes were seen in the two treatment groups. Hot flashes occurred in both groups, placebo—N = 525 (59.0%) versus tamoxifen—N = 620 (69.6%) (51).

UK/ANZ DCIS Trial

This trial had a 2 × 2 factorial design, and 1,701 women were randomly assigned to radiation + tamoxifen, radiation alone, tamoxifen alone, or to no adjuvant treatment.

RESULTS

After a median follow-up of 12.7 years (IQR 10.9–14.7), 376 (163 invasive [122 ipsilateral vs. 39 contralateral], 197 DCIS [174 ipsilateral vs. 17 contralateral], and 16 of unknown invasiveness or laterality) breast cancers were diagnosed. Radiation reduced the incidence of all new breast events (HR 0.41; $P < .0001$), reducing the incidence of ipsilateral invasive disease (0.32; $P < .0001$) as well as ipsilateral DCIS (0.38; $P < .0001$). Tamoxifen reduced the incidence of all new breast events (HR 0.71; $P = .002$), reducing recurrent ipsilateral DCIS (0.70; $P = .03$) and contralateral tumors (0.44; $P = .005$), but had no effect on ipsilateral invasive disease (0.95; $P = .8$). Data on adverse events except cause of death was not collected for this trial (16).

A systematic review and meta-analysis of postoperative tamoxifen following surgical resection of DCIS using a fixed effect model was done (52).

Data on local DCIS recurrence, new invasive breast cancer, distant disease, mortality, and adverse effects were extracted from RCTs comparing tamoxifen after surgery for DCIS (regardless of ER status), with or without adjuvant radiotherapy; 2 RCTs (16,51) were included. Tamoxifen after surgery for DCIS reduced recurrence of ipsilateral DCIS (HR 0.75; 95% CIs [0.61, 0.92]) and contralateral DCIS (RR 0.50; 95% CIs [0.28, 0.87]). Contralateral invasive breast cancer was reduced (RR 0.57; 95% CIs [0.39, 0.83]), and there was a trend toward decreased ipsilateral invasive breast cancer (HR 0.79; 95% CIs [0.62, 1.01]). The number needed to treat in order for tamoxifen to have a protective effect against all breast events is 15. There was no evidence of a difference in all-cause mortality (RR 1.11; 95% CIs [0.89, 1.39]).

Aromatase Inhibitors Versus Tamoxifen

IBIS-II DCIS- was a double-blind, multicenter, randomized placebo-controlled trial. Women with locally excised, hormone-receptor-positive DCIS were eligible and randomly assigned in a 1:1 ratio to receive anastrozole 1 mg daily or tamoxifen 20 mg daily for 5 years. The primary end point was all recurrence, including recurrent DCIS and new contralateral tumors; 2,980 postmenopausal women from 14 countries were randomly assigned to receive anastrozole (1,449 analyzed) or tamoxifen (1,489 analyzed) (53).

RESULTS

With a median follow-up of 7.2 years (IQR 5.6–8.9), 144 breast cancer recurrences were seen, there was a statistically significant difference in overall recurrence (67 recurrences for anastrozole vs. 77 for tamoxifen; HR 0.89; 95% CIs [0.64, 1.23]). Anastrozole treatment was noninferior but not superior to tamoxifen (upper 95% CI <1.25). There was no difference in deaths between the two treatment groups (53).

ADVERSE EVENTS

The number of any adverse events was similar between anastrozole (1,323 women, 91%) and tamoxifen (1,379 women, 93%). As expected, the side-effect profiles of the two drugs were different. More fractures, musculoskeletal events, hypercholesterolemia, and strokes were observed with anastrozole, while more muscle spasm, gynecological cancers and symptoms, vasomotor symptoms, and deep vein thromboses were observed with tamoxifen (53).

National Surgical Adjuvant Breast and Bowel Project B-35

Postmenopausal women with hormone positive DCIS treated by lumpectomy with clear resection margins and WBI were enrolled and randomly assigned (1:1) to receive tamoxifen 20 mg per day (with matching placebo) or anastrozole 1 mg per day (with matching placebo) for 5 years. Randomization was stratified by age (<60 vs. ≥60 years). The primary outcome was breast-cancer-free interval, defined as time from randomization to any breast cancer event (local, regional, or distant recurrence, or contralateral breast cancer, invasive disease, or DCIS), analyzed by intention to treat (54).

RESULTS

In total, 3,104 women were randomized to the two treatment groups (1,552—tamoxifen and 1,552—anastrozole); with median follow-up of 9 years (IQR 8.2–10.0); 212 breast-cancer-free interval events occurred: 122 in the tamoxifen group and 90 in the anastrozole group (HR 0.73, 95% CIs [0.56, 0.96]; *P* = .0234). There was also a significant interaction between treatment and age group (*P* = .0379), showing that anastrozole was superior only in postmenopausal women younger than 60 years of age. In this trial, compared to tamoxifen, anastrozole treatment provided a significant improvement in breast-cancer-free interval, mainly in women younger than 60 years of age (54).

ADVERSE EVENTS

Adverse events were similar between anastrozole and tamoxifen, except for thrombosis or embolism; 17 grade 4/5 events in the tamoxifen versus 4 in the anastrozole group were noted.

➤ MANAGEMENT PEARLS

Surgery

Patients with DCIS may be treated with BCS or mastectomy with excellent long-term survival. A 2-mm margin is currently recommended in patients with pure DCIS undergoing BCS.

Radiation

Following BCS for DCIS, adjuvant radiotherapy reduces the risk of IBE by ~50%, an effect independent of prognostic factors. Approximately half of local failures are DCIS and half are invasive breast cancer. Survival and breast-cancer-related mortality are not affected by local failure rates in randomized trials. For well-selected patients, BCS alone results in LR rates of 1% to 2% per year. These rates do not plateau through 12 years of follow-up.

Systemic Therapy

Unless bilateral mastectomy is done, for patients with completely excised ER-positive DCIS, we recommend tamoxifen 20 mg daily for 5 years if premenopausal and anastrozole 1 mg daily or tamoxifen 20 mg daily for 5 years if postmenopausal.

REFERENCES

1. Virnig BA, Tuttle TM, Shamliyan T, Kane RL. Ductal carcinoma in situ of the breast: a systematic review of incidence, treatment, and outcomes. *J Natl Cancer Inst.* 2010;102(3):170.
2. Baxter NN, Virnig BA, Durham SB, Tuttle TM. Trends in the treatment of ductal carcinoma in situ of the breast. *J Natl Cancer Inst.* 2004;96:443–448.
3. Zujewski JA, Harlan LC, Morrell DM, et al. Ductal carcinoma in situ: trends in treatment over time in the US. *Breast Cancer Res Treat.* 2011;127:251. doi:10.1007/s10549-010-1198-z
4. Fisher B, Dignam J, Wolmark N, et al. Lumpectomy and radiation therapy for the treatment of intraductal breast cancer: findings from National Surgical Adjuvant Breast and Bowel Project B-17. *J Clin Oncol.* 1998;16:441–452.
5. Wapnir IL, Dignam JJ, Fisher B, et al. Long-term outcomes of invasive ipsilateral breast tumor recurrences after lumpectomy in NSABP B-17 and B-24 randomized clinical trials for DCIS. *J Natl Cancer Inst.* 2011;103:478–488.

6. Silverstein MJ, Lagios MD, Groshen S, et al. The influence of margin width on local control of ductal carcinoma in situ of the breast. *N Engl J Med.* 1999;340:1455–1461.

7. Bijker N, Peterse JL, Duchateau L, et al. Risk factors for recurrence and metastasis after breast conserving therapy for ductal carcinoma-in-situ: analysis of European organization for research and treatment of cancer trial 10853. *J Clin Oncol.* 2001;19:2263–2271.

8. Dunne C, Burke JP, Morrow M, Kell MR. Effect of margin status on local recurrence after breast conservation and radiation therapy for ductal carcinoma in situ. *J Clin Oncol.* 2009;27(10):1615–1620. doi:10.1200/JCO.2008.17.5182

9. Stuart KE, Houssami N, Taylor R, et al. Long-term outcomes of ductal carcinoma in situ of the breast: a systematic review, meta-analysis and meta-regression analysis. *BMC Cancer.* 2015;15:890. doi:10.1186/s12885-015-1904-7

10. Carlson GW, Page A, Johnson E, et al. Local recurrence of ductal carcinoma in situ after skin-sparing mastectomy. *J Am Coll Surg.* 2007;204:1074–1078; discussion 1078–1080.

11. Romics L, Chew BK, Weiler-Mithoff E, et al. Ten-year follow-up of skin-sparing mastectomy followed by immediate breast reconstruction. *Br J Surg.* 2012;99:799–806. doi:10.1002/bjs.8704

12. Leclere FM, Panet-Spallina J, Kolb F, et al. Nipple-sparing mastectomy and immediate reconstruction in ductal carcinoma in situ: a critical assessment with 41 patients. *Aesthetic Plast Surg.* 2014;38:338–343.

13. Peled AW, Foster RD, Stover AC, et al. Outcomes after total skin-sparing mastectomy and immediate reconstruction in 657 breasts. *Ann Surg Oncol.* 2012;19(11):3402–3409.

14. Wärnberg F, Garmo H, Emdin S, et al. Effect of radiotherapy after breast-conserving surgery for ductal carcinoma in situ: twenty-year follow-up in the randomized SweDCIS trial. *J Clin Oncol.* 2014;32:3613–3618.

15. Donker M, Litière S, Werutsky G, et al. Breast-conserving treatment with or without radiotherapy in ductal carcinoma in situ: 15-year recurrence rates and outcome after a recurrence, from the EORTC 10853 randomized phase III trial. *J Clin Oncol.* 2013;31:4054–4059.

16. Cuzick J, Sestak I, Pinder SE, et al. Effect of tamoxifen and radiotherapy in women with locally excised ductal carcinoma in situ: long-term results from the UK/ANZ DCIS trial. *Lancet Oncol.* 2011;12(1):21–29. doi:10.1016/S1470-2045(10)70266-7

17. Early Breast Cancer Trialists' Collaborative Group. Overview of the randomized trials of radiotherapy in ductal carcinoma in situ of the breast. *J Natl Cancer Inst Monogr.* 2010:162–177.

18. Rakovitch E, Pignol JP, Paszat L, et al. Significance of multifocality in ductal carcinoma in situ: outcomes of women treated with breast-conserving therapy. *J Clin Oncol.* 2007;25:5591–5596.

19. Lagios M, Page DL. Lagios experience. In: Silverstein MJ, Lagios MD, Poller DN, et al, eds. *Ductal Carcinoma In Situ of the Breast.* Baltimore, MD: William & Wilkins; 1997:361–365.

20. Silverstein MJ, Lagios MD. Choosing treatment for patients with ductal carcinoma in situ: fine tuning the University of Southern California/Van Nuys prognostic index. *J Natl Cancer Inst Monogr.* 2010;2010:193–196.

21. Di Saverio S, Catena F, Santini D, et al. 259 patients with DCIS of the breast applying USC/Van Nuys prognostic index: a retrospective review with long term follow up. *Breast Cancer Res Treat.* 2008;109:405–416.

22. Solin LJ, Gray R, Baehner FL, et al. A multigene expression assay to predict local recurrence risk for ductal carcinoma in situ of the breast. *J Natl Cancer Inst.* 2013;105:701–710.

23. Lazzeroni M, Guerrieri-Gonzaga A, Botteri E, et al. Tailoring treatment for ductal intraepithelial neoplasia of the breast according to Ki-67 and molecular phenotype. *Br J Cancer*. 2013;108:1593–1601.

24. Narod SA, Iqbal J, Sun P, et al. Breast cancer mortality after a diagnosis of ductal carcinoma in situ. *JAMA Oncol*. 2015;1(7):888–896.

25. Solin LJ, Gray R, Hughes L, et al. Surgical excision without radiation for ductal carcinoma in situ of the breast: 12-year results from the ECOG-ACRIN E5194 Study. *J Clin Oncol*. 2015;33:3938–3944.

26. Wong JS, Chen YH, Gadd MA, et al. Eight-year update of a prospective study of wide excision alone for small low- or intermediate-grade ductal carcinoma in situ (DCIS). *Breast Cancer Res Treat*. 2014;143:343–350.

27. McCormick B, Winter K, Hudis C, et al. RTOG 9804: a prospective randomized trial for good-risk ductal carcinoma in situ comparing radiotherapy with observation. *J Clin Oncol*. 2015;33:709–715.

28. Recht A. Are the randomized trials of radiation therapy for ductal carcinoma in situ still relevant? *J Clin Oncol*. 2014;32:3588–3590.

29. Nilsson C, Valachis A. The role of boost and hypofractionation as adjuvant radiotherapy in patients with DCIS: a meta-analysis of observational studies. *Radiother and Oncol*. 2015;114:50–55.

30. Omlin A, Amichetti M, Azria D, et al. Boost radiotherapy in young women with ductal carcinoma in situ: a multicentre, retrospective study of the rare cancer network. *Lancet Oncol*. 2006;7:652–656.

31. Whelan TJ, Pignol JP, Levine MN, et al. Long-term results of hypofractionated radiation therapy for breast cancer. *N Engl J Med*. 2010;362(6):513–520.

32. Haviland JS, Owen JR, Dewar JA, et al. The UK standardization of breast radiotherapy (START) trials of radiotherapy hypofractionation for treatment of early breast cancer: 10-year follow-up results of two randomized controlled trials. *Lancet Oncol*. 2013;14(11):1086–1094.

33. Vicini F, Shah C. Ductal carcinoma in situ: review of the role of radiation therapy and current controversies. *Am J Heme/Oncol*. 2015;11(2):23–27.

34. Lalani N, Paszat L, Sutradhar R, et al. Long-term outcomes of hypofractionation versus conventional radiation therapy after breast-conserving surgery for ductal carcinoma in situ of the breast. *Int J Radiat Oncol Biol Phys*. 2014;90(5):1017–1024.

35. Wai ES, Lesperance ML, Alexander CS, et al. Effect of radiotherapy boost and hypofractionation on outcomes in ductal carcinoma in situ. *Cancer*. 2011;117:54–62.

36. Williamson D, Dinniwell R, Fung S, et al. Local control with conventional and hypofractionated adjuvant radiotherapy after breast conserving surgery for ductal carcinoma in-situ. *Radiother Oncol*. 2010;95:317–320.

37. Wong P, Lambert C, Agnihotram RV, et al. Ductal carcinoma in situ–the influence of the radiotherapy boost on local control. *Int J Radiat Oncol Biol Phys*. 2012;82:e153–e158.

38. Polgar C, Fodor J, Major T, et al. Breast-conserving therapy with partial or whole breast irradiation: ten-year results of the Budapest randomized trial. *Radiother Oncol*. 2013;108(2):197–202.

39. Smith BD, Arthur DW, Buchholz TA, et al. Accelerated partial breast irradiation consensus statement from the American Society for Radiation Oncology (ASTRO). *Int J Radiat Oncol Biol Phys*. 2009;74(4):987–1001.

40. Shah C, Vicini F, Wazer DE, et al. The American Brachytherapy Society consensus statement for accelerated partial breast irradiation. *Brachytherapy.* 2013;12(4):267–277.

41. Ribeiro GG, Magee B, Swindell R, et al. The Christie Hospital breast conservation trial: an update at 8 years from inception. *Clin Oncol (R Coll Radiol).* 1993;5(5):278–283.

42. Jeruss JS, Kuerer HM, Keisch M, et al. Update on DCIS outcomes from the American Society of Breast Surgeons accelerated partial breast irradiation registry trial. *Ann Surg Oncol.* 2011;18(1):65–71.

43. Stull TS, Goodwin M, Gracely EJ, et al. A single-institution review of accelerated partial breast irradiation in patients considered "cautionary" by the American Society for Radiation Oncology. *Ann Surg Oncol.* 2012;19(2):553–559.

44. Israel PZ, Vicini F, Robbins AB, et al. Ductal carcinoma in situ of the breast treated with accelerated partial breast irradiation using balloon-based brachytherapy. *Ann Surg Oncol.* 2010;17(11):2940–2944.

45. Kamrava M, Kuske RR, Anderson B, et al. Outcomes of breast cancer patients treated with accelerated partial breast irradiation via multicatheter interstitial brachytherapy: the pooled registry of multicatheter interstitial sites (PROMIS) experience. *Ann Surg Oncol.* 2015;22(suppl 3):S401–S411.

46. Hammond ME, Hayes DF, Wolff AC, et al. American Society of Clinical Oncology/College of American Pathologists guideline recommendations for immunohistochemical testing of estrogen and progesterone receptors in breast cancer. *J Oncol Pract.* 2010;6(4):195–197.

47. Page DL, Dupont WD, Rogers LW, et al. Continued local recurrence of carcinoma 15–25 years after a diagnosis of low grade ductal carcinoma in situ of the breast treated only by biopsy. *Cancer.* 1995;76(7):1197–1200.

48. Kerlikowske K, Molinaro A, Cha I, et al. Characteristics associated with recurrence among women with ductal carcinoma in situ treated by lumpectomy. *J Natl Cancer Inst.* 2003;95:1692–1702.

49. Miller WR. Aromatase inhibitors: mechanism of action and role in the treatment of breast cancer. *Semin Oncol.* 2003;30(4, suppl 14):3–11.

50. Brodie A, Lu Q, Liu Y, Long B. Aromatase inhibitors and their antitumor effects in model systems. *Endocrine-Related Cancer.* 1999;6:205–210.

51. Fisher B, Dignam J, Wolmark N, et al. Tamoxifen in treatment of intraductal breast cancer: National Surgical Adjuvant Breast and Bowel Project B-24 randomised controlled trial. *Lancet.* 1999;353:1993–2000.

52. Staley H, McCallum I, Bruce J. Postoperative tamoxifen for ductal carcinoma in situ: cochranesystematic review and meta-analysis. *Breast.* 2014;23(2014):546–551.

53. Forbes JF, Sestak I, Howell A, et al. Anastrozole versus tamoxifen for the prevention of locoregional and contralateral breast cancer in postmenopausal women with locally excised ductal carcinoma in situ (IBIS-II DCIS): a double-blind, randomized controlled trial. *Lancet.* 2016;387:866–873.

54. Margolese RG, Cecchini RS, Julian TB, et al. Anastrozole versus tamoxifen in postmenopausal women with ductal carcinoma in situ undergoing lumpectomy plus radiotherapy (NSABP B-35): a randomised, double-blind, phase 3 clinical trial. *Lancet.* 2016;387:849–856.

SUPPLEMENTAL READING

Al-Ghazal SK, Fallowfi eld L, Blamey RW. Comparison of psychological aspects and patient satisfaction following breast conserving surgery, simple mastectomy and breast reconstruction. *Eur J Cancer.* 2000;36:1938–1943.

Allred DC, Anderson SJ, Paik S, et al. Adjuvant tamoxifen reduces subsequent breast cancer in women with estrogen receptor-positive ductal carcinoma in situ: a study based on NSABP protocol B-24. *J Clin Oncol.* 2012;30:1268.

Allred DC. Ductal carcinoma in situ: terminology, classifi cation, and natural history. *J Natl Cancer Inst Monogr.* 2010;2010(41):134–138.

Carter D, Schnitt SJ, Millis RR. The breast. In: Mills SE, ed. *Sternberg's Diagnostic Surgical Pathology.* 5th ed. Philadelphia, PA: Lippincott Williams & Wilkins; 2010:285–350.

Chagpar AB, Killelea BK, Tsangaris TN, et al. A randomized, controlled trial of cavity shave margins in breast cancer. *N Engl J Med.* 2015;373:503–510.

Chin-Lenn L, Mack LA, Temple W, et al. Predictors of treatment with mastectomy, use of sentinel lymph node biopsy and upstaging to invasive cancer in patients diagnosed with breast ductal carcinoma in situ (DCIS) on core biopsy. *Ann Surg Oncol.* 2014;21: 66–73.

Claus EB, Chu P, Howe CL, et al. Pathobiologic fi ndings in DCIS of the breast: morphologic features, angiogenesis, HER-2/neu and hormone receptors. *Exp Mol Pathol.* 2001;70(3):303.

Ernster VL, Barclay J, Kerlikowske K, et al. Incidence of and treatment for ductal carcinoma in situ of the breast. *JAMA.* 1996;275:913–918.

Eusebi V, Mai KT, Taranger-Charpin A. Tumours of the nipple. In: Lakhani SR, Ellis IO, Schnitt SJ, et al, eds. *WHO Classifi cation of Tumours of the Breast.* 4th ed. Geneva, Switzerland: World Health Organization; 2012:104–106.

Fitzgibbons PL, Dillon DA, Alsabeh R, et al. Template for reporting results of biomarker testing of specimens from patients with carcinoma of the breast. http://www.cap.org/ShowProperty?nodePath=/UCMCon/Contribution%20Folders/WebContent/pdf/cp-breast-biomarker-template-14.pdf. Published 2014.

Francis AM, Haugen CE, Grimes LM, et al. Is sentinel lymph node dissection warranted for patients with a diagnosis of ductal carcinoma in situ? *Ann Surg Oncol.* 2015;22:4270–4279.

Garwood ER, Moore D, Ewing C, et al. Total skin-sparing mastectomy: complications and local recurrence rates in 2 cohorts of patients. *Ann Surg.* 2009;249:26–32.

Greenway RM, Schlossberg L, Dooley WC. Fift een-year series of skin-sparing mastectomy for stage 0 to 2 breast cancer. *Am J Surg.* 2005;190:918–922.

Guillot E, Vaysse C, Goetgeluck J, et al. Extensive pure ductal carcinoma in situ of the breast: identifi cation of predictors of associated infi ltrating carcinoma and lymph node metastasis before immediate reconstructive surgery. *Breast.* 2014;23:97–103.

Intra M, Rotmensz N, Veronesi P, et al. Sentinel node biopsy is not a standard procedure in ductal carcinoma in situ of the breast: the experience of the European Institute of Oncology on 854 patients in 10 years. *Ann Surg.* 2008;247:315–319.

Jones V, Linebarger J, Perez S, et al. Excising additional margins at initial breastconserving surgery (BCS) reduces the need for re-excision in a predominantly African American population: a report of a randomized prospective study in a public hospital. *Ann Surg Oncol.* 2015;23:456–464.

Kroll SS, Schusterman MA, Tadjalli HE, et al. Risk of recurrence aft er treatment of early breast cancer with skin-sparing mastectomy. *Ann Surg Oncol.* 1997;4:193–197.

Lester SC. The breast. In: Kumar V, Abbas AK, Fausto N, Aster JC, eds. *Robbins and Cotran Pathologic Basis of Disease.* 8th ed. Philadelphia, PA: Saunders; 2010:1065–1095.

Lester SC, et al. Protocol for the examination of specimens from patients with ductal carcinoma in situ (DCIS) of the breast. http://www.cap.org/ShowProperty?nodePath=/UCMCon/Contribution%20Folders/WebContent/pdf/cp-breast-dcis-13protocol-3200.pdf. Published 2013.

Lyman GH, Temin S, Edge SB, et al. Sentinel lymph node biopsy for patients with early-stage breast cancer: American Society of Clinical Oncology clinical practice guideline update. *J Clin Oncol.* 2014;32:1365–1383.

Melstrom LG, Melstrom KA, Wang EC, et al. Ductal carcinoma in situ: size and resection volume predict margin status. *Am J Clin Oncol.* 2010;33:438–442.

Merrill AL, Coopey SB, Tang R, et al. Implications of new lumpectomy margin guidelines for breast-conserving surgery: changes in reexcision rates and predicted rates of residual tumor. *Ann Surg Oncol.* 2015.

Moore KH, Sweeney KJ, Wilson ME, et al. Outcomes for women with ductal carcinoma-in-situ and a positive sentinel node: a multi-institutional audit. *Ann Surg Oncol.* 2007;14:2911–2917.

Moran MS, Schnitt SJ, Giuliano AE, et al. Society of Surgical Oncology-American Society for Radiation Oncology consensus guideline on margins for breast-conserving surgery with whole-breast irradiation in stages I and II invasive breast cancer. *Ann Surg Oncol.* 2014;21:704–716.

Ouldamer L, Lechaux E, Arbion F, et al. What should be the width of radiological margin to optimize resection of non-palpable invasive or in situ ductal carcinoma? *Breast.* 2014;23:889–893.

Pang JM, Gorringe KL, Fox SB. Ductal carcinoma in situ—update on risk assessment and management. *Histopathology.* 2016;68(1):96–109.

Prendeville S, Ryan C, Feeley L, et al. Sentinel lymph node biopsy is not warranted following a core needle biopsy diagnosis of ductal carcinoma in situ (DCIS) of the breast. *Breast.* 2015;24:197–200.

Rubio IT, Mirza N, Sahin AA, et al. Role of specimen radiography in patients treated with skin-sparing mastectomy for ductal carcinoma in situ of the breast. *Ann Surg Oncol.* 2000;7:544–548.

Sagara Y, Mallory MA, Wong S, et al. Survival benefi t of breast surgery for low-grade ductal carcinoma in situ: a population-based cohort study. *JAMA Surg.* 2015;150:739–745.

Slavin SA, Schnitt SJ, Duda RB, et al. Skin-sparing mastectomy and immediate reconstruction: oncologic risks and aesthetic results in patients with early-stage breast cancer. *Plast Reconstr Surg.* 1998;102:49–62.

Spiegel AJ, Butler CE. Recurrence following treatment of ductal carcinoma in situ with skin-sparing mastectomy and immediate breast reconstruction. *Plast Reconstr Surg.* 2003;111:706–711.

Sumner WE, 3rd, Koniaris LG, Snell SE, et al. Results of 23,810 cases of ductal carcinoma-in-situ. *Ann Surg Oncol.* 2007;14:1638–1643.

Tavassoli FA, Hoefl er H, Rosai R, et al. Intraductal proliferative lesions. In: Lakhani SR, Ellis IO, Schnitt SJ, et al, eds. *WHO Classifi cation of Tumours of the Breast.* 4th ed. Geneva, Switzerland: World Health Organization; 2012:63–73.

Veronesi P, Intra M, Vento AR, et al. Sentinel lymph node biopsy for localised ductal carcinoma in situ? *Breast.* 2005;14:520–522.

Voltura AM, Tsangaris TN, Rosson GD, et al. Nipple-sparing mastectomy: critical assessment of 51 procedures and implications for selection criteria. *Ann Surg Oncol.* 2008;15:3396–3401.

Wang F, Peled AW, Garwood E, et al. Total skin-sparing mastectomy and immediate breast reconstruction: an evolution of technique and assessment of outcomes. *Ann Surg Oncol.* 2014;21:3223–3230.

Wilke LG, McCall LM, Posther KE, et al. Surgical complications associated with sentinel lymph node biopsy: results from a prospective international cooperative group trial. *Ann Surg Oncol.* 2006;13:491–500.

Wong JS, Kaelin CM, Troyan SL, et al. Prospective study of wide excision alone for ductal carcinoma in situ of the breast. *J Clin Oncol.* 2006;24:1031–1036.

Paula Rosenblatt, J. W. Snider III, Steven J. Feigenberg, Neha Bhooshan,
Sally B. Cheston, Susan B. Kesmodel, Lindsay Hessler, Julia Terhune,
Olga Ioffe, Rachel White, Yang Zhang, Ina Lee, Krista Chain, Chad Tarabolous,
Rawand Faramand, Angela DeRidder, Jennifer Ding, and Katherine H. R. Tkaczuk

EPIDEMIOLOGY/GENERAL CHARACTERISTICS

In the United States, one in eight women will develop breast cancer (BC) in their lifetime. In 2015, 231,840 new cases of invasive breast carcinoma were diagnosed, representing 14% of all new cancer cases (1). While rates for new BC cases have been stable over the last 10 years, death rates have been falling on average 1.9% each year. Still, approximately 40,000 BC-related deaths occur in the United States annually (1). Early-stage presentation is most common in this country due to screening, with 61% of women presenting with localized (confined to the primary site) BC and an additional 32% with regional (spread to regional lymph nodes) BC (1). Five-year survival is excellent following standard treatments for patients with localized (98.6%) and regional (84.9%) involvement at presentation (1). With more extensive local–regional involvement, such as skin, chest wall, or internal mammary and supraclavicular lymph nodes, outcomes are significantly worse.

Risk Factors for Breast Cancer

Risks include personal history of breast disease, family history of BC, hormonal exposures, and life exposures. Specifics are contained in Box 5.1.

Symptoms and Signs

In the United States nearly 60% of patients with early-stage BC present due to an abnormal screening mammogram. The other 40% present with a palpable breast mass, change in breast contour, or nipple discharge (26,27). Only 2% to 7% of patients with a malignant mass initially present with breast pain (28). Physical exam findings concerning for malignancy include: a hard, irregular, or nodular breast lump; skin tethering; nipple inversion; dilated veins; ulceration; peau d'orange; and nipple changes (inversion or excoriation). Metastatic BC can spread to the bones, liver, lungs, brain, and other organs (29). The route of spread for BC is via local lymphatic channels and hematogenous. A thorough history and physical exam looking for signs and symptoms of metastatic disease is warranted in anyone with a concerning breast mass.

Box 5.1 Risks for Breast Cancer Include Both Modifiable and Nonmodifiable Factors

Nonmodifiable Factors That Increase Risk of Breast Cancer

- Known genetic mutation (for details, see Chapter 9)
- Gender—100:1 female:male incidence BC (1)
- Age—age <50, risk 1:53; age >70 to death, risk 1:15 (1)
- Personal history of breast disease
  - Dense breast—4–5 × risk BC vs. women with less dense tissue (2,3)
  - Atypical ductal hyperplasia—up to 30% risk of BC at 25 years (4)
  - LCIS—1% risk of invasive disease per year; RR 2–8 depending on study (5–7)
  - DCIS—at 20 years, 6.2% risk of invasive disease, higher with younger age at diagnosis (8)
  - Invasive BC—4% risk of contralateral BC at 7.5 years (9)
- Family history
  - Age of first degree relative diagnosis—RR 2.1 for mother diagnosed before age 40 (95% CIs [1.6, 2.8]) as opposed to 1.5 after age 70 (95% CIs [1.1, 2.2]) (10)
  - Number of first degree relatives—the risk ratios were 1.80, 2.93, and 3.90, respectively, for one, two, and three or more affected first degree relatives ($P < .0001$ each) (11)
- Hormonal factors
  - Age of menarche—menarche at age ≥15 vs. <13%–24% decreased ER/PR+ BC and 16% decreased HR– BC (HR 0.76, 95% CIs [0.68, 0.85] and HR 0.84, CIs [0.69, 1.03]) (12)
  - Null parity and increasing age at childbirth associated with increased risk—cumulative incidence up to age 70 years was about 20% lower, 10% lower, or 5% higher for parous vs. nulliparous women if their first birth was at age 20, 25, or 35 years, respectively (13,14)

Modifiable—Lifestyle Risk Factors That Increase BC Risk

- Postmenopausal long hormone replacement therapy term (>3 y) (15)
- Alcohol consumption—dose response starting at three drinks per week: RR 1.15 (95% CIs [1.06, 1.24]) (16)
- Weight gain—NHS gains of 25.0 kg since age 18: RR 1.45 (95% CIs [1.27, 1.66]; $P < .001$) and 10 kg since menopause: RR 1.18 (95% CIs [1.03, 1.35]; $P = .002$) (17)
- IGF-1 and endogenous insulin levels—IGF-1 concentration of highest versus the lowest fifth OR 1.28 (95% CIs [1.14, 1.44]; $P < .0001$) (18,19)
- Postmenopausal obesity although premenopausal obesity NOT associated (20)
- Chest radiation exposure—highest risk with adolescence exposure: RR 15–25; each Gray unit received by any breast increased the excess relative risk of BC by 0.13 (21,22)

(continued)

> **Box 5.1 Risks for Breast Cancer Include Both Modifiable and Nonmodifiable Factors (*continued*)**
>
> **Modifiable Risk Factors That Decrease BC Risk**
>
> - Exercise—regular physical exercise reduced the risk of BC by 25%, especially among postmenopausal women: reduced serum estrogens, insulin, and IGF-1 levels (23)
> - Breastfeeding—for every 12 months of breastfeeding, there was a 4.3% reduction in the relative risk of BC although data confounded by parity (24,25)
>
> BC, breast cancer; DCIS, ductal carcinoma in situ; ER/PR, hormone receptors, estrogen-ER, progesterone-PR; HR, hazard ratio; IGF-1, insulin growth factor-1; LCIS, lobular carcinoma in situ; NHS, Nurses' Health Study; RR, relative risk.

Diagnosis and Workup of Breast Cancer

As discussed in Chapter 1, the majority of patients can be diagnosed utilizing nonsurgical image-guided breast and axillary biopsies. In most cases, image-guided core needle biopsy (CNB) provides tissue to confirm the diagnosis of noninvasive or invasive BC and to obtain tissue markers, estrogen receptor (ER), progesterone receptor (PR), human epidermal growth factor receptor 2 (HER2)/neu expression, and Ki-67 by immunohistochemical (IHC) stains.

> ➤ We recommend that all patients with clinically or mammographically suspicious breast abnormalities be assessed with nonsurgical core needle biopsy approaches first before surgical excision for diagnosis.

Multidisciplinary evaluation **of every patient at the time of diagnosis is standard.** We review the pathology slides and imaging studies with a team, which includes specialists in breast imaging, pathology, breast surgical oncology, radiation oncology, medical oncology, and genetic counseling. Our nurse navigator, research nurses, and nurse coordinators are also present during our multidisciplinary conference and clinic to assist the patient and providers and ensure seamless and comprehensive care.

Pretreatment workup should include a full history and physical examination with discussion of symptoms (bone pains, breathing problems, nausea, abdominal pains, and headaches) and bilateral breast exam and examination of the regional nodal basins (axillary, infraclavicular, supraclavicular, and cervical).

Initial laboratory tests include a complete blood count (CBC) and comprehensive metabolic panel (CMP), which include liver function and alkaline phosphatase.

Local/regional staging: We recommend additional imaging of the axilla and biopsy of abnormal lymph nodes. This approach is helpful in determining the extent and type of axillary surgery. Women who have biopsy-proven positive axillary lymph nodes are usually recommended a level 1 and 2 lymph node dissection as opposed to a sentinel lymph node biopsy (SLNB).

Systemic imaging of clinically asymptomatic patients with presumed stage 1 and 2 disease is NOT necessary and we recommend against routine systemic imaging (30). In our practice, patients with stage 3 BC undergo staging with CT of chest/abdomen/pelvis with intravenous contrast and bone scan or a fludeoxy-glucose (FDG) PET/CT to rule out distant metastasis. Additional systemic imaging is considered based on clinical symptoms. For instance, if new headaches or neurologic symptoms are present, a contrast-enhanced CT or MRI of the brain should be performed to rule out intracranial involvement. In patients with new back pain and/or unilateral leg weakness or urinary/fecal incontinence, additional contrast-enhanced imaging (preferably MRI) of the entire spine should be done to rule out spinal cord involvement.

Psychosocial assessment of patients' comorbidities, social situation, family support, financial concerns, and ability to understand the risks and benefits of the treatment should be assessed at this initial evaluation. These variables should factor into the recommended surgery and adjuvant treatments. We encourage family and friends to be present during our multidisciplinary consultations. In addition, we work closely with American Cancer Society (ACS) certified patient advocates who often sit in on the consultations and help patients to understand the proposed treatments.

General Staging

Currently, staging is based on the seventh edition of the American Joint Commission on Cancer (AJCC) Tumor, Nodes, Metastasis (TNM) staging system (Tables 5.1 and 5.2).

Clinical staging includes tumor size and lymph node assessment by clinical breast exam and breast/systemic imaging.

Pathological staging is the assessment of tumor size and locoregional lymph node involvement by the pathologist after breast surgery is completed.

Neoadjuvant systemic therapy staging: Patients who are offered systemic treatment before surgery will have clinical staging prior to therapy and pathologic response after neoadjuvant therapy, designated as ypTNM.

(*text continues on page 80*)

AJCC Staging—TNM

Table 5.1 TNM Classification for Breast Cancer	
Primary tumor (T)	
TX	Primary tumor cannot be assessed
T0	No evidence of primary tumor
Tis	Carcinoma in situ
Tis (DCIS)	Ductal carcinoma in situ
Tis (LCIS)	Lobular carcinoma in situ
Tis (Paget)	Paget disease of the nipple NOT associated with invasive carcinoma and/or carcinoma in situ (DCIS and/or LCIS) in the underlying breast parenchyma. Carcinomas in the breast parenchyma associated with Paget disease are categorized based on the size and characteristics of the parenchymal disease, although the presence of Paget disease should still be noted

(continued)

Table 5.1 TNM Classification for Breast Cancer (*continued*)	
T1	Tumor ≤20 mm in greatest dimension
T1mi	Tumor ≤1 mm in greatest dimension
T1a	Tumor >1 mm but ≤5 mm in greatest dimension
T1b	Tumor >5 mm but ≤10 mm in greatest dimension
T1c	Tumor >10 mm but ≤20 mm in greatest dimension
T2	Tumor >20 mm but ≤50 mm in greatest dimension
T3	Tumor >50 mm in greatest dimension
T4	Tumor of any size with direct extension to the chest wall and/or to the skin (ulceration or skin nodules)
T4a	Extension to chest wall, not including only pectoralis muscle adherence/invasion
T4b	Ulceration and/or ipsilateral satellite nodules and/or edema (including peau d'orange) of the skin, which do not meet the criteria for inflammatory carcinoma
T4c	Both T4a and T4b
T4d	Inflammatory carcinoma
Regional lymph nodes (N)	
Clinical	
NX	Regional lymph nodes cannot be assessed (eg, previously removed)
N0	No regional lymph node metastasis
N1	Metastasis to movable ipsilateral level I, II axillary lymph node(s)
N2	Metastases in ipsilateral level I, II axillary lymph nodes that are clinically fixed or matted or in clinically detected* ipsilateral internal mammary nodes in the *absence* of clinically evident axillary lymph node metastasis
N2a	Metastases in ipsilateral level I, II axillary lymph nodes fixed to one another (matted) or to other structures
N2b	Metastases only in clinically detected* ipsilateral internal mammary nodes and in the *absence* of clinically evident level I, II axillary lymph node metastases
N3	Metastases in ipsilateral infraclavicular (level III axillary) lymph node(s), with or without level I, II axillary node involvement, or in clinically detected* ipsilateral internal mammary lymph node(s) and in the *presence* of clinically evident level I, II axillary lymph node metastasis; or metastasis in ipsilateral supraclavicular lymph node(s), with or without axillary or internal mammary lymph node involvement
N3a	Metastasis in ipsilateral infraclavicular lymph node(s)

(*continued*)

Table 5.1 TNM Classification for Breast Cancer (*continued*)	
N3b	Metastasis in ipsilateral internal mammary lymph node(s) and axillary lymph node(s)
N3c	Metastasis in ipsilateral supraclavicular lymph node(s)
*"Clinically detected" is defined as detected by imaging studies (excluding lymphoscintigraphy) or by clinical examination and having characteristics highly suspicious for malignancy or a presumed pathologic macrometastasis on the basis of fine needle aspiration (FNA) biopsy with cytologic examination.	
Pathologic (pN)*	
pNX	Regional lymph nodes cannot be assessed (eg, previously removed, or not removed for pathologic study)
pN0	No regional lymph node metastasis identified histologically. *Note:* Isolated tumor cell clusters (ITCs) are defined as small clusters of cells ≤0.2 mm, or single tumor cells, or a cluster of <200 cells in a single histologic cross-section; ITCs may be detected by routine histology or by immunohistochemical (IHC) methods; nodes containing only ITCs are excluded from the total positive node count for purposes of N classification but should be included in the total number of nodes evaluated
pN0(i–)	No regional lymph node metastases histologically, negative IHC
pN0(i+)	Malignant cells in regional lymph node(s) ≤0.2 mm (detected by hematoxylin–eosin [H&E] stain or IHC, including ITC)
pN0(mol–)	No regional lymph node metastases histologically, negative molecular findings (reverse transcriptase polymerase chain reaction [RT-PCR])
pN0(mol+)	Positive molecular findings (RT-PCR) but no regional lymph node metastases detected by histology or IHC
pN1	Micrometastases; or metastases in 1–3 axillary lymph nodes and/or in internal mammary nodes, with metastases detected by sentinel lymph node biopsy but not clinically detected[†]
pN1mi	Micrometastases (>0.2 mm and/or >200 cells, but none >2.0 mm)
pN1a	Metastases in 1–3 axillary lymph nodes (at least 1 metastasis >2.0 mm)
pN1b	Metastases in internal mammary nodes, with micrometastases or macrometastases detected by sentinel lymph node biopsy but not clinically detected[†]
pN1c	Metastases in 1–3 axillary lymph nodes and in internal mammary lymph nodes, with micrometastases or macrometastases detected by sentinel lymph node biopsy but not clinically detected[†]
pN2	Metastases in 4–9 axillary lymph nodes or in clinically detected[‡] internal mammary lymph nodes in the absence of axillary lymph node metastases

(*continued*)

Table 5.1 TNM Classification for Breast Cancer (*continued*)	
pN2a	Metastases in 4–9 axillary lymph nodes (at least 1 tumor deposit >2.0 mm)
pN2b	Metastases in clinically detected[‡] internal mammary lymph nodes in the absence of axillary lymph node metastases
pN3	Metastases in ≥10 axillary lymph nodes; or in infraclavicular (level III axillary) lymph nodes; or in clinically detected[‡] ipsilateral internal mammary lymph nodes in the presence of ≥1 positive level I, II axillary lymph nodes; or in >3 axillary lymph nodes and in internal mammary lymph nodes, with micrometastases or macrometastases detected by sentinel lymph node biopsy but not clinically detected[†]; or in ipsilateral supraclavicular lymph nodes
pN3a	Metastases in ≥10 axillary lymph nodes (at least 1 tumor deposit >2.0 mm); or metastases to the infraclavicular (level III axillary lymph) nodes
pN3b	Metastases in clinically detected[‡] ipsilateral internal mammary lymph nodes in the presence of ≥1 positive axillary lymph nodes; or in >3 axillary lymph nodes and in internal mammary lymph nodes, with micrometastases or macrometastases detected by sentinel lymph node biopsy but not clinically detected[†]
pN3c	Metastases in ipsilateral supraclavicular lymph nodes

*Classification is based on axillary lymph node dissection, with or without sentinel lymph node biopsy. Classification based solely on sentinel lymph node biopsy without subsequent axillary lymph node dissection is designated (sn) for "sentinel node"—for example, pN0(sn).

[†]"Not clinically detected" is defined as not detected by imaging studies (excluding lymphoscintigraphy) or not detected by clinical examination.

[‡]"Clinically detected" is defined as detected by imaging studies (excluding lymphoscintigraphy) or by clinical examination and having characteristics highly suspicious for malignancy or a presumed pathologic macrometastasis on the basis of FNA biopsy with cytologic examination.

Distant metastasis (M)	
M0	No clinical or radiographic evidence of distant metastasis
cM0(i+)	No clinical or radiographic evidence of distant metastases, but deposits of molecularly or microscopically detected tumor cells in circulating blood, bone marrow, or other nonregional nodal tissue that are no larger than 0.2 mm in a patient without symptoms or signs of metastases
M1	Distant detectable metastases as determined by classic clinical and radiographic means and/or histologically proven >0.2 mm

TNM, tumor, nodes, metastasis.

Source: Used with permission of the American Joint Committee on Cancer (AJCC), Chicago, Illinois. From Ref. (31). Edge S, Byrd DR, Compton CC, et al. *AJCC Cancer Staging Handbook: From the AJCC Cancer Staging Manual.* 7th ed. New York, NY: Springer Science + Business Media; 2010.

Table 5.2 TNM Anatomic Stages/Prognostic Groups

Stage	T	N	M
0	Tis	N0	M0
IA	T1	N0	M0
IB	T0	N1mi	M0
	T1	N1mi	M0
IIA	T0	N1	M0
	T1	N1	M0
	T2	N0	M0
IIB	T2	N1	M0
	T3	N0	M0
IIIA	T0	N2	M0
	T1	N2	M0
	T2	N2	M0
	T3	N1	M0
	T3	N2	M0
IIIB	T4	N0	M0
	T4	N1	M0
	T4	N2	M0
IIIC	Any T	N3	M0
IV	Any T	Any N	M1

TNM, tumor, nodes, metastasis.

Source: Used with permission of the American Joint Committee on Cancer (AJCC), Chicago, Illinois. From Ref. (31). Edge S, Byrd DR, Compton CC, et al. *AJCC Cancer Staging Handbook: From the AJCC Cancer Staging Manual.* 7th ed. New York, NY: Springer Science + Business Media; 2010.

PATHOLOGY

Invasive breast carcinomas are the most common type of breast malignancy. The pathologic evaluation of these tumors includes the determination of multiple important prognostic and predictive factors. Most powerful among these are pathologic tumor stage (tumor size, lymph node status) (32,33), histologic type, histologic grade, lymphatic vascular space invasion, margin status, and the results of prognostic/predictive marker analysis.

Pathologic Tumor Stage

Pathologic staging is the gold standard and consists of tumor–lymph node–metastasis (TNM) components. Tumor size (T) is measured both grossly and microscopically; microscopic tumor size is most accurate. T1 tumors are ≤20 mm, T2 tumors are >20 mm but ≤50 mm, and T3 tumors are >50 mm in greatest dimension. T4 tumor stage is reserved for tumors of any size that exhibit direct extension into the chest wall and/or skin. Staging of tumors is extremely important for prognosis, and studies have shown a direct relationship between the size of breast tumors, the frequency of axillary nodal involvement, and patient survival (32).

Nodal status is a powerful prognostic factor (33). Nodal stage (N) increases with the number of involved axillary lymph nodes. A tumor is stage N1a when 1 to 3 axillary lymph nodes are involved, N2a when 4 to 9 axillary lymph nodes are involved, and N3a when 10 or more axillary lymph nodes are involved. Isolated tumor cells, which are malignant cells in regional lymph node(s) ≤0.2 mm, are referred to a N0 (i+). Micrometastasis are 0.2 mm to 2 mm and are designated as N1mic (Table 5.1). Isolated tumor cells in lymph nodes behave similar to node-negative cancers (34,35).

Histologic Types of Invasive Breast Carcinoma

BC, like many other malignancies, is often viewed as a single pathological entity, but in fact, this disease encompasses numerous histologic types. The histologic type imparts unique features to BC and often determines its behavior and impacts management. According to the World Health Organization (WHO) classification, there are up to 21 distinct histological types on the basis of cell morphology, growth, and architecture pattern. The most common and clinically significant histologic types of BC are invasive ductal carcinoma (IDC), lobular carcinoma, medullary carcinoma, mucinous carcinoma, tubular carcinoma, micropapillary carcinoma, and metaplastic carcinoma.

Invasive Ductal Carcinoma

IDC, sometimes referred to as invasive carcinoma of no special type, comprises 70% to 80% of breast carcinomas (Figure 5.1). If an IDC is well differentiated (histologic grade 1), the cells resemble cells lining normal breast ducts and lobules. These tumors typically form cohesive cell nests, which can mimic the architecture of normal breast tissue, forming glands and tubules. Typical gross appearance of IDC is that of a stellate firm mass with a fibrotic center. When IDC metastasize, they spread most frequently to the lymph nodes, liver, and central nervous system (36).

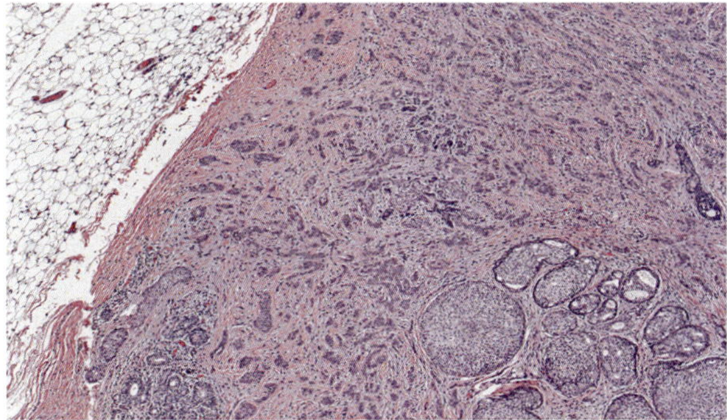

Figure 5.1 Invasive ductal carcinoma associated with ductal carcinoma in situ (lower right).

Invasive Lobular Carcinoma (ILC)

Invasive lobular carcinoma (ILC) accounts for approximately 10% of BC. Despite the implication of their name, lobular carcinomas arise from the same terminal duct/lobular cells as IDCs (Figure 5.2). The defining characteristic of lobular carcinomas is their loss of expression of intercellular adhesion protein E-cadherin (Figure 5.3), which can be confirmed with the aid of IHC stain. Although the prognosis of this histological type is similar to that of IDC, its clinicopathologic features differ considerably. Unlike IDC, lobular carcinoma cells infiltrate the surrounding tissue diffusely, by single cells, files, or in sheets (37). This diffuse pattern of infiltration makes early detection more difficult, as the cancer may not be visible on imaging or palpable on physical exam (38). Lobular carcinomas are more frequently multifocal (MF) and bilateral. MRI of the breast will often be performed to fully evaluate the extent of ILC given its underestimation on mammography. ILC may be more challenging to remove by breast conserving surgery (BCS) as it is often more extensive than expected. ILC will more frequently have positive surgical margins than ductal carcinomas (39). In addition, lobular carcinomas are more likely than ductal carcinomas to spread to the gastrointestinal organs, gynecologic organs, peritoneum, and meninges (36).

Pleomorphic lobular carcinoma is a very rare and aggressive variant of lobular carcinoma (accounting for <1% of all invasive mammary carcinomas) that frequently presents with lymphovascular invasion and at advanced stage (40). The growth pattern of this tumor is identical to that seen in classical lobular carcinoma but the pleomorphic variant is composed of cells with more evidence of nuclear atypia and pleomorphism. HER2 is overexpressed in up to 30% of the cases of pleomorphic lobular carcinoma metastasis (40).

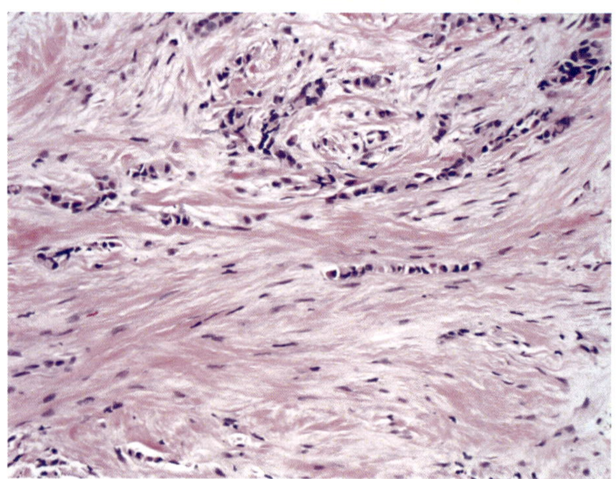

Figure 5.2 Invasive lobular carcinoma. The tumor cells are very small and bland, and infiltrate as single cells and cell files.

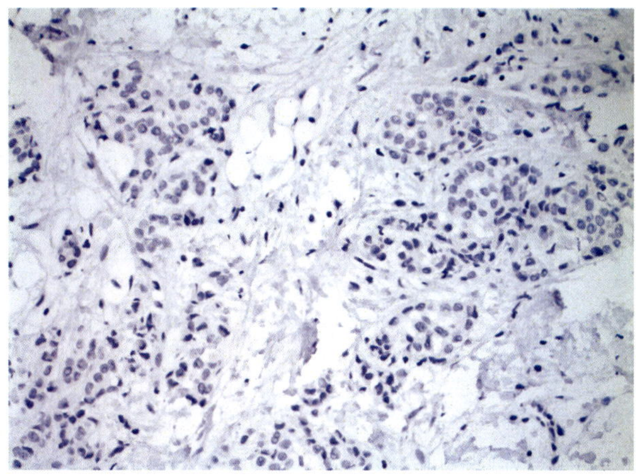

Figure 5.3 Invasive lobular carcinoma, negative E-cadherin immunostain.

Other Histological Types

Medullary carcinomas account for 1% to 7% of BC. The tumors usually present as a discrete lobulated mass (41). The tumors are well circumscribed and exhibit overtly malignant morphology and high degree of cytologic atypia and mitotic activity. The histologic grade of these tumors is always high. Notably, medullary carcinomas are often infiltrated with immune cells, such as lymphocytes and plasma cells. These features must be present in the entire tumor for the diagnosis of classical medullary carcinoma. Cases that do not fulfill all these criteria are defined as atypical medullary carcinoma or carcinoma with medullary features. Medullary carcinomas are usually triple negative and have high Ki-67 index but are less likely to spread to the lymph nodes. Patients with medullary carcinoma have a more favorable prognosis compared to those with ductal or lobular carcinoma (42). An association of medullary carcinomas with BRCA1 mutations has been reported.

Mucinous carcinomas, tubular and cribriform carcinomas account for a small percentage of well-differentiated BCs. Mucinous carcinomas occur most frequently in older patients and are low grade, with clusters of bland cells floating in lakes of mucin (Figure 5.4). Tubular and cribriform carcinomas more often affect younger women and can be MF. The tumor cells are very bland and form angulated tubules or cribriform, sieve-like nests. Mucinous, cribriform, and tubular carcinomas have a favorable prognosis as compared to the other histologic types of BC; they typically are low grade, strongly express ER and PR, are negative for HER2, and have a low proliferation rate (43).

Invasive micropapillary carcinoma is a tumor with a peculiar appearance characterized by rounded tumor nests surrounded by empty spaces (Figure 5.5). These tumors tend to be very aggressive, with massive lymph node metastases and extensive lymphatic vascular space invasion resulting in intramammary tumor spread with MF and multicentric (MC) tumors (44).

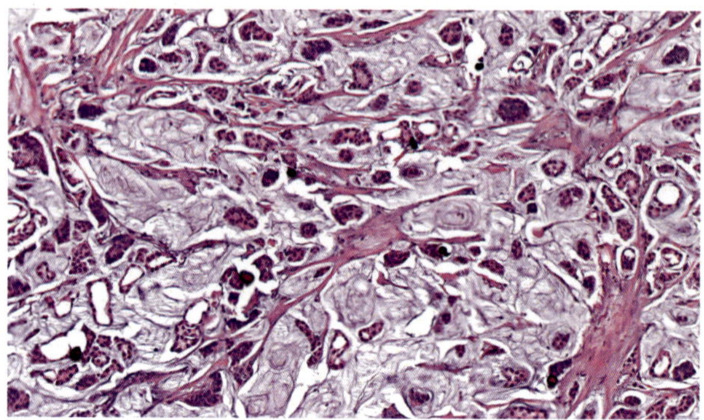

Figure 5.4 Invasive mucinous (colloid) carcinoma. Neoplastic nests of cells floating in lakes of extravasated mucin.

Metaplastic carcinomas are a heterogeneous group of tumors characterized by aberrant differentiation of the neoplastic epithelium into squamous or mesenchymal phenotype. The WHO classifies these as squamous cell carcinoma, spindle cell carcinoma, and metaplastic carcinoma with mesenchymal differentiation (also called matrix-producing carcinomas). These tumors are high grade, triple negative, and have a high Ki-67 index. The metaplastic carcinoma group also includes low-grade adenosquamous carcinomas and fibromatosis-like metaplastic carcinomas that are associated with a more favorable prognosis.

Histologic Grade

The most widely utilized histologic grading system for invasive carcinomas of the breast is the Nottingham combined histologic grade (Table 5.3). The variables

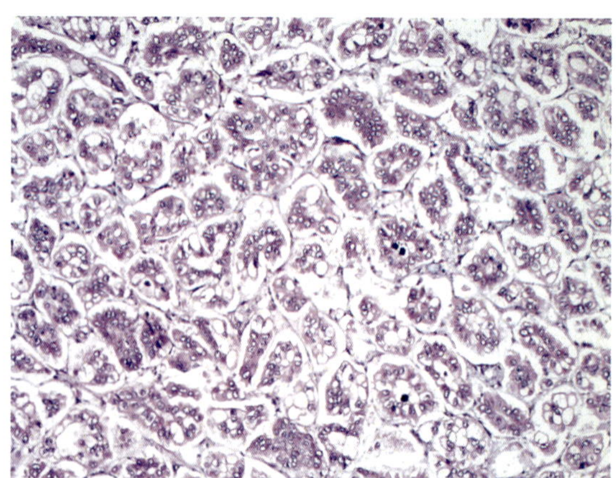

Figure 5.5 Invasive micropapillary carcinoma. Tumor cell nests grow as small papillary clusters surrounded by retraction artifact.

Table 5.3 Nottingham Combined Histologic Grade
Glandular/tubular differentiation
Score 1: >75% of tumor area forming glandular/tubular structures
Score 2: 10%–75% of tumor area forming glandular/tubular structures
Score 3: <10% of tumor area forming glandular/tubular structures
Nuclear atypia
Score 1: tumor nuclei similar to normal breast epithelial cell nuclei
Score 2: intermediate nuclei with moderate variability in size and shape, visible nucleoli
Score 3: large nuclei with marked variation in size and shape, prominent nucleoli
Mitotic rate (per 10 HPF with 40 × objective and field area of 0.196 mm²)
Score 1: 0–7 mitoses
Score 2: 8–14 mitoses
Score 3: 15 or more mitoses
Overall grade
Grade 1 (well differentiated): total score of 3, 4, or 5
Grade 2 (moderately differentiated): total score of 6 or 7
Grade 3 (poorly differentiated): total score of 8 or 9
HPF, high powered fields.

measured in this system include the degree of glandular/tubular differentiation, the extent of nuclear atypia, and the mitotic rate (number of mitotic figures per 10 high-power fields). Each of the three parameters is scored on a scale of 1 to 3, and the final Nottingham grade (Table 5.3) is the sum of these three scores. All invasive carcinomas of the breast, regardless of histologic type (Figure 5.6), should be graded, as histologic grade has been shown to be strongly associated with overall survival (OS) (45). Figure 5.6 illustrates an example of a high grade tumor.

Prognostic Markers

Over the last few decades, the use of immunophenotyping to stratify patients for prognostication and treatment selection has become the mainstay of workup of all newly diagnosed BC. The basic prognostic/predictive panel for invasive carcinomas of the breast includes IHC stains for **ER, PR, HER2, and Ki-67 proliferative index.**

ER/PR: Approximately 75% of all invasive breast carcinomas are positive for hormone receptors (HRs), with slightly more tumors being ER-positive than PR-positive. While ER and PR are weak favorable prognostic factors, they serve as strong predictive factors for how well a tumor will respond to hormonal therapy (46). Guidelines published by the College of American Pathologists (CAP) in 2010 state that BC demonstrating **ER or PR immunoreactivity in at least 1% of tumor cells should be classified as receptor-positive** (Figure 5.7) (47).

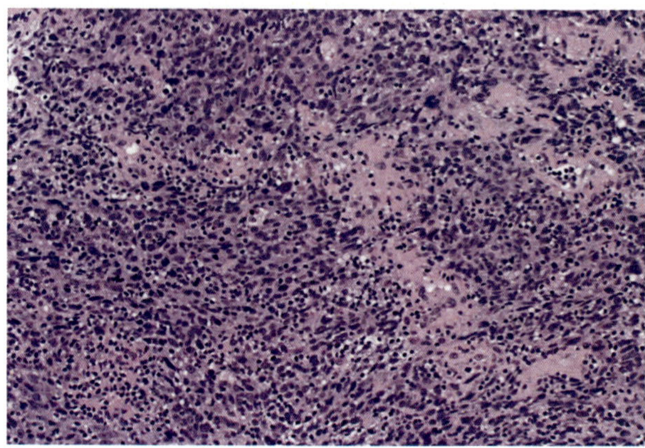

Figure 5.6 Basal-like invasive carcinoma. The tumor is high grade, grows as solid sheets, and is associated with lymphoid infiltrate.

HER2, also known as ERB-B2, is a signaling molecule that is upregulated in approximately 20% of invasive BC, and confers a worse prognosis. In addition, it is important to detect amplification of HER2 gene/overexpression of HER2 protein in BC (Figure 5.8) in order to identify patients who will benefit from anti-HER2 therapy. Immunohistochemistry and fluorescence in situ hybridization (FISH) are methods to detect HER2 overexpression. According to American Society of Clinical Oncology (ASCO)/CAP guidelines, HER2 status should be determined in all patients with invasive BC on the basis of one or more HER2 test results (negative, equivocal, or positive); if the initial HER2 test is equivocal, reflex testing should

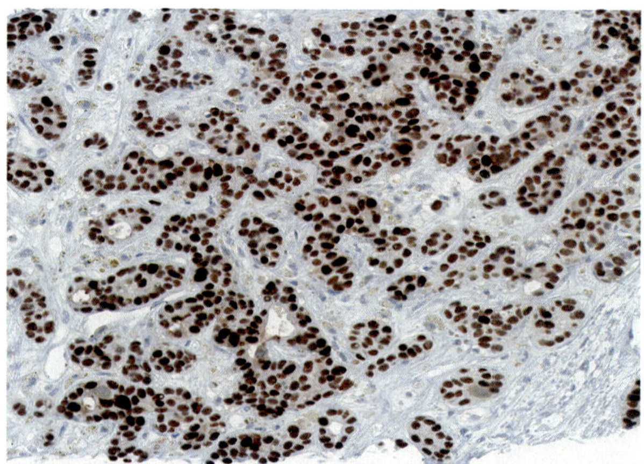

Figure 5.7 Estrogen receptor (ER) immunostain: most (>90%) of the tumor cells are strongly positive.

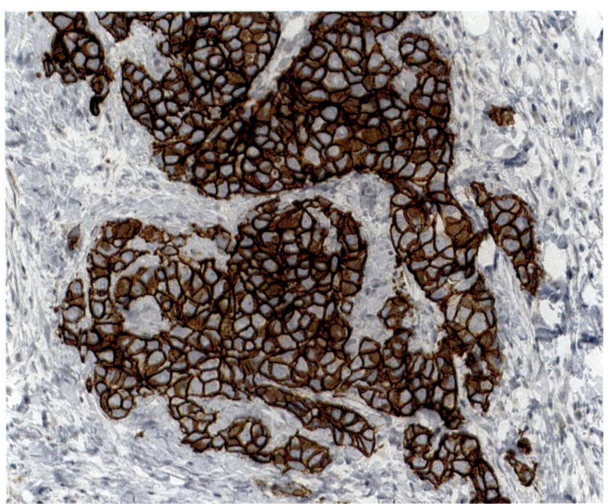

Figure 5.8 Strongly positive (3+) HER2/neu immunostain.

be performed on the same specimen using the alternative test or on an alternative specimen. Patients who were previously HER2-negative in the primary tumor and present with recurrent disease should have the metastatic site retested for HER2.

HER2 Testing Guidelines (ASCO/CAP 2013) (48)

HER2 TESTING BY IHC

- Score 0 (negative)—no staining or only incomplete, faint membrane staining in ≤10% of tumor cells
- Score 1+ (negative)—incomplete, faint membrane staining in >10% of tumor cells
- Score 2+ (equivocal)—incomplete and/or weak to moderate circumferential membrane staining occurs in >10% of tumor cells or complete, intense, circumferential in ≤10% of tumor cells
- Score 3+ (positive) is to be reported when complete, intense, circumferential staining is demonstrated in >10% of tumor cells

FLUORESCENCE IN SITU HYBRIDIZATION (FISH), HER POSITIVITY

- Single-probe average HER2 copy number ≥6.0 signals/cell
- Dual-probe HER2/CEP17 ratio ≥2.0 with an average HER2 copy number ≥4.0 signals per cell
- Dual-probe HER2/CEP17 ratio ≥2.0 with an average HER2 copy number <4.0 signals/cell
- Dual-probe HER2/CEP17 ratio <2.0 with an average HER2 copy number ≥6.0 signals/cell

Ki-67 is a nuclear protein expressed in dividing cells; it is a reliable marker of cell proliferation and has been shown to correlate with tumor grade. Moreover, studies have shown that the Ki-67 index is an independent prognostic factor, correlating significantly with disease-free and overall survival in BC patients (49). In 2009, the Saint Gallen consensus conference determined cutoffs for the Ki-67 index. It was recommended that a Ki-67 proliferative index of less than 15% be considered low/favorable, a Ki-67 proliferative index of 16% to 30% be deemed "not useful for decision," and an index greater than 30% be considered unfavorable.

Prognostic and Predictive Multigene Tests

In the recent past, tumor biomarker tests have pursued a single target. However, the past decade has seen huge advances in –omics-based technology, in which numerous analytes (eg, expression of several genes) are measured. Commercially available multigene tests and their clinical validation trials are discussed later in the chapter (Table 5.8). These multigene tests have been used for prognostics and prediction of benefit from chemotherapy and extended hormone therapy.

Other Cancers Presenting in the Breast

While metastasis of extramammary malignancies to the breast accounts for a rare minority of breast lesions (50,51), a wide range of primary tumor sites and histological types giving rise to secondary breast lesions have been reported in both women and men. Lymphomas are the most frequent culprits, with melanoma; carcinomas of the lung, gastrointestinal tract, genitourinary tract, and gynecological tract; and sarcomas of the uterus also featuring prominently (52–56).

To distinguish primary breast tumors from extramammary metastases, the constellation of gross examination, cellular morphology, tissue architecture, IHC staining, patient history, and clinical presentation must be considered. Typical metastatic lesions are solitary, round, well-circumscribed nodules in a background of fibrotic breast tissue, with absence of in situ mammary carcinoma. In contrast, primary breast tumors often have spiculated borders that infiltrate the breast parenchyma and feature elastosis and calcification (53,57). Microscopically, features characteristic of specific tissue origin are often observed within metastases and certain pathognomonic clues may be adequate in some cases to render a diagnosis (58,59). Comparison with pathological specimens of previously diagnosed primary tumors, when available, can be particularly helpful.

Immunophenotype of a breast lesion, determined by a panel of carefully chosen antibody markers, plays a supporting role in augmenting or refuting the identification of a metastasis to the breast. For poorly differentiated metastatic tumors in patients lacking a diagnosis of a primary malignancy or metastases that mimic primary BCs or benign breast lesions, immunochemistry may form the cornerstone for diagnosis (60). For example, high-grade serous carcinoma of the ovary metastatic to the breast is frequently misdiagnosed as a primary breast carcinoma due to overlapping morphologic and IHC features (53). While both malignancies may have an estrogen receptor +/progesterone receptor +/cytokeratin 7 +/cytokeratin 20– expression profile, PAX8 and Wilms tumor (WT-1) can be used to distinguish between breast and ovarian origin. Ovarian tumors tend to be PAX8+/WT-1+, while breast tumors are typically PAX8–/WT-1– (57).

SURGERY

Historical Perspective

Described by William Stewart Halsted in 1894, the radical mastectomy was the standard of care for operable BC throughout most of the 20th century (61). The procedure involved removal of the entire breast, ipsilateral pectoralis muscles, and axillary lymph nodes and was associated with significant morbidity (61). Over the past several decades, a number of key clinical trials have prompted major advances in the surgical management of early-stage invasive BC. Radical mastectomy has been replaced by modified radical mastectomy (sparing the pectoralis muscles as well as decreasing the extent of the axillary dissection with removal of only level 1 and 2 lymph nodes) and then by BCS toward the end of the 20th century as several clinical trials have shown that less extensive surgical procedures provide equivalent oncologic outcomes and result in lower morbidity (62).

Management of the Breast

Surgery for BC consists of removal of the tumor by either BCS or mastectomy and simultaneous evaluation of the regional lymph nodes by sentinel lymph node biopsy (SLNB) or axillary lymph node dissection (ALND).

Breast Conserving Surgery

BCS, also referred to as a lumpectomy, partial mastectomy, segmentectomy, quadrantectomy, and wide local excision, involves removal of the primary tumor with a surrounding rim of normal breast tissue while preserving the remainder of the breast. Since the majority of breast tissue is left intact, the incision is closed primarily and no reconstruction is required. This approach is routinely combined with adjuvant radiation therapy (RT) to reduce the incidence of local recurrence (LR), which translates into a survival advantage described further in the radiation section. Table 5.4 summarizes the prospective trials that compared BCS with radiation to mastectomy.

MARGINS

There has been significant controversy over the years regarding adequate margin width in patients undergoing BCS for invasive BC. The most recent data demonstrate no significant difference in LR rates when negative margins, defined as "no tumor on ink," are achieved in patients undergoing BCS and whole breast irradiation (WBI) and who receive appropriate adjuvant systemic therapy (69,70). However, patients with multifocal (MF) close margins with "no tumor on ink" may still need to be considered for reexcision. This may be particularly important in patients with an extensive intraductal component. Therefore, it is essential to review each patient's pathology individually to ensure that adequate margins are obtained.

> ➤ We currently consider "no tumor on ink" as an adequate margin in patients with invasive BC. In patients with a combination of invasive BC and DCIS, while "no tumor on ink" is considered an adequate margin, reexcision may be necessary depending on the extent of DCIS.

Table 5.4 Prospective Trials Comparing Breast Conserving Surgery to Mastectomy Prior to Modern Systemic Therapy

Study	Local treatment	Local recurrence (LR) (%)	Overall survival (OS) (%)	Follow-up (y)
NSABP B-06 (63)	BCS + Radiation	14	46	20
	Mastectomy	8	47	
Milan Cancer Institute (64)	BCS + Radiation	9	58	20
	Mastectomy	2	59	
National Cancer Institute (65)	BCS + Radiation	22	54	18
	Mastectomy	10	58	
Institute Gustave-Roussy (66)	BCS + Radiation	13	73	15
	Mastectomy	18	65	
EORTC (67)	BCS + Radiation	20	65	10
	Mastectomy	12	66	
Danish Breast Cancer Group (68)	BCS + Radiation	3	79	6
	Mastectomy	4	82	

BCS, breast conserving surgery; EORTC, European Organisation for Research and Treatment of Cancer; NSABP, National Surgical Adjuvant Breast and Bowel Project.

BCS ELIGIBILITY

Absolute contraindications include diffuse suspicious or malignant appearing calcifications on imaging, persistently positive margins after multiple excisions, multicentric (MC) disease (two foci of disease in different quadrants) that cannot be removed with a single excision, early pregnancy, and prior thoracic radiation.

Relative contraindications include large tumors that will lead to poor cosmesis, very large breast size, patients who are not candidates for postoperative RT and multifocal (MF) disease (two foci in the same quadrant). For patients with large tumors who desire BCS, neoadjuvant systemic therapy may be considered to reduce tumor size and increase eligibility for BCS.

Although the use of BCS in MF or MC disease is controversial, a study from the European Institute of Oncology in Milan, in which 421 patients with MF cancer and 55 with MC cancer were treated with BCS, demonstrated a 5-year cumulative incidence of LR of 5.1% (71). For patients with one of these relative contraindications, a full disclosure of risks and benefits of each option should be discussed.

Mastectomy

Mastectomy removes the entire breast. This procedure may be considered in patients with all stages of BC. Mastectomy is often combined with breast reconstruction in patients who are candidates.

TYPES OF MASTECTOMY

Simple mastectomy (total mastectomy): complete removal of the breast including the nipple–areolar complex (NAC).

Modified radical mastectomy: removal of the breast, NAC, and level 1 and 2 axillary lymph nodes.

Skin-sparing mastectomy: removal of all breast tissue and the NAC with preservation of the skin envelope of the breast.

Nipple-sparing mastectomy (NSM): removal of all breast tissue while preserving the entire skin envelope of the breast including the NAC. This approach is often used for prophylactic mastectomy in high-risk patients or for patients with small BCs located away from the NAC (Figure 5.9).

Skin-sparing mastectomy outcomes. The majority of patients in studies of skin-sparing mastectomy had early-stage disease (stage 0–II) and the reported LR rates ranged from 1.9% to 7% with follow-up times of 49 to 118 months (72–77). Patients are generally considered eligible for skin-sparing mastectomy if they have early-stage BC, stage 0–II. While this procedure has been examined in patients with more advanced BC (stage IIB and III), the studies are small and the oncologic safety cannot be confirmed (78–80).

NSM outcomes. Factors associated with NAC involvement include larger tumors, smaller distance between the tumor and NAC, MC disease, lymph node involvement, higher tumor grade, and HER2 amplification. NSM was initially utilized in high-risk patients undergoing prophylactic mastectomy for risk reduction. However, the procedure has since been expanded to patients with small, unifocal tumors (<2–3 cm) that are at least 1 to 2 cm from the NAC (81–83). In studies that have evaluated the procedure in patients with BC, NAC involvement was seen in 8% to 33% of cases (84). Relative contraindications to the procedure include significant ptosis in the breasts, large breasts, smoking, diabetes, and obesity (84). Small studies that examined oncologic outcomes in patients undergoing NSM showed LR rates of 2% to 3% at follow-up times of 28 to 60 months (81–83).

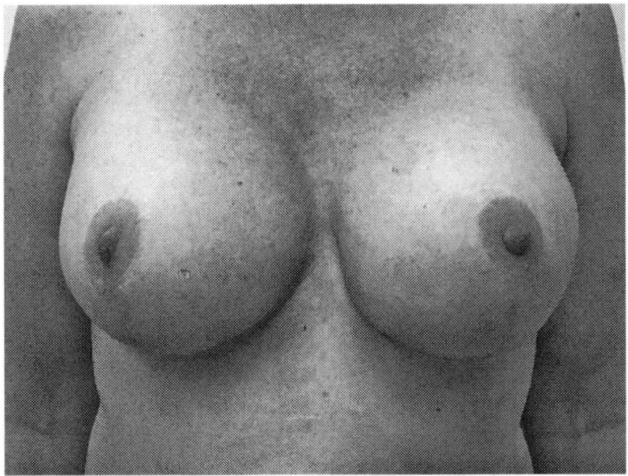

Figure 5.9 Bilateral nipple sparing mastectomy with implant reconstruction.

> ➤ Currently, we consider NSM for patients with unifocal BCs that are <3 cm in size and at least 1 to 2 cm away from the NAC.

Surgical Staging of Lymphatics

Following the trend toward less invasive and morbid procedures, surgical management of the axilla has moved away from the extensive axillary dissections to targeted removal of axillary lymph nodes through lymphatic mapping and SLNB.

Surgical Options

SLNB is a less morbid alternative to ALND for staging of the regional lymph nodes in patients with BC with clinically negative lymph nodes (85,86). This technique involves the targeted identification and removal of the first draining lymph nodes of the breast, which are located in the axilla in the majority of cases. The mapping procedure uses a radiolabeled tracer and/or blue dye, which is injected into the breast tissue (either intradermal, peritumoral, periareolar, or subareolar), and then travels through the lymphatics and accumulates in the sentinel node(s) (85–89). The sentinel lymph nodes (SLNs) may be detected at the time of surgery by visualization of blue dye or by radioactivity detection using a gamma probe. The combination of dye and radiotracer results in an SLN detection rate of over 95% with false-negative rates (FNRs) reported between 0% and 10% (88–90). After a negative SLNB without ALND, axillary recurrence rates are extremely low (91).

> ➤ We recommend SLNB in patients with early-stage, clinically node-negative invasive BC, and in patients with DCIS undergoing mastectomy.

Patient Eligibility for SLNB

Clinical situations in which there is insufficient data to support SLNB include patients with T3/T4 BC, locally advanced disease, inflammatory BC, DCIS when BCS is planned, and pregnancy. We typically consider SLNB in patients with T3 tumors. In pregnant patients with early-stage BC, we consider SLNB with the use of radiolabeled tracer alone. In addition, in patients with DCIS, we perform SLNB in patients with a large area of involvement (>5 cm), a palpable mass, imaging findings concerning for an invasive BC, and in cases where SLNB may not be successful after BCS due to location of disease.

AXILLARY LYMPH NODE DISSECTION

This procedure is utilized for patients with clinically positive lymph nodes or in patients with multiple positive SLNs. It involves removal of the level 1 and 2 axillary lymph nodes. Level 3 lymph nodes are only removed when they are grossly positive, although this may significantly increase morbidity due to an increase in lymphedema. This procedure provides regional disease control in patients.

Management of Clinically Negative Axillary Lymph Nodes

The **National Surgical Adjuvant Breast and Bowel Project (NSABP) B-32 trial** examined and confirmed the efficacy of SLNB in patients with early-stage BC. This study included patients with clinically negative lymph nodes who were randomized to either SLNB with ALND or SLNB alone (with ALND only if the SLN was positive). In patients who had pathologically negative SLNs, outcomes were statistically equivalent between the two groups, including 8-year OS (91.8% SLNB + ALND vs. 90.3% SLNB alone; P = .12), disease-free survival (DFS) (82.4% vs. 81.5%; P = .54) and regional disease control (0.4% vs. 0.7%; P = .22) (91).

> ➤ For patients with clinically negative axillary nodes and pathologically negative SLNs, no further axillary surgery is needed.

The **American College of Surgeons Oncology Group (ACOSOG) Z0011 trial** examined the need for ALND in patients with early-stage BC and one or two positive SLNs who were planning to undergo BCS followed by systemic therapy and WBI (92,93). Patients were randomized to either ALND or SLNB alone. The trial accrued slowly and closed early, but demonstrated no significant difference between ALND and SLNB at 5 years in terms of LR (3.1% vs. 1.6% SLNB; P = .11), regional recurrence (0.5% vs. 0.9%; P = .45), DFS (82.2% vs. 83.9%; P = .14), and OS (91.8% vs. 92.5%; P = .25) (92,93). For patients with clinically negative axillary nodes with one or two pathologically positive SLNs, no further axillary dissection is necessary as long as whole breast radiation and appropriate adjuvant systemic therapy is planned.

> ➤ The 2014 ASCO guidelines now recognize that patients with one or two positive SLNs who undergo BCS and receive appropriate adjuvant systemic therapy and WBI do not require ALND.

One caveat to this study was that the volume irradiated was not standardized, as standard tangential radiation does not cover the entire volume that would be encompassed in a level 1/2 axillary dissection, such that some patients received larger radiation volumes to the entire axilla (ie, high tangents in 50% of patients on Z0011) or received radiation to the entire axilla and supraclavicular fossa (19% of patients on Z0011).

The **IBCSG-23-01 trial** also compared SLNB and ALND to SLNB alone in patients with positive SLNs and included patients with T1/2 N0 disease and the presence of one or more SLNs with micrometastases (<2 mm) (94). Unlike Z0011, patients undergoing mastectomy were also included and comprised about 10% of the patient population and did not undergo radiotherapy. The 5-year DFS was similar between those who underwent ALND (84.4%) and SLNB alone (87.8%), P = .16 (94).

The **AMAROS trial evaluated** radiation targeting the axilla (levels 1–3) and supraclavicular fossa as an alternative to ALND in patients with clinical T1/2 N0 BC with positive SLNs (95). Patients with at least one positive SLN were randomized to external radiation therapy (XRT) or ALND. The 5-year results showed similar axillary recurrence rates in the two groups (ALND 0.54% vs. XRT 1.03%)

(95). The lymphedema rates were lower in those patients undergoing axillary XRT, with clinical signs of lymphedema in ALND 23% versus XRT 11% ($P < .0001$) and with an arm circumference increase of >10% in ALND 13% versus XRT 5% ($P < .0009$) (95).

Clinical Node-Negative, SLN Positive, Candidates for ALND

Completion ALND (levels 1 and 2) may be offered to some patients with positive SLNs. This includes patients who do not meet criteria for ACOSOG Z0011 or the IBCSG-23-01 trial.

- Patients who have more than two positive SLNs.
- Patients undergoing mastectomy who have macrometastatic disease in SLNs and will not receive adjuvant XRT.
- Patients who receive neoadjuvant therapy.
- Patients who cannot receive recommended adjuvant systemic therapy and RT.

Management of Clinically Positive Axillary Nodes

> **We recommend axillary ultrasound (US) and FNA or core biopsy of clinically palpable or mammographically/US/MRI suspicious lymph nodes to confirm involvement.**

If biopsy is negative, SLNB should be performed at surgery for appropriate staging.

If biopsy is positive, ALND at surgery or neoadjuvant systemic therapy may be considered. In patients who will receive neoadjuvant systemic therapy we recommend core biopsy and clip placement so that the biopsied lymph node may be localized and removed at the time of surgery.

Conclusions

The surgical management of early-stage invasive BC has changed significantly over the past several decades. Based on the outcomes from a number of pivotal clinical trials, clinicians are able to offer increasingly less extensive surgical procedures while maintaining oncologic outcomes. While the surgical management of primary tumors and lymph nodes is constantly evolving, the overall goal of improving patient outcomes through multimodality therapy remains the same.

RADIATION THERAPY IN THE ADJUVANT SETTING FOLLOWING SURGERY

RT complements surgery by reducing the incidence of local and regional failures. In the modern era of systemic therapy, these reductions in local–regional disease have had an impact on reducing distant metastases, as certain regional disease can act as a harbinger of distant disease, and have also had an impact on survival (96). In addition, the delivery of radiation has improved substantially with novel technologies that reduce the morbidity and mortality of therapy, causing an overall improvement in quality of life for patients with BC.

RADIATION THERAPY AS AN ADJUVANT TO BCS FOR EARLY-STAGE BC

Comparison of BCS to Modified Radical Mastectomy (MRM) for Women With Tumors <5 cm in Size

As reviewed in Table 5.4, six randomized trials were performed several decades ago comparing BCS and whole breast radiation versus mastectomy. The results of the studies demonstrated similar local control, DFS, and OS between the two approaches. Due to psychological and quality of life benefits of BCS, the National Cancer Institute (NCI)/National Institutes of Health (NIH) Consensus described BCS as the **"preferable" strategy** in managing early-stage BC in eligible and appropriate patients (97).

BCS Without Radiation in an Unselected Population

In an attempt to improve quality of life further, many trials have tried to forgo radiation completely following BCS. In the unselected population, the absence of radiation was associated with recurrence and detriments in survival as described in the following.

NSABP B-06 accrued 1,851 women with primary tumors <4 cm who were randomized to total mastectomy versus wide local excision and radiation versus wide local excision alone (98). While there was no OS benefit with the addition of radiation, there was substantial (39.2% vs. 14.3%; $P < .001$) reduction in ipsilateral BC recurrence. There were, however, suggestions in this trial that adjuvant radiotherapy may affect survival in that BC deaths were reduced marginally (hazard ratio [HR] 0.82; $P = .04$) with the addition of radiation to lumpectomy. This effect was somewhat offset by competing all-cause deaths, later attributed to the negative cardiac effects of radiotherapy. However, it should be noted that WBI in this trial was delivered with what would now be considered antiquated techniques and current radiation volumes to the heart are significantly lower.

The **Early Breast Cancer Trialists' Collaborative Group (EBCTCG)** subsequently published an overview encompassing 78 randomized trials, 42,000 women, and 15-year results (99). With the increased power from the large sample size, **an OS benefit of 5.3% ($P = .005$) was realized with the addition of radiotherapy to lumpectomy**. For every four local, in-breast recurrences prevented with radiotherapy, one woman was saved from death from BC. Importantly, this analysis demonstrated that interventions affecting a 10% or more improvement in local control at the primary site at 5 years resulted in a reduction in BC mortality at 15 years.

BCS Without Radiation in a Selected Population

EBCTCG asserts that interventions with minimal local control benefit fail to yield a survival benefit (100). A meta-analysis including 17 randomized trials, 10,801 women, and 15 years of follow-up sought to identify individual prognostic factors that could identify patients who benefit minimally from adjuvant radiotherapy. Despite examining age, tumor size, tumor grade, ER status, additional therapy, and surgical procedure extent, no subgroup was identified in which it was completely safe to omit radiotherapy without a decrease in local control.

NSABP B-21: Investigators then postulated that hormonal therapy might replace RT in an unselected population and randomized 1,009 women with tumors less than 1 cm in diameter and node-negative disease to one of three arms following lumpectomy—tamoxifen alone, RT and placebo, or RT and tamoxifen (101). Eight-year follow-up showed no difference in distant failure or OS between the three groups. RT reduced recurrences more than tamoxifen alone (16.5% vs. 9.3% at 8 years), but the best in-breast control was seen with the combination of RT and tamoxifen (2.8% at 8 years).

The Cancer and Leukemia Group B (CALGB) 9343 trial was more selective and enrolled 636 low-risk patients who were **70 years of age or older with ER+ (99% of cases) disease** with tumors that were <2 cm (98% of cases) in maximum dimension who were treated with lumpectomy and tamoxifen. The randomization was between radiation and no radiation with the primary end point being a difference in local control (102). The 12-year update showed a significant improvement in local control (10% without radiation vs. 2% with radiation) (103) without a difference in OS. This trial is often mistakenly identified as demonstrating a lack of benefit of radiotherapy. Nonetheless, this treatment approach has emerged as a reasonable, but not necessarily preferred, option for women over 70 with the most favorable BC characteristics.

The PRIME II study has served to affirm the efficacy of this strategy despite relatively short follow-up (104). With a similar randomization of women 65 and older, ipsilateral BC recurrence in the 5-year report was 1.3% versus 4.1% with and without radiotherapy, respectively, similar to the 5-year results of the CALGB trial.

These findings are the best to date in identifying a group that may be able to forgo adjuvant radiation without detriment to survival. However, it should be noted that these trials consistently demonstrate a benefit in local–regional control with the addition of radiotherapy, even in highly selected populations. For women older than 70 electing to forgo radiation based on the previous data, consideration of a "trial period" for women electing to proceed with adjuvant hormone therapy alone can be employed. If either tolerance or compliance is poor at 3 to 4 months following surgery, radiotherapy could be employed at this juncture, either in place of or along with continued medical therapy.

> ➤ **For patients who refuse or cannot tolerate hormonal therapy or have a life expectancy of 10 years or more, radiotherapy is recommended.**

Techniques of Radiation

Deep inspiratory breath-hold requires the patient to inspire deeply and hold her breath while individual fields of radiotherapy are administered. This technique moves the heart medially and inferiorly, substantially reducing the heart dose without sacrificing breast tissue coverage (see Figures 5.10A and 5.10B). For many patients, this is a relatively simple procedure with reliable reproducibility when the stability of the breath can be monitored during radiation (105).

Prone breast radiation allows for the breast to fall away from the chest wall. In women with larger breasts, this approach can be particularly advantageous in reducing redundant breast folds, which can lead to more substantial acute skin toxicity, as well as improving dose homogeneity, which can reduce both acute and long-term side effects (see Figure 5.11). This technique can also aid in reducing the dose to the heart and lungs (106,107). However, this technique is not utilized when treatment

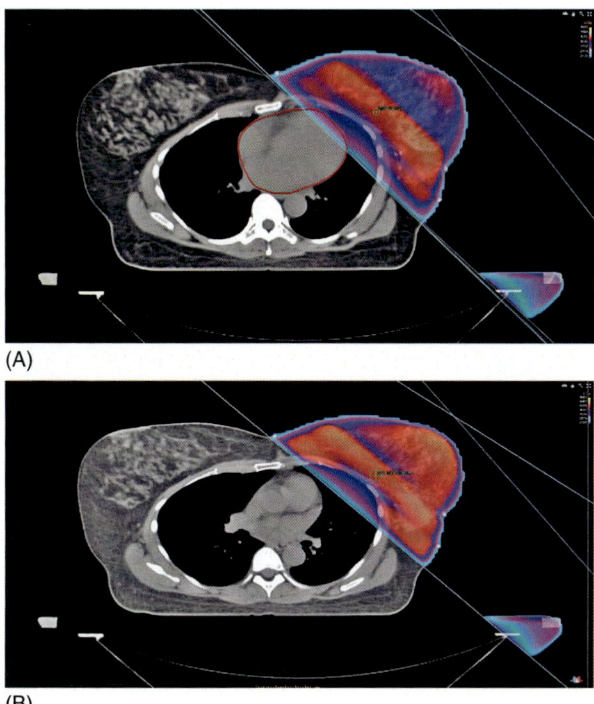

(A)

(B)

Figure 5.10 (A) Techniques of radiation—free breathing. (B) Techniques of radiation—deep inspiration breath-hold. Standard breast positioning; redundant breast folds can cause increased skin toxicity.

of the regional nodes is necessary. There is also concern that the chest wall can be underdosed with this approach and should be used with caution for patients in whom chest radiation may be of benefit (ie, triple negative BC).

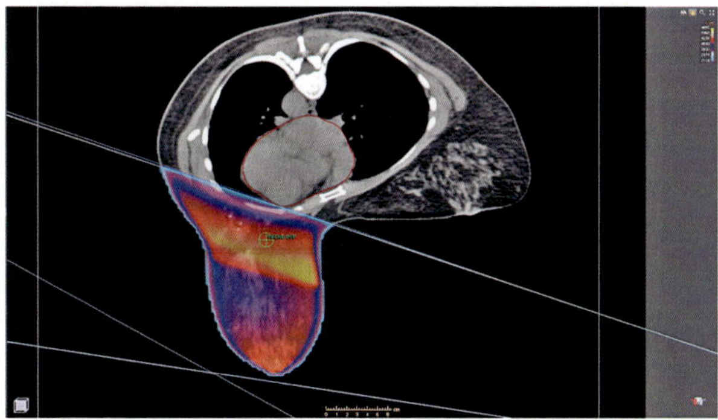

Figure 5.11 Prone breast radiation allows the breast to fall away from the chest wall.

Intensity-modulated radiation therapy (IMRT) is a sophisticated method of radiation delivery used for BC in two situations. In early-stage disease, it is used to make the dose delivery more homogeneous, which has been shown in randomized clinical trials to reduce acute grade 2–3 toxicity compared to conventional RT (108,109). The second approach is used in more advanced disease to conform the high doses of radiation around nearby critical structures. The largest experience in early disease was published from Fox Chase Cancer Center, which demonstrated the superiority of using breast IMRT compared to conventional radiation (110). The series included 804 consecutive women with early-stage BC who were treated with BCS and radiation from 2001–2006, where 399 had received photon IMRT. The maximum toxicity (grade 2 and higher) was significantly reduced using IMRT, 75% for conventional radiotherapy and 52% for IMRT ($P < .0001$). In addition, the duration (percentage of treatment weeks) patients spent experiencing grade 2 and higher dermatitis was substantially reduced from 71% for conventional radiation versus 18% for those who received IMRT ($P < .0001$). Two smaller retrospective series demonstrated similar benefits with decreased acute skin toxicity grade 2 or 3 (39% vs. 52%; $P = 0.047$) (111) and reduced grade 2 or greater breast edema (0% vs. 36%; $P < .001$) (112). There is also improvement in late effects with reduction in the risk of developing chronic grade 2 or greater breast edema (3% vs. 30%; $P = .007$) (112) and improved cosmesis (113).

In a randomized phase III prospective trial from Canada of 358 patients, conventional radiation was compared to IMRT. It was found that IMRT was associated with improved dose homogeneity and reduced moist desquamation (31% vs. 48%; $P = .0019$) (109). This translated into a quality of life benefit for those patients who experienced moist desquamation. A randomized trial from the United Kingdom compared standard radiotherapy to IMRT in patients with early-stage BC and 240 of 306 patients were able to be evaluated by photographs for change in breast appearance (108). There was a negative change in breast appearance in 58% of patients randomized to conventional treatment compared to 40% randomized to IMRT. Two-dimensional (2D) RT was 1.7 times more likely to have a change in breast appearance than IMRT ($P = .008$).

WHOLE BREAST IRRADIATION—FRACTIONATION

Standard adjuvant radiotherapy for BC has traditionally incorporated 5 to 5.5 weeks of WBI followed by a "boost" delivered over 1 to 1.5 additional weeks to the lumpectomy cavity. The whole breast is targeted to ensure full coverage of the postsurgical cavity as well as occult MC disease within the remainder of the breast (114). Results from randomized trials have suggested that radiotherapy may be hypofractionated in early-stage BC—delivering a radiobiologically similar dose over 3 to 4 weeks (115–121).

The UK Standardization of Breast Radiotherapy (START) A and START B trials were intended to elucidate inherited radiobiologic differences between normal breast tissue and BC such that similar cell kill could be achieved through a shorter course of RT without altering acute or late effects. Multiple randomized phase III trials have tested this concept in comparison to conventional fractionation.

START A included 2,236 women with early-stage BC treated with partial mastectomy and then split them into three treatment groups to receive either 50 Gy in

25 fractions (2 Gy per fraction), 41.6 Gy in 13 fractions (3.2 Gy per fraction), or 39 Gy in 13 fractions (3 Gy per fraction) (115). At 5-year follow-up, all three arms had similar local control. There was a slightly higher rate of failures in the 39 Gy arm, although this was not statistically significant.

START B randomized 2,215 women to 50 Gy in 25 fractions or 40 Gy in 15 fractions (2.67 Gy per fraction) given over 3 weeks (116). Again, at 5 years, local–regional relapse was not significantly different between the 50 Gy (2.2%) and 40 Gy (3.3%) cohorts. At 10-year follow-up, these results have held, further solidifying shortened regimens as viable options in this disease (122). Concerns regarding the potential for increased late toxicity with higher doses per fraction have proven to be unfounded at 10 years of follow-up.

The Ontario Clinical Oncology Group (OCOG) performed a randomized trial in the mid-1990s with similar structure and intent to shorten duration (118,119,121). This effort enrolled 1,234 women with T1 or T2, node-negative BC treated with BCS who were randomized to whole breast RT, either 50 Gy in 25 fractions or 42.5 Gy in 16 fractions. The 10-year results showed comparable rates of local control (6.7% vs. 6.2%) with nearly identical rates of good to excellent cosmesis (71.3% vs. 69.8%). Two recent reports suggesting improvements in acute toxicity with hypofractionation should further bolster this effect (123,124).

> ➤ With this evidence, the American Society for Radiation Oncology (ASTRO) strengthened its stance through the Choosing Wisely campaign to highly recommend consideration of hypofractionation in appropriately selected women over the age of 50 (125). Currently, we routinely use 40 Gy in 15 fractions or 42.5 Gy in 16 fractions for most women with the exception of high-grade tumors (specifically triple negative and HER2+) based on the subset analysis of the OCOG trial, which showed a detriment in this subset of patients treated with the hypofractionated regimens.

THE ROLE OF A LUMPECTOMY CAVITY BOOST IRRADIATION

WBI is commonly followed by a "boost" to the lumpectomy cavity. The rationale for such an approach arose from multiple series indicating the perilumpectomy tissue as the highest risk area for recurrence and the most likely to harbor substantial pockets of subclinical disease (126–128). Two large, randomized trials completed in the 1990s demonstrated a local control benefit of a boost (129–132).

The European Organisation for Research and Treatment of Cancer (EORTC) 22881-10882 trial included 5,318 BC patients. Whole breast radiotherapy to 50 Gy was followed by randomization to a 16 Gy boost versus no boost (130–132). At 5-year follow-up, the boost reduced local failure rates (7.3% vs. 4.3%; $P < .001$; HR 0.59). Younger women benefited the most, while the oldest patients received the least benefit. With 10 years of follow-up, the absolute benefit widened to 4%. The use of a boost reduced salvage mastectomies by 41%, while significant fibrosis was increased.

Following these results, conventionally fractionated whole breast radiation followed by **a lumpectomy cavity boost to approximately 60 to 66 Gy has become the standard**. With the advent of hypofractionation, the utility and safety of the boost have again come into question. Results of the Royal Marsden and START experiences, which permitted a boost, are reassuring and make the addition of an approximate 10 Gy boost (usually at 2.5 Gy per fraction) to either the European or Canadian fractionation schema a reasonable option (115–117,122).

> ➤ ER+ BC patients over the age of 65, who only have a 10% risk of recurrence at 12 years without radiation, are not routinely offered a boost if whole breast radiation is recommended, unless hormonal therapy is omitted.

Partial Breast Irradiation

This approach is vastly different than whole breast radiation by focusing only on the lumpectomy cavity such that smaller volumes can be irradiated in treatments of 1 week or less. This approach was initially developed to reduce the logistical burdens that adjuvant therapy places on patients and caregivers, likely improving compliance (133,134). Over the last several decades, this approach has been shown to be safe and effective, and six phase III trials have completed accrual in comparison to whole breast radiation. Early results have shown similar outcomes for BC patients treated with interstitial brachytherapy (135), while two studies using intraoperative approaches have demonstrated less favorable results (136,137). The long-term results of all of these trials are needed to ensure equivalence of partial breast irradiation (PBI), but will take years to emerge.

As the field awaits the oncologic results, there is also growing evidence that PBI has worse cosmesis (138–140) and potentially a worse quality of life related to increased pain, fat necrosis, and postoperative infections in comparison to whole breast radiation (141). Following the publication of multiple prospective experiences demonstrating the oncologic equivalence of PBI to whole breast radiotherapy, ASTRO published consensus guidelines in 2009 dividing patients into "suitable," "cautionary," and "unsuitable" cohorts for consideration of PBI off-study (142).

PBI can be offered to patients in the suitable group that includes those who meet the following criteria: age ≥60, negative for *BRCA* mutation, tumor size ≥2 cm, negative margins, negative for lymphovascular space invasion, ER+, LN−, unicentric, clinically unifocal, invasive ductal or other favorable histology, negative for extensive intraductal component, invasive disease (not DCIS), and not receiving neoadjuvant therapy. Recently, there has been further discussion of loosening these recommendations to be more inclusive of younger patients (143) and those with pure ductal carcinoma in situ (144).

PBI can be delivered by a number of techniques that include external beam radiotherapy, intraoperative radiotherapy, multicatheter brachytherapy, single-entry intracavitary device brachytherapy, and stereotactic radiotherapy. However, external beam radiotherapy remains by far the most commonly utilized due to its familiarity among oncologists, ease of application, wide availability, and noninvasive nature (145).

Investigational Radiation Devices

GammaPod is a novel, noninvasive breast-specific stereotactic radiotherapy device that has been developed which addresses many of the challenges encountered with three-dimensional conformal radiation therapy (3D-CRT) or IMRT techniques. With GammaPod, the patient's breast is placed under a slight negative pressure inside a custom-designed breast immobilization cup, which can reduce the planning target volume (PTV) expansion from 10 to 3 mm. The patient is treated in the prone position on a translating couch. The device employs 36 noncoplanar, nonoverlapping ^{60}Co beams in a dynamic dose-painting fashion to effect highly conformal distributions akin to intracavitary brachytherapy applications with less heterogeneity and better control of dose fall-off at the skin in comparison to all Food and Drug Administration (FDA) approved intracavitary devices (146–148). Relative to traditional 3D-CRT and IMRT PBI techniques, this device has demonstrated significant improvements in sparing of normal tissues using a similar noninvasive approach (149). Currently this device is being tested in the pre-FDA approved setting under an investigational device exemption. Once FDA approved, this device will also be tested in the neoadjuvant setting, permitting ablative radiotherapy (150,151).

Role of Radiation for Patients Undergoing BCS With Node-Positive Cancer

Historically, when regional lymph nodes are involved there is concern that the patterns of failure can change, increasing the risk of failure in the axilla and the infraclavicular/supraclavicular region, as well as the internal mammary lymph nodes, based on the postmastectomy literature (152–155). Three recently published randomized trials using modern systemic therapy drive therapy decisions regarding regional nodal radiotherapy in this population.

The **ACOSOG Z0011 trial** was intended to address the role of completion ALND in patients with one or two positive SLNs (156). A total of 891 patients were randomized and no improvement in oncologic outcomes was realized with the completion ALND after SLNB. Of note, participating institutions were instructed to utilize only tangential-field whole breast radiotherapy following surgical intervention. As the two arms were equivalent, it was concluded by the authors, and assumed by many clinicians, that tangent-only radiotherapy was adequate in patients similar to this cohort. Unfortunately, review of delivered radiation fields revealed a high rate of deviation from treating with tangents alone (157). Of 228 patients with RT records, over half received high tangents, which encompass 75% to 95% of the level 1 and 2 lymph nodes typically resected, while another 18.9% received directed regional nodal radiotherapy to the axilla and infraclavicular/supraclavicular region. Though departures from the tangent's directive were balanced between the arms, the heterogeneity of employed fields complicates interpretation of this trial as to the ideal radiation approach.

EORTC 22922 enrolled 4,004 women with either lymph node negative, medial/inner quadrant tumors, or axillary involvement who had undergone BCS or mastectomy (158). Patients were randomized to receive regional nodal irradiation (defined as internal mammary and medial supraclavicular lymph node regions) or not. Women who underwent a lumpectomy received whole breast radiation in both arms. It is important to note that systemic therapy was widely utilized in this study with 99% of LN+ patients and 66.3% of LN− patients receiving chemotherapy. At 10-year follow-up, DFS (72.1% vs. 69.1%; $P = .04$), distant DFS (78.0% vs. 75.0%; $P = .02$), and BC mortality (12.5% vs. 14.4%; $P = .02$) were all significantly improved with the addition of regional nodal radiation **with the largest benefit surprisingly seen in the node-negative cohort**. There was a trend toward a survival benefit (82.3% vs. 80.7%; $P = .06$).

The **MA.20 trial** was concurrently published (159). This study enrolled patients with invasive BC who underwent BCS and SLNB or ALND. Eligible patients were those with positive axillary nodes (N1 only) or lymph node negative but with high-risk features (≥5 cm primary; ≥2 cm primary with fewer than 10 axillary nodes removed and at least one of the following: grade 3 disease, ER-negativity, or lymphovascular space invasion [LVI+]). Patients were randomized to receive WBI with or without regional nodal radiotherapy defined as the internal mammary, supraclavicular, and axillary basins. At 10 years of follow-up, nodal irradiation improved DFS by 5% (absolute, 82% vs. 77%; $P = .01$), representing a relative improvement of 24%. Local–regional DFS was improved from 92.2% to 95.2% ($P = .009\%$), and distant metastasis DFS improved from 82.4% to 86.3% ($P = .03$). OS was not statistically significantly improved ($P = .38$). On a preplanned subgroup analysis, patients with ER-negative disease receiving comprehensive irradiation did achieve an improvement in survival (81.3% vs. 73.9%; $P = .05$). There was slightly higher radiation dermatitis, pneumonitis, and lymphedema with the additional nodal radiotherapy, though the rates of grade 3 toxicity remained very low.

Recommendations: These results demonstrate the greater importance of treating the subclinical disease in the **infraclavicular/supraclavicular and internal mammary regions** as opposed to the axilla alone when lymph nodes are pathologically involved. However, the authors believe the benefit is primarily related to the infraclavicular and supraclavicular region due to the rarity of internal mammary node recurrence.

Internal Mammary Node Radiation

The **Danish Breast Cancer Cooperative Group** prospective, population-based cohort study with over 3,000 women has suggested a survival benefit to internal mammary nodal irradiation (160). Due to the concern of heart irradiation (161), internal mammary nodal radiation was only delivered to women with right-sided BC. The results were strikingly similar to the benefits seen in **MA.20 and EORTC 22922** with a 2.5% absolute reduction in distant metastases ($P = .07$), 2.5% absolute reduction in BC mortality ($P = .03$), and a 3.7% improvement in survival ($P = .005$) without any detriment in heart disease with a median follow-up of 8 years. The only group of patients who may not have benefitted was the subgroup with lateral tumors with 1 to 3 lymph nodes involved.

> ➤ We recommend nodal radiation, including the internal mammary nodes, in all patients with macroscopic nodal involvement except for patients with shorter life expectancies or elderly, otherwise favorable risk patients (ER+ with less than four lymph nodes involved).

Postmastectomy Radiation (PMRT): Historically, PMRT was used to prevent LRs, which were very disabling and rarely curable. With the advent of first generation chemotherapy, the use of PMRT did not just reduce recurrences but had an impact on BC-specific and overall survival.

Techniques for Treatment With PMRT

"Step and shoot" IMRT, volumetric-modulated arc therapy (VMAT), and field-within-field forward planned 3D-CRT can each be applied to augment target coverage, reduce dose to normal structures, and improve dose homogeneity in BC treatments. Technique selection must be undertaken on a case-by-case basis dependent upon anatomical and individual patient considerations. These approaches can decrease the volume receiving high dose as a cost of delivering lower dose to a larger volume.

Proton radiotherapy will likely increase in utilization, particularly when internal mammary lymph node radiation is considered beneficial. The finite range associated with the proton radiotherapy due to Bragg peak effect lends this technique to sparing of deep tissues such as the heart and lungs, which receive lower doses than incurred with IMRT and VMAT (Figures 5.12A and 5.12B), which may be clinically important (161). Pencil beam or spot scanning proton delivery allows for further improvements in dose conformity and normal tissue protection. Emerging clinical trials will likely help to elucidate the magnitude of benefit to this approach.

The **Danish 82b trial** evaluated high-risk premenopausal patients (positive axillary lymph nodes, tumor size >5 cm, and invasion of skin or pectoral fascia) while **Danish 82c** focused on postmenopausal patients (152,153). In the Danish 82b trial, 1,708 premenopausal patients underwent MRM and were then randomized to adjuvant CMF chemotherapy alone or PMRT plus chemotherapy. With a

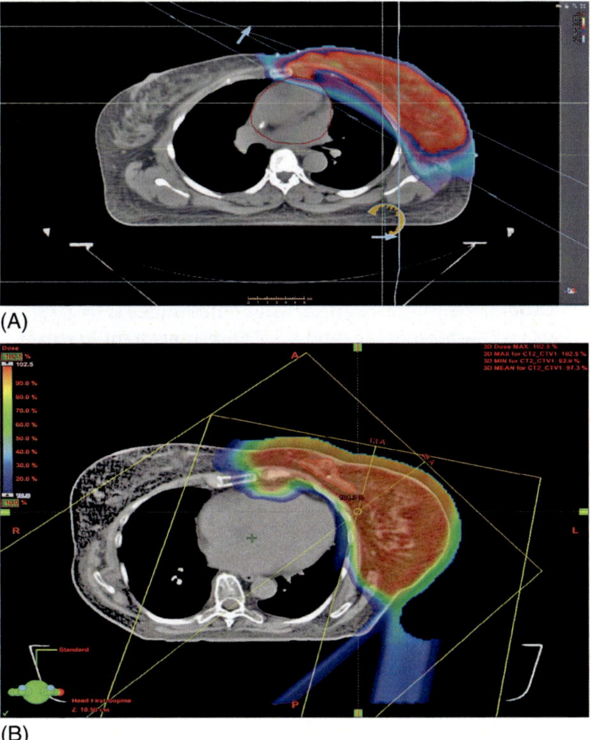

(A)

(B)

Figure 5.12 (A) Volumetric-modulated arc therapy treatment planning. (B) Proton radiotherapy treatment planning.

median follow-up of 114 months, PMRT improved local–regional failure (LRF) from 32% to 9% and increased 10-year DFS from 34% to 48% and 10-year OS from 45% to 54%. On multivariable analysis, PMRT improved DFS and OS irrespective of number of positive lymph nodes, tumor size, or grade. The Danish 82c trial demonstrated a similar benefit to PMRT in 1,406 postmenopausal patients.

The **British Columbia trial** included 318 premenopausal patients status post-MRM with pathologically positive lymph nodes with a similar design to the Danish 82b trial (154). With a median follow-up of 20 years, PMRT decreased LRF from 26% to 10% while increasing BC-specific survival from 38% to 53% and OS from 37% to 47%. However, these trials have been criticized due to the higher axillary failure rates due to the limited axillary dissections performed.

To answer this criticism, a reanalysis of the Danish 82b/82c patients who had at least 8 LN dissected was performed (162). In patients with four or more positive LNs, radiation significantly decreased the 15-year LRF rate from 51% to 10% and improved 15-year survival from 12% to 21%. Similar results were seen in the patients with one to three positive lymph nodes; 15-year LRF significantly improved from 27% to 4% and 15-year survival from 48% to 57% with the use of radiation.

EBCTCG published an update to address the criticisms of the 2005 meta-analysis and to provide longer follow-up results (162). Women were classified as having axillary dissection if the protocol mandated or if the median number of lymph nodes removed was at least 10. Women were otherwise classified as having axillary sampling. In the 22 trials for which data was available, radiotherapy was given to the chest wall and the supraclavicular fossa and/or the axilla. In 20 of 22 trials, radiation to the internal mammary nodes was also administered. With a median follow-up of 9.4 years, 8,135 women received radiation to the chest wall and regional nodes and the extent of axillary surgery was known in 98% of patients.

Altogether, 3,131 women had positive lymph nodes following a mastectomy and ALND and the use of **PMRT** significantly reduced 10-year overall recurrence risk from 62.5% to 51.9% and 20-year BC mortality by 8.1% from 66.4% to 58.3%. In the 1,314 patients with one to three involved lymph nodes following mastectomy and ALND, a significant benefit in local–regional control, overall control, and BC mortality was seen with PMRT. The authors also looked at pN1+ patients, and RT still significantly decreased local–regional recurrence and overall recurrence.

Large Node Negative Breast Cancer

Patients with large tumors (T3) but negative lymph nodes is a rare subset of patients who remain a controversial group to treat with PMRT. The Danish 82b trial showed that radiation improved 10-year LRF from 17% to 3% and 10-year survival from 70% to 82%, while Danish 82c showed a similar benefit to local control (6%–23%) but failed to show a survival benefit (152,153). However, follow-up retrospective studies demonstrated a low recurrence risk of about 7% in the NSABP series in this subset of patients (163). A recent Surveillance, Epidemiology, and End Results (SEER) analysis of T3N0 patients treated with MRM by Johnson et al (164) found that PMRT significantly improved OS (HR 0.63) and cause specific survival (CSS) (HR 0.77), suggesting that PMRT would be of use in T3N0 patients. Some compromise and offer radiation only to the chest wall, although we recommend radiation to the chest wall and regional nodes, especially in light of the MA.20 and EORTC studies described here.

Other Factors That Predict for Local–Regional Relapse

In addition to axillary status and tumor size, it is also important to consider other clinical, histologic, and pathological factors when deciding on the use of PMRT. Kyndi et al demonstrated that ER-negative and PR-negative receptor status and HER2-positive receptor status were risk factors (165). In node-negative patients, risk factors such as LVI, tumor size >2 cm (especially medially located tumors), premenopausal status, grade, and use of systemic therapy have been identified (166–168). Truong et al (169) focused on pT1-2N0 patients, and in addition to LVI and T stage, determined that grade and use of systemic therapy were also significant risk factors. Jagsi et al (167) demonstrated that 10-year local–regional recurrence (LRR) rate increased with the number of risk factors from 10% with one risk factor to 40.6% with three risk factors in the node-negative population.

Kyndi et al evaluated 1,000 patients from the PMRT Danish trials in whom receptor status was determined and generated three prognostic groups: "good" was defined by at least four of five factors (≤ 3 LN+, tumor size <2 cm, grade 1, ER- or PR-positive, HER2-negative) while "poor" was defined by at least two of three factors (>3 positive nodes, tumor size >5 cm, grade 3). Interestingly, the "poor" prognosis group had the largest absolute reduction in 5-year LR probability by 36%. However, this LR reduction did not translate into any reduction in 15-year BC mortality (168), suggesting that the patients with the lowest risk of distant disease had the greatest benefit in survival (96).

International Breast Cancer Study Group evaluated 8,106 patients from 13 trials treated with mastectomy (170). Age, number of positive lymph nodes, and number of uninvolved lymph nodes were all significant risk factors.

> ➤ When examining recurrence by site, they found negative ER status, larger tumor size, LVI, and grade 3 are risk factors for supraclavicular recurrence while tumor size, positive ER status, and LVI are risk factors for LR.

Several retrospective reviews have also investigated the role of positive and close surgical margins. Freedman et al (171) published on 789 patients and found that patients less than 50 years old with clinical T1–T2 tumor size and 0 to 3 positive nodes who have a close (<5 mm) or positive mastectomy margin have a 8-year recurrence risk of 28% despite the use of systemic therapy and, therefore, should be considered for PMRT.

Truong et al (169) focused on pT1-2 pN0 BC patients and determined in a population of 2,570 patients, of which 94 had positive margins, that local–regional recurrence rates were approximately 20% with positive margins with the addition of at least one of the following factors: age <50 years, tumor size 2 to 5 cm, grade III, or LVI.

Childs et al (172) investigated 397 patients status postmastectomy and no radiation and found 5-year LRR of 6.2%, 1.5%, and 1.9% in patients with positive, close (≤2 mm), and negative margins, respectively. Thus, surgical margins need to be considered in conjunction with other clinical and histological factors.

In summary, PMRT is offered to all patients with macroscopic lymph node metastases as well as all patients with T3 and T4 disease. In the node-negative patients with tumor size <5 cm, other factors are considered including clinical MC disease (173), young age, higher grade, T2 (especially medial location), triple negative, LVI, and close or positive margins as significant predictors of LR.

These patients would likely benefit from discussion in a multidisciplinary setting to determine optimal treatment or at least warrant consultation with a radiation oncologist.

SYSTEMIC ADJUVANT THERAPY

Adjuvant systemic therapy has been shown to reduce the risk of recurrence of early-stage BC (174–178). Adjuvant therapy can consist of hormonal therapy, cytotoxic chemotherapy, and/or biologic therapy. EBCTCG analysis showed that standard early generation chemotherapy (CMF or AC) reduced 2-year relative recurrence rates by 50% and in the next 8 years by 33% compared to no chemotherapy. Furthermore, BC mortality rates were reduced by 20% to 25% (179). For ER+ disease, 5 years of adjuvant hormone therapy (tamoxifen) reduces the annual BC death rate by 31% (180). Accordingly, for women with ER+ disease, the BC mortality rate throughout the 15 years after diagnosis could be approximately halved by 6 months of anthracycline-based chemotherapy followed by 5 years of adjuvant tamoxifen. Third generation chemotherapy regimens, HER2 targeting agents, and aromatase inhibitors (AIs) further improve survival outcomes in early-stage BC.

There are multiple guidelines for prescribing systemic adjuvant therapy. We recommend being familiar with the **National Comprehensive Cancer Network (NCCN), ASCO, and the St. Gallen International Expert Consensus. The NCCN** (www.nccn.org) is well known for their flow chart type recommendations with comprehensive review for each cancer. The **St. Gallen International Expert Consensus** meets every other year to review new studies and update recommendations (181). The **ASCO** publishes its cancer guidelines (www.asco.org/practice-guidelines/quality-guidelines/guidelines/breast-cancer). We recommend all cancer providers be familiar with the previous guidelines and incorporate them in clinic. In the following sections, we review adjuvant hormone therapy followed by adjuvant chemotherapy. We examine the clinical trials that support the use of these therapies. Table 5.5 summarizes our recommendations.

Hormonal Therapy

WHO SHOULD BE CONSIDERED FOR ADJUVANT (CMF OR AC) ENDOCRINE (HORMONAL) THERAPY?

As per ASCO/CAP guidelines, a breast tumor is considered hormone-receptor-positive if IHC staining for estrogen-ER and/or progesterone-PR (ER/PR) is ≥1% (47). We recommend adjuvant hormonal therapy (HT) for nearly all women with ER and/or PR ≥1% invasive BC, but studies have shown that benefit is increased for higher expression of ER/PR. There are few circumstances of limited life expectancy when we may defer treatment. Our practice is to start HT immediately after completion of adjuvant chemotherapy; but others start after the completion of radiation. If HER2 targeted therapy is needed, HT is given concurrently with HER2 therapy but after completion of chemotherapy.

The choice of the agent(s) depends primarily on **the menopausal status at the time of initiation of adjuvant chemotherapy.** For women with an intact uterus, we use >12 months of no menstruation for determining if the patient is postmenopausal. For women who have undergone a hysterectomy, we check follicle-stimulating hormone (FSH) and estradiol levels prior to chemotherapy. Women who are premenopausal before chemotherapy and stop menstruating

Table 5.5 Suggested Systemic Adjuvant Treatment Recommendations by Clinicopathologic (CP) and Tumor Genomic Factors (GF)

Gene expression	Clinicopathologic factors	Recommended treatment	Comments
ER/PR+ HER2–	T < 0.5 cm, N0	Hormonal therapy	
	T 0.5–1 cm, N0	Hormonal therapy	Consider MammaPrint or OncotypeDx (we typically do not order these tests if grade 1, low Ki-67, and strongly ER/PR+)
	T > 1–5 cm, N0	Hormonal therapy +/– chemotherapy	MammaPrint or OncotypeDx test for decision on chemotherapy, we consider chemotherapy risk/benefit, consider a non-anthracycline regimen
	Any T, 1–3 LN+	Chemotherapy followed by hormonal therapy	For older patients and those with multiple comorbid conditions, we consider chemotherapy risks/benefits and may use MammaPrint or OncotypeDx to guide decisions
	Any T, ≥ 4LN+	Chemotherapy followed by hormonal therapy	Anthracycline regimen preferred
ER/PR+ HER2+	T ≤ 0.5 cm, N0	Hormonal therapy	We typically do not recommend chemotherapy + trastuzumab
	T 0.6–1 cm, N0	Hormonal therapy +/– chemotherapy + trastuzumab	MammaPrint can be considered to risk stratify, we use P × 12 wks + trastuzumab × 12 mos as our preferred regimen if high risk by MammaPrint
	T > 1 cm, N0	Chemotherapy + trastuzumab followed by hormonal therapy	TCH is preferred or although may use P × 12 wks with H × 12 mos for patients with smaller tumors

(continued)

Table 5.5 Suggested Systemic Adjuvant Treatment Recommendations by Clinicopathologic (CP) and Tumor Genomic Factors (GF) (*continued*)

Gene expression	Clinicopathologic factors	Recommended treatment	Comments
	Any T size, LN+	Chemotherapy + trastuzumab followed by hormonal therapy	TCH is preferred, we have used H + P to complete 12 mos of antiHER2 therapy
ER/PR– HER2+	T ≤ 0.5 cm, N0	No chemotherapy	
	T < 0.6–1 cm, N0	Chemotherapy + trastuzumab can be considered	Consider risk/benefits in choosing regimen –P × 12 wks with H × 12 mos or TCH
	T ≥ 1 cm, N0	Chemotherapy + trastuzumab	TCH is preferred, although may use T × 12 wks with H × 12 mos for pts with smaller tumors, especially if not medically fit
	Any T size, LN+	Chemotherapy + trastuzumab	TCH is preferred regimen; we have used H + P to complete 12 mos of therapy
ER/PR– HER2–	T ≤ 0.5 cm, N0	No chemotherapy	
	T < 0.6–1 cm, N0	Chemotherapy can be considered	Can forgo chemotherapy if elderly or multiple comorbid conditions, consider non-anthracycline regimens
	T ≥ 1 cm, N0	Chemotherapy	Anthracycline regimens preferred unless medically ineligible
	Any T, LN+	Chemotherapy	Anthracycline regimens preferred

Definitions of Regimens

TCH-H-Docetaxel/Carboplatin/Trastuzumab every 3 wks then Trastuzumab every 3 wks for a total of 12 mos of adjuvant antiHER2 therapy.

P+H-weekly paclitaxel × 12 wks concurrently with weekly Trastuzumab × 12 wks, then Trastuzumab every 3 wks to complete 12 mos of antiHER2 therapy.

T+P-Trastuzumab/Pertuzumab every 3 wks to complete 12 mos of antiHER2 therapy.

during chemotherapy should **not** be considered postmenopausal even if the FSH and estradiol levels are in postmenopausal range after chemotherapy treatment. Studies show that after anthracycline- and taxane-based adjuvant chemotherapy, ovarian function may resume later in up to 85% of women ≤40 years old (182). **Tamoxifen is the preferred hormonal agent in premenopausal women, while very young women <35 years old or premenopausal after adjuvant chemotherapy benefit additionally from ovarian suppression + tamoxifen or exemestane.**

ADJUVANT HORMONE TREATMENTS FOR BREAST CANCER

Tamoxifen is a selective estrogen receptor modulator with both antagonist and agonist receptor functions depending on the site of action. It functions as an antagonist of the estrogen receptor in BC cells, inhibiting translocation and nuclear binding of the ER, and ultimately altering transcriptional and posttranscriptional events (183–185). It is an ER agonist in the endometrium; therefore, increased risk of endometrial cancer (ECA) has been observed.

Aromatase inhibitors (AIs) block aromatase, the enzyme that converts the androgens (androstenedione/testosterone) to the estrogens (estrone/estradiol). Aromatase is found predominantly in peripheral tissues (eg, skin, muscle, fat) and leads to low, but stable levels of estrogen (183). In postmenopausal women, AIs can lead to almost complete blockade of the pathway for estrogen production. **In premenopausal women, due to negative feedback, AIs can cause an increase in estrogen levels hence it is important to never use AIs in premenopausal women.** AIs are divided into steroidal (eg, exemestane) and nonsteroidal (eg, anastrozole, letrozole) categories.

Ovarian suppression is the practice of making a premenopausal woman effectively postmenopausal by eliminating ovarian function. This can be accomplished surgically with oophorectomy, medically with the use of gonadotropin-releasing hormone agonists, or through the use of radiation to the ovaries.

TAMOXIFEN THERAPY

An EBCTCG meta-analysis of over 21,000 women from 20 prospective trials compared at least 3 to 5 years of tamoxifen therapy to no tamoxifen (186). ER-positive patients who received tamoxifen had half the recurrence rate during years 0 to 4 and a reduction by a third during years 5 to 9, with an overall recurrence rate reduction of 39% (RR 0.61; $P < .00001$) compared to those who did not receive tamoxifen (186). **This demonstrates the carryover effect of tamoxifen after 5 years, even after it is discontinued.**

TAMOXIFEN DURATION

The benefits of tamoxifen in ER/PR+ patients are duration-dependent.

- **EBCTCG** completed a meta-analysis, which showed that 1 to 2 years of therapy with tamoxifen was inferior to 5 years of tamoxifen adjuvant treatment for recurrence ($P < .00001$) and for BC mortality ($P = .0001$) (180).
- **NSABP B-14** enrolled patients with ER+, lymph node negative BC, and randomized women who remained disease-free at 5 years to an additional 5 years of tamoxifen or placebo. In this study, the extension of tamoxifen to 10 years initially showed a detriment in DFS for patients who continued tamoxifen for 10 years (187,188). However, given that tamoxifen has a carryover effect with

mortality benefits increasing to at least 15 years, it was felt longer follow-up was needed before definitive conclusions could be drawn regarding trials extending tamoxifen treatment beyond 5 years.

- **ATLAS** was an open-label, international study conducted in 36 countries from 1996 to 2005 that randomized women after 5 years of tamoxifen to receive 5 more years of tamoxifen or to stop therapy.
- **Results:** With 3,428 ER+ women in the continued tamoxifen arm and 3,418 ER+ women in the completion at 5 years arm, patients assigned to tamoxifen for 10 years had a reduced risk of recurrence (617 vs. 711 recurrences; P = .002), BC mortality (331 vs. 397 deaths; P = .01), and overall mortality (639 vs. 722 deaths; P = .01) (189). Absolute BC mortality reduction was 2.8% (12.2% vs. 15%) from years 5 to 14. The differences in recurrence and BC mortality effects were noted in the second decade after diagnosis. The difference in risk ratios for BC mortality for years 5 to 9 compared to after year 10 was significant (RR 0.97 vs. 0.71; P = 0.04) (189).
- **Side effects:** Tamoxifen-related adverse events included increased risk for pulmonary embolus (1.87; P = .01) and endometrial cancer ECA (1.74; P = .0002). There was no mortality difference from pulmonary embolus (0.2% in both groups), and there was a nonsignificant 0.2% difference (0.4% vs. 0.2%) in mortality from ECA. There did seem to be some cardiovascular protective effect from continuing tamoxifen, as that group had a reduction in the incidence of ischemic heart disease (RR 0.76; P = .02), with a trend toward improved mortality from heart disease without recurrence (P = .1) (189).
- **Adjuvant Tamoxifen—To offer more? (aTTom):** This was a UK-based multicenter trial conducted from 1991 to 2005 enrolling almost 7,000 women. Similar to ATLAS, women were randomized after 5 years of tamoxifen to complete 10 years of tamoxifen therapy or to stop therapy. More than 60% of patients had ER-unknown status.
- **Results:** Patients who continued tamoxifen had significantly reduced BC recurrence (580/3,468 vs. 672/348; P = .003) and BC mortality (392 vs. 443 deaths; P = .05) (190). Overall mortality was reduced but was not significant (P = .1). As in the ATLAS trial, reductions in BC recurrence and mortality, as well as overall mortality, were more pronounced in the later years (190).
- **Side effects:** In aTTom, there was an increased risk of ECA (RR 2.20; P < .0001) and death from ECA (37 vs. 20 deaths, absolute hazard 0.5%; P = .02).
- When results from ATLAS and aTTom were combined, improvement in OS was significant (P = .005) (190).

AROMATASE INHIBITORS

AI trials have taken three main approaches:

1. Upfront: AI versus tamoxifen
2. Sequential: 1 to 3 years of tamoxifen followed by an AI versus tamoxifen to complete 5 years
3. Extended adjuvant: 5 years of tamoxifen followed by 5 years of an AI or 10 years of adjuvant AI versus 5 years of AI or 5 years of tamoxifen followed by 10 years of an AI.

Recent analysis from the EBCTCG of 31,920 postmenopausal women with ER+ early-stage BC in the randomized trials of (a) 5 years of AI versus 5 years of tamoxifen, (b) 5 years of AI versus 2–3 years of tamoxifen followed by AI to complete 5 total years, and (c) 5 years of tamoxifen versus 2–3 years of tamoxifen followed by AI confirmed the benefit of upfront or any time exposure to adjuvant AI therapy in early-stage BC (191). AIs reduce recurrence rates by about 30% (proportionately) compared to tamoxifen during treatment, but not thereafter. BC mortality was reduced overall with 5 years of an AI therapy, reducing 10-year BC mortality rates by 15% compared to 5 years of tamoxifen and 40% (proportionately) compared to no hormone therapy (191). There were fewer endometrial cancers with AI than tamoxifen (10-year incidence 0.4% vs. 1.2%; RR 0.33, 0.21–0.51) but more bone fractures (5-year risk 8.2% vs. 5.5%; RR 1.42, 1.28–1.57). Non-breast-cancer mortality was similar (191).

Aromatase inhibitors upfront versus tamoxifen: Multiple studies show the benefit of AI over tamoxifen as frontline adjuvant therapy for early-stage BC.

- **The Arimidex, Tamoxifen, Alone or in Combination (ATAC) trial** was one of the first large-scale adjuvant hormonal phase III trials to show the benefits of an AI, anastrozole, in postmenopausal women (192). This was a three-arm, double-blind placebo-controlled study with patients with operable BC randomized after primary surgery and chemotherapy (if indicated) to adjuvant upfront tamoxifen (TAM) alone + placebo, anastrozole (ANA) alone + placebo, or concurrent tamoxifen + anastrozole (TAM+ANA).
- **Results:** The primary end point of DFS at 3 years showed that the absolute benefit of ANA was 2% greater than TAM (89.4% vs. 87.4%) and 2.2% compared to TAM+ANA (89.4% vs. 87.2%), indicating that the combination is not more effective than ANA alone. 10-year updated results showed continued DFS improvement in the ANA group compared to TAM, with a 10-year DFS benefit in ER/PR+ patients of 4.3% (193). However, there was no OS difference between the TAM or ANA alone groups, even when evaluating only ER/PR+ patients.
- **BIG 1-98** was a four-arm, double-blind trial of over 8,000 women with operable ER/PR+ BC who were assigned to 5 years of TAM monotherapy, 5 years of letrozole (LET) monotherapy, 2 years of TAM followed by 3 years of LET, or 2 years of LET followed by 3 years of TAM (194).
- **Results:** Comparisons of LET alone to TAM alone favored LET, with 5-year DFS estimates of 84.0% versus 81.4% (DFS HR 0.81; 0.70–0.93); however, there was no OS difference between the two treatments (194).

Sequential Therapy

- **BIG 1-98:** Subsequent analysis of the sequential treatment groups compared to LET alone showed no difference in DFS or OS between either of the sequentially treated groups and the LET alone group, providing evidence that both upfront and sequential treatment with LET are acceptable treatment strategies.
- **Results:** Updated OS data of LET versus TAM alone showed a trend toward benefit with LET, with absolute 5-year OS differences of 91.8% versus 90.9% (HR 0.87; 0.75–1.02; $P = .08$) (195).

- **The Tamoxifen Exemestane Adjuvant Multinational (TEAM):** The amended study enrolled women with operable ER/PR+ BC in an open-label randomized trial comparing upfront exemestane (EXE) for 5 years to TAM for 2 to 3 years followed by EXE to complete 5 years of treatment.
- **Results:** No differences in DFS or OS were seen between the two groups (196).
- **The Intergroup Exemestane Study (IES)** randomized over 4,000 women with operable, ER/PR+ BC after 2 to 3 years of TAM to either continue TAM or switch to EXE to complete 5 years of therapy (197).
- **Results:** The primary end point of DFS was significantly better in the group that switched to EXE, with DFS rates 3 years after randomization of 91.5% versus 86.8%. Updated OS results showed a benefit with EXE when 122 ER-negative patients were excluded from analysis (17% relative risk reduction of death; $P = .05$) (198).
- **MA.17** was a double-blind, placebo-controlled trial that randomized over 5,000 women with operable ER/PR+ BC after 4.5 to 6 years of TAM to LET or placebo for 5 more years (199).
- **Results:** The primary end point of DFS was significantly better for the LET group, with 4-year DFS of 93% in the LET group and 87% in the placebo group. There was no OS difference between the groups in the first analysis. However, exploratory multivariable analysis showed a significant OS benefit with LET for patients with axillary LN+ disease, tumors positive for both ER and PR, and for all patients when adjusting for women who crossed over to LET after unblinding (199–201). MA.17 patients randomized to receive placebo after TAM were unblinded and offered LET. The median time after completing TAM was 2.8 years. Patients who accepted LET had significantly improved DFS and OS when compared to patients who continued in the placebo group, showing that exposure to LET, even after a prolonged time had elapsed from TAM use, was still beneficial (202).
- **NSABP B-33:** Similar to MA.17, women with early-stage, operable ER/PR+ BC were randomized after 5 years of TAM to either EXE or placebo for 5 more years.
- **Results:** The MA.17 trial results showing the benefits of extended adjuvant LET necessitated the early termination of patient accrual and unblinding of treatment groups; 44% of patients in the placebo group crossed over to receive EXE. In the intention-to-treat analysis, 4-year DFS trended toward improvement with EXE (91% vs. 89%; $P = .07$) and recurrence-free survival (RFS) was significantly improved in the EXE group (96% vs. 94%; $P = .004$), even in this underpowered study (due to early termination) with significant crossover of the placebo group to active treatment (203).
- **MA17R-trial:** The MA17R trial extended adjuvant AI therapy to 10 years and accrued 1,918 women with ER/PR+ early stage BC to an additional 5 years of treatment with letrozole or placebo, after 5 years of tamoxifen+5 years of an AI or 5 years of AI adjuvant therapy. After a median follow-up of 6.3 years, there were 165 events involving disease recurrence or the occurrence of contralateral BC (67 with letrozole and 98 with placebo) and there was no difference in the number of deaths in each group. The 5-year DFS rate was 95% (95% CI 93–96) with letrozole and 91% (95% CI 89–93) with placebo. The annual incidence rate of contralateral BC in the letrozole group was 0.21% (95% CI 0.10–0.32), and 0.49% (95% CI

0.32–0.67) in the placebo group (HR 0.42; *P* = .007). Letrozole-treated patients had higher incidence of bone pain, bone fractures, and new-onset osteoporosis, but no significant differences were observed in scores measuring quality of life (204).

Aromatase inhibitor comparisons: Because ANA, LET, and EXE all showed benefit over TAM as adjuvant therapy in postmenopausal women, and absolute DFS benefits were similar between AIs, they have generally been considered to have similar efficacies. Direct comparisons between AIs have been attempted to confirm this.

- **NCIC CTG MA.27** compared EXE to ANA as upfront adjuvant therapy in an open-label phase III study.
- **Results:** At a median follow-up of 4.1 years, the primary end point of event-free survival (EFS) at 4 years was no different between patients taking EXE versus ANA (205).
  Femara versus Anastrozole Clinical Evaluation (FACE) trial compared LET to ANA. In total, 4,136, ER+, LN+ postmenopausal women with early-stage BC were randomized.
  Results showed the estimated 5-year DFS rates were similar, 84.9% for LET versus 82.9% for ANA (HR 0.93; P = NS), and OS was not statistically different between arms (HR 0.98; *P* = NS). Due to the low number of events, the study was terminated in September 2014 (206).

Extended adjuvant AI therapy: Similiar to tamoxifen, the recommended length of AI therapy has been a topic of research.

- **MA17.R trial:** This was a phase III randomized, double-blinded, placebo controlled trial evaluating 5 years of extended letrozole therapy following 4.5–6 years of adjuvant AI therapy. After a median follow up of 6.3 years, the 5-year DFS rate was 95% with extended therapy and 91% with placebo (HR = 0.66, *P* = .01). There was increased risk of bone fractures and osteoporosis in the extended therapy but no difference in quality of life scales (204).

Ovarian ablation and suppression: Postmenopausal women may have better oncologic outcomes than premenopausal women (180). Many studies that evaluate ovarian suppression to induce a postmenopausal state have been performed.

- **EBCTCG analysis** involving patients who received ovarian ablation or suppression (OAS) versus those that did not showed 15-year recurrence and BC mortality rates were improved (47.3% vs. 51.6%; *P* = .00001 and 40.3% vs. 43.5%; *P* = .004, respectively) (180). The impact was greatest in trials comparing OAS to no adjuvant chemotherapy.
- **The Tamoxifen and Exemestane Trial (TEXT)** randomized premenopausal women with ER/PR+ BC to EXE 25 mg daily or TAM 20 mg daily for 5 years with OAS (triptorelin, an injectable luteinizing-hormone-releasing hormone [LHRH] agonist) every 4 weeks for 5 years, oophorectomy, or ovarian radiation. Adjuvant chemotherapy was allowed.
- **The Suppression of Ovarian Function trial (SOFT)** randomized 3,066 premenopausal women with ER/PR+ BC to EXE 25 mg daily + OAS, TAM 20 mg daily + OAS, or TAM 20 mg daily alone for 5 years of therapy. Adjuvant chemotherapy was allowed.

- **Results:** After a median follow-up of 67 months, no significant difference in the TAM alone arm versus the OAS arms for the unselected population was noted (DFS—86.6% vs. 84.7%, respectively, HR 0.83; $P = .10$) (207). However, further analysis did show a significant DFS improvement when adjusting for prognostic factors. Multivariable analysis for prognostic factors found a benefit with TAM + OAS compared to TAM alone in younger patients and those receiving chemotherapy (HR, 0.78; 95% CIs [0.62, 0.98]) (207). Most recurrences occurred in women who had received prior standard chemotherapy, which is generally given to the higher risk population. In the chemotherapy population at 5 years, the rate of freedom from BC was 85.7% in the EXE + OAS group, 82.5% in TAM + OAS, and 78% in TAM alone. The EXE + OAS versus TAM was statistically significant with HR 0.65 (95% CIs [0.49, 0.87]), a 35% reduction in the events in favor of the EXE + OAS arm (207).
- **Side effects:** Hot flashes, sweating, decreased libido, vaginal dryness, insomnia, depression, musculoskeletal symptoms, hypertension, and glucose intolerance (diabetes) were reported more frequently in the TAM + OAS than in the TAM group. Osteoporosis was reported in 5.8% in TAM + OAS versus 3.5% in TAM alone group.
- **TEXT and SOFT trials:** The primary analysis of OAS treatment arms was published and combined data from 4,690 patients in the two trials.
- **Results:** After 68 months median follow-up, DFS at 5 years was excellent for both treatment groups, 91.1% in EXE + OAS and 87.3% in the TAM + OAS group with a 28% reduction in the events in the EXE + OAS group (HR = 0.72; $P = .0002$) (207). With only 194 deaths (4.1%), this analysis did not show an OS advantage with EXE + OAS compared to TAM + OAS. The 4% absolute difference in DFS in favor of EXE + OAS versus TAM + OAS was statistically significant at 5 years and reflected reductions in local, regional, distant, and contralateral BC events. It should be noted that the majority (60%) of the first recurrence events involved recurrences at a distant site and may affect survival with longer follow-up (208).

  The TEXT and SOFT trials provide evidence that OAS combined with either TAM or EXE can provide clinical benefit in select premenopausal, early-stage patients with a higher risk of recurrence such as women who are younger than 35 years of age and women who received chemotherapy and did not become menopausal. However, OS differences are currently lacking at this time for both TEXT and SOFT trials.

Tables 5.6 and 5.7 summarize key adjuvant hormone studies with our recommendations for adjuvant hormone therapy in Box 5.2.

Adjuvant Chemotherapy

WHO SHOULD BE CONSIDERED FOR ADJUVANT CHEMOTHERAPY?

The benefit from adjuvant chemotherapy in terms of reduction in the risk of BC recurrence and improvements in BC specific and OS has been demonstrated in the EBCTCG analysis, but the side effects such as cytopenias, nausea, vomiting, gastrointestinal toxicities, fever/neutropenia, sensory neuropathy, heart dysfunction/failure,

(text continues on page 121)

Table 5.6 Key Adjuvant Hormonal Therapy Early-Stage BC Trials, Treatment for ≤5 Years

Study	Design	Key eligibility criteria/N = patients	Primary end point results	OS difference and other study end points	Toxicities
ATAC (192)	Upfront A vs. upfront T vs. A + T Placebo-controlled	HR+/− No neo-adj chemo; N = 9,366	DFS; A > T HR: 0.83 (P = .013) A > A + T HR: 0.81 (P = .006) A + T = T HR: 1.02 (P = .8)	No A = T HR: 0.95 (P = .4), 3 yr DFS (%) A > T > AT: 89.4 vs. 87.4 vs. 87.2 A > T DFS in HR+ HR: 0.86 (P = .003) A > T ARR: 4.3% at 10 yr	T > A: hot flushes, vaginal discharge and bleeding, CVA, VTE, ECA A > T: MSK d/o, fractures (mainly spine)
ARNO 95 (209)	Sequential: T × 2 yr, then A or T to finish 5 yr	HR+ pT1-3, pN0-2 No chemo; N = 979	DFS; A > T HR: 0.66 (P = .049)	Yes—A > T HR: 0.53 (P = .045); 3 yr DFS absolute diff 4.2%	Fewer AEs (%) in A (22.7) vs. T (30.8)
ABCSG 8 (210)	Sequential: T × 2 yr, then A or T to finish 5 yr	HR+, G1-2 No chemo Low-int risk; N = 3,714	RFS; A = T HR: 0.80 (P = .06) When compensating for crossover: A > T HR: 0.76 (95% CIs [0.60, 0.97])	No—A = T HR: 0.87 (P = .34); DRFS 22% risk reduction (HR 0.78; 0.60–0.99)	More bone pain in A vs. T (3.6% diff, P < .02) More uterine d/o in T vs. A (20.2% vs. 14.1%, P < .001)
ITA (211)	Sequential: T × 2–3 yr, then A or T to finish 5 yr	ER+, LN+; N = 448	DFS; A > T HR: 0.35 (P = .001)	No—A = T HR: 0.79 (P = .3); 3 yr diff in RFS 5.8%	More AE in A vs. T (203 vs. 150, P = .04) More SAE (%) in T (22 vs. 13.9, P = .04) More GYN changes (%) in T (11.3 vs. 1, P = .0002) Sig more GYN problems in T (8 ECA vs. 1)

(continued)

Table 5.6 Key Adjuvant Hormonal Therapy Early-Stage BC Trials, Treatment for ≤5 Years (*continued*)

Study	Design	Key eligibility criteria/N = patients	Primary end point results	OS difference and other study end points	Toxicities
ABCSG 8 + ARNO 95 (212)	Planned, event-driven combined analysis	HR+ No chemo; N = 3,224	EFS; A > T HR: 0.60 (*P* = .0009)	No—3 year OS A vs. T: 97% vs. 96%, *P* = .16; 3 yr DFS (%) A > T: 95.8 vs. 92.7	Sig A > T fractures, nausea, trend toward bone pain Sig T > A thromboses, trend toward emboli and ECA
ABCSG 8 + ARNO 95 + ITA (211)	Meta-analysis	N = 4,006	DFS; A > T HR: 0.59 (*P* < .0001)	Yes—A > T HR: 0.71 (*P* = .0377); A > T EFS HR: 0.55 (*P* < .0001) A > T DRFS HR: 0.61 (*P* = .0015)	
BIG 1-98 (194)	Upfront T vs. upfront L Double-blind	HR+; N = 8,010	DFS; L > T HR: 0.81 (*P* = .003)	No—L=T HR: 0.87 (*P* = .08); 5 yr DFS (%) estimates 84 vs. 81.4	Sig L > T: fractures (5.7% vs. 4%), grade 3–5 cardiac events, arthralgia, cholesterol elevation Sig T > L: VTE, GYN bleeding, ECA (0.3% vs. 0.1%), hot flashes

(*continued*)

Table 5.6 Key Adjuvant Hormonal Therapy Early-Stage BC Trials, Treatment for ≤5 Years *(continued)*

Study	Design	Key eligibility criteria/N = patients	Primary end point results	OS difference and other study end points	Toxicities
BIG 1-98 (195)	Sequential T/L or L/T vs. L alone	HR+; N = 6,182	DFS; T/L = L HR: 1.05 (0.84–1.32) L/T = L HR: 0.96 (0.76–1.21)	No—T/L = L HR: 1.13 (0.83–1.53); L/T = L HR: 0.90 (0.65–1.24); T/L vs. L/T vs. L 5 yr DFS (%): 86.2 vs. 87.6 vs. 87.9; T/L vs. L/T vs. L 5 yr OS (%): 92.4 vs. 93.7 vs. 93.4	Sig T > L: VTE, GYN bleeding, hot flashes, night sweats Sig L > T: HLD, arthralgia, myalgia, fractures
IES (198)	Sequential: T × 2–3 yr, then E vs. T to finish 5 yr Double-blind	ER+ or unknown; N = 4,742	DFS; E > T HR: 0.68 (*P* < .001)	No E=T HR: 0.85 (*P* = .08) ER (–) excluded HR: 0.83 (*P* = .05); 3 yr DFS (%) 91.5 vs. 86.8	Sig E > T: arthralgia, diarrhea, osteoporosis, visual disturbances Sig T > E: GYN sxs, vag bleed, muscle cramps, VTE, 2nd primary nonbreast CA
TEAM (196)	E alone × 5 yr vs. after T × 2–3 yr for 5 yr (amended after IES results)	HR+; N = 9,766	DFS; E = T/E HR: 0.97 (*P* = .6)	No—5 year OS 91% in both (HR 1.00); no difference in distant mets T/E vs. E DFS (%) 5 yr: 85 vs. 86 T/E vs. E RFS (%) 5 yr: 11 vs. 10 (*P* = .29)	T/E > E: GYN sxs, VTE, endometrial abn E > T/E: MSK AEs, osteoporosis, fractures, HTN, HLD, CHF

(continued)

Table 5.6 Key Adjuvant Hormonal Therapy Early-Stage BC Trials, Treatment for ≤5 Years (*continued*)

Study	Design	Key eligibility criteria/N = patients	Primary end point results	OS difference and other study end points	Toxicities
SOFT (207)	T vs. T + OS vs. E + OS for 5 yr	HR+, premenopausal after chemotherapy N = 1021 T, 1024 T + OS, 1021 E + OS	DFS; T vs. T + OS HR 0.83 (*P* = .1)	No—E + OS vs. T recurrence HR 0.65; 95% CIs [0.49, 0.87]	OS > hot flashes, sweating, GYN, osteoporosis, insomnia, depression, musculoskeletal symptoms, hypertension,
TEXT + SOFT (208)	T + OS vs. E + OS for 5 yr	HR+, premenopausal N = 4,719	DFS; T + OS < E + OS (HR 0.72; *P* < .001)	No—E + OS = T + OS	E + OS > fractures, musculoskeletal symptoms, GYN sx T + OS > VTE, hot flashes, sweating, and urinary incontinence

A, anastrozole; abn, abnormalities; adj, adjuvant; AE, adverse events; AG, aminoglutethimide; ARR, absolute reduction of recurrence; ax, axillary; A+T, anastrozole and tamoxifen concurrently; BC, breast cancer; CA, cancer; chemo, chemotherapy; CHF, congestive heart failure; CVA, cerebrovascular accident; d/o, disorders; diff, difference; DFS, disease-free survival; DRFS, distant relapse free survival; E, exemestane; ECA, endometrial cancer; EFS, event-free survival; G1–2, grade 1–2; GYN, gynecologic; HLD, hyperlipidemia; HR, hazard ratio; HR+/−, hormone receptor; int, intermediate; L, letrozole; LN, lymph node; L/T, letrozole followed by tamoxifen; MSK, musculoskeletal; OS, ovarian suppression; plac, placebo; SAE, serious adverse events; sig, significant; sxs, symptoms; T, tamoxifen; T/E, tamoxifen followed by exemestane; T/L, tamoxifen followed by letrozole; VTE, venous thromboembolism.

Table 5.7 Key Extended Adjuvant Hormonal Therapy Early Breast Cancer Trials, Treatment for >5 Years

Study	Design	Key eligibility criteria	N = patients	Primary end point/results	OS difference	Other end points	Toxicities
ATLAS (189)	Tam × 5 yr vs. 10 yr	HR+/− Disease-free at 5 yr	6,846	OS; T >none ERR: 0.87 (P = .01)	Yes—639 vs. 722 deaths		10 yr T: ECA, pulmonary embolus. Protective on ischemic heart disease
aTTom (190)	Tam × 5 yr vs. 10 yr	ER+ or unknown	6,953	BC recurrence; T >none: 580 vs. 672 (P = .003)	No Overall mortality: 849 vs. 910 deaths (P = .1)	Reduction in BC recurrence, mortality, and overall mortality increased with time	10 yr T: ECA (RR = 2.20), ECA deaths (absolute hazard 0.5%, P = .02)
ABCSG 6a (213)	Extended: Tam or Tam + AG × 5 yr then A or nothing × 3 yr	HR+ stage I or II pT1-3a, N+/−	1,135	RFS; T + A > T HR: 0.62 (P = .031)	No T + A = T HR: 0.89 (P = .57)	Distant mets only significant difference (16 vs. 35 events, P = .034) 10 yr recurrence (%) T + A vs. T: 7.1 vs. 11.8	Significant T + A > T hot flushes, asthenia, somnolence, allergy, skin rash/toxicity, hair loss, nausea (all grade 1)

(continued)

Table 5.7 Key Extended Adjuvant Hormonal Therapy Early Breast Cancer Trials, Treatment for >5 Years (*continued*)

Study	Design	Key eligibility criteria	N = patients	Primary end point/results	OS difference	Other end points	Toxicities
MA17 (199)	Extended after Tam × 4.5–6 yr, L vs. plac × 5 more yr; double-blind, placebo-controlled	HR+	5,187	DFS; L > plac HR: 0.57 (P = .00008)	Yes, in ER+/PR+ L > plac HR: 0.58 (0.37–0.90) Yes, in LN+ L > plac HR: 0.61 (P = .04)	4 yr DFS L vs. plac: 93% vs. 87% P < .001 No OS diff in ITT analysis OS diff when factoring for crossover	Sig L > P: hot flashes, arthritis, arthralgia, myalgia Sig P > L: vaginal bleeding Trend toward more osteoporosis with L (P = .07)
NSABP B-33 (197)	Extended: after Tam × 5 yr, then E vs. plac × 5 more yr Double-blind, stopped early	HR+ T1-3, N0-1	1,598	DFS; E = plac HR: 0.68 (P = .07)	No Not enough deaths to draw conclusions	E vs. plac 4 yr DFS (%): 91 vs. 89 E vs. plac 4 yr RFS (%): 96 vs. 94, RRR 56% P = .004	Grade 3 toxicity (%) higher in E vs. plac (9 vs. 6)

A, anastrozole; DFS, disease-free survival; E, exemestane; ECA, endometrial cancer; ER, estrogen receptor; HR, hormone receptor; L, letrozole; LN, axillary lymph node; OS, overall survival; plac, placebo; RFS, recurrence-free survival; RRR, relative risk or recurrence; Tam, tamoxifen.

> ### Box 5.2 Recommendation for Adjuvant Hormonal Treatment by Menopausal Status
>
> **Premenopausal women**
> - Tamoxifen 20 mg daily for 5 to 10 years
> - Very young premenopausal women ($\leq$35 or requiring adjuvant chemotherapy)—consider luteinizing-hormone-releasing hormone (LHRH) agonist every 4 weeks (triptorelin, Lupron, or Zoladex monthly injections) with tamoxifen or exemestane for 5 years (207). Given that premenopausal women may have increased estrogen with AI, AI should be started approximately 6 weeks after LHRH to allow full ovarian suppression.
>
> **Postmenopausal women**
> - Up front aromatase inhibitor for 5–10 years is the most common treatment.
> - Sequential tamoxifen for 5 years followed by AI for 5–10 years can be considered.
> - If unable to tolerate AI up front, use tamoxifen for 10 years.

and leukemia may be substantial (179). The individual patient's absolute benefit from adjuvant chemotherapy depends on the pathologic prognostic factors (tumor size, number of positive lymph nodes, ER/PR and HER2 status, Ki-67, genomic tests) as well as the patient's comorbidities and life expectancy. The final decision to "give or not give" chemotherapy is based on assessment of the patient's risk of recurrence and death from intercurring malignancy, the patient's medical "fitness" to tolerate chemotherapy, and overall personal goals.

> ➤ Patients with an ECOG performance status of 3 or 4, life expectancy of less than 2 to 5 years, and severe comorbid conditions are not good candidates for adjuvant chemotherapy.

TUMOR GENOMIC MULTIGENE ASSAYS

With increased understanding of tumor biology and genomics, multiple gene-based tumor assays have been developed to estimate the likelihood of BC recurrence and the benefit of hormonal therapy or chemotherapy + hormonal therapy. As more data are gathered, these tests have had an increasingly prominent role in assessing prognosis and predicting benefit of therapy. In Table 5.8, we summarize the genomic tumor tests and indications for use.

Genomic Tests for Extended Hormone Therapy

Hormone receptor positive BC is known for late recurrences (214). Given that there are many side effects (hot flashes, sweats, bone loss, endometrial pathology, and ECA) of extended HT, identification of those patients who will benefit from extended HT is a goal of molecular diagnostics. Breast Cancer Index and EndoPredict are two genomic tests that assess the risk for late recurrence. At this time, our recommendations are to consider these tests in select patients.

Table 5.8 Genomic Tests for Breast Cancer

Test name	Company	Number of genes	FDA approved	Recommending organizations	Appropriate candidate/purpose	Prognostic/predictive	Score	Prospective clinical trials
Oncotype Dx 21 gene recurrence score	Genomic Health	21	No	NCCN ASCO ESMO St. Gallen NICE	ER+, HER2– Node negative 1–3 Node positive	Prognostic and predictive of adjuvant chemotherapy	Low <18, intermediate 18–30, high 31+	TAILORx, RxPonder
MammaPrint Amsterdam 70 gene profile	Agendia	70	Yes	ESMO St. Gallen	Any receptor pattern Node negative 1–3 Node positive	Prognostic and predictive of adjuvant chemotherapy	Low or high risk	Raster, MINDACT
Prosigna Predictor Analysis of Microarray 50 gene	NanoString	50	Yes	St. Gallen	ER+ Node negative 1–3 Node positive	Prognostic	Low, intermediate, high risk of recurrence	
Breast Cancer Index	BioTheranostics	Molecular Grade Index and H/I (HOXB13: IL17BR) ratio	No	St. Gallen	ER+	Prognostic for risk of late distant recurrence Predictive for benefit of prolonged hormone therapy	Low (<5) or high (>5)	
EndoPredict	Sividon/ Myriad	qPCR-based 12 gene	No	St. Gallen	ER+, HER2– Node negative 1–3 Node positive	Prognostic for late distant metastasis	EPclin score low or high	

Genomic Tests for Addition of Chemotherapy to Hormonal Therapy

The developers of these tests initially relied upon retrospective analysis of large prospective randomized trials conducted several decades ago. More recently, two prospective randomized genomics driven trials (**TAILORx and MINDACT**) in patients with early-stage BC using two different sets of cancer-associated genes have been reported (215,216). These tests are expensive, and while most are covered by insurance, consideration of the indication and usefulness of the information should be considered prior to ordering. We discourage ordering more than one genomic test for the same purpose on the same tumor and additionally recommend careful assessment of baseline clinicopathologic tumor factors before considering any one of these tests (217).

Genomic Tests and Their Validation Trials

ONCOTYPE DX TRIALS

The Oncotype Dx assay (Genomic Health, Redwood, California) is a 21-gene tumor tissue assay that uses optimized RT-PCR technology for quantifying gene expression in formalin-fixed, paraffin-embedded tumor tissue to provide an individualized prediction of the benefit of adjuvant chemotherapy and the rate of BC recurrence at 10 years. Sixteen cancer-related genes, associated with distant recurrence free survival and five control genes, were used to provide a recurrence score (RS) from 0 to 100 as a continuous variable, which can then be used to predict the chance of recurrence in patients with early-stage LN–/1-3LN+, ER+, HER2– BC. Low RS (<18) conveys an average risk of recurrence of 6.8%, intermediate RS (18–31)—14.3% and high RS (>31)—30.5% at 10 years (218,219). This multigene expression assay is incorporated into various guidelines (ASCO, NCCN, ESMO, St Gallen).

The **NSABP B-20 trial** was used to evaluate the ability of Oncotype Dx to predict distant recurrence in patients with **ER+ LN negative BC** who were treated with TAM alone or TAM + cyclophosphamide, methotrexate, and 5-fluorouracil (CMF). Patients with a tumor RS of ≥31 experienced a large benefit from chemotherapy (HR 0.26, 95% CIs [0.13, 0.53]; absolute decrease in 10-year distant recurrence rate: mean 27.5%), while patients with a RS of ≤18 had no benefit from chemotherapy (218,219). Patients with an intermediate RS did not appear to experience a benefit from chemotherapy; however, due to the small number of patients in this subgroup, a modest benefit could not be excluded (218,220).

SWOG 8814 was used to generate the predictive clinical validity of Oncotype Dx in women with **ER+, 1–3 lymph node positive** BC who were either treated with TAM alone or chemotherapy + TAM. The study suggests that patients with 1 to 3 lymph node positive with low RS ≤18 do not seem to benefit from adjuvant chemotherapy (HR 1.02, 95% CIs [0.54, 1.93]), whereas those with a high RS ≥31 show an improvement in DFS, independent of the number of positive nodes (HR 0.59, 95% CIs [0.35, 1.101]) (221).

> ➤ The decision to use Oncotype Dx in patients with ER+ HER2– BC with 1 to 3 positive nodes can be discussed with patients.

The Trial Assigning Individualized Options in Treatment (TAILORx) NCT00310180 is a large phase III trial of more than 10,000 women with ER+,

LN negative disease and prospectively evaluates the role of Oncotype Dx 21 gene expression assay in making a decision for adjuvant systemic therapy (222). The investigators used different RS cutoffs in this study: "low risk" ≤10, "intermediate risk" 11 to 25, and high risk >25. Patients with a **low-risk** score received HT only. The data on outcome from the low-risk group have been analyzed and show that at 5 years, the rate of invasive BC DFS was 93.8% (95% CIs [92.4, 94.9]), the rate of freedom from recurrence of BC at a distant site was 99.3% (95% CIs [98.7, 99.6]), and the rate of OS was 98% (95% CIs [97.1, 98.6]) on HT alone (216).

> ➤ The TAILORx results confirm the predictive ability of Oncotype Dx in the "low risk" (RS ≤10), ER/PR+ HER2–, LN– BC patients who should receive hormonal treatment alone.

Patients with **intermediate risk** scores were randomized to HT alone or chemotherapy + HT. These intermediate risk patients are still being followed and results are not yet available. The findings from this trial will help clarify the benefit of treating patients at intermediate risk with adjuvant chemotherapy.

MAMMAPRINT TRIALS

MammaPrint (Agendia, Irvine, California) is a microarray-based test that uses paraffin-embedded tumor tissue to determine expression levels of 70 cancer-associated genes to assess distant recurrence risk in early-stage BC, irrespective of ER or HER2 expression (223). In 2007, the FDA cleared the MammaPrint test for use in the United States for LN– BC patients of all ages, with ER– or ER+, tumors <5 cm. The test is resulted in a binary fashion as low risk or high risk of BC recurrence. A "low-risk" MammaPrint result conveys an average 10% chance of BC recurrence while a "high-risk" MammaPrint conveys a 29% chance of BC recurrence within 10 years without any additional adjuvant treatment, either hormonal therapy or chemotherapy (224). The 5-year distant recurrence free interval (DRFI) probabilities for low-risk and high-risk BC patients were 97.0% and 91.7% (225). In a univariate analysis looking at other clinical pathologic factors, MammaPrint's prognostic value is highly statistically significant ($P = .002$) (225).

The **microarRAy-prognoSTics-in-breast-cancER (RASTER)** study prospectively evaluated the performance of MammaPrint in 427 BC patients with T 1–3, LN– tumors with 5-year DRFIs as the primary outcome measure (225). The 5-year DRFI probabilities were compared between subgroups based on MammaPrint and Adjuvant! Online, and adjuvant chemotherapy was used based on doctors' and patients' preferences of following gene array or clinicopathologic indices. As compared to standard clinicopathological classification, MammaPrint restratified 20% of clinical high-risk patients to low risk. After a median follow-up time of 61.6 months, the 124 patients who were classified as low risk by MammaPrint and high risk by Adjuvant! Online, of whom 94 (76%) chose not to receive adjuvant chemotherapy, had a 5-year DRFI of 98.4%.

> ➤ The RASTER study suggests that MammaPrint low-risk patients can safely forgo chemotherapy.

TransBig trial was a validation study. Patients (n = 307, with 137 events after a median follow-up of 13.6 years) were divided into high- and low-risk groups based on the MammaPrint 70 gene signature classification and on clinicopathologic risk classification (226). Hazard ratios were computed for time to distant metastases, DFS, and OS in high- versus low-risk groups. In this study the 70-gene tissue test was better than the clinicopathologic risk assessment in predicting all end points. For OS, the 70-gene signature had an unadjusted HR = 2.79 (95% CIs [1.60, 4.87]), while the clinicopathologic risk had an HR = 1.67 (95% CIs [0.93, 2.98]). This confirmed that the 70-gene MammaPrint test had independent prognostic value.

MIcroarray for 0–3 Node+ Disease may Avoid Chemotherapy Trial (MINDACT), EORTC 10041, BIG 3-04 was a large-scale international prospective randomized study. The study participants were divided into four risk groups, based on the risk of recurrence assessed by clinical pathologic risk (C) (modified version Adjuvant! Online) and genomic (G) risk by MammaPrint. G-low/C-low recieved no chemotherapy, G-high/C-high received chemotherapy, and the G-low/C-high and G-high/C-low were randomized to chemotherapy or no chemotherapy. The results were presented at the AACR 2016 Plenary Session by Piccart et al. (215). Patients who received treatments guided by genomic tumor assessment with MammaPrint had a 5-year distant metastasis-free survival (DMFS) for the discordant G-low/C-high-risk group (48% LN+) over 94% whether they received chemotherapy or not (227). Of note, the G-low/C-high whom received chemotherapy had a DMFS of 96%, but the 1.5% difference was not statistically significant. Among the patients in the clinical high-risk group (C-high), the use of MammaPrint genomic testing was associated with 46% reduction in the use of adjuvant chemotherapy. Approximately 14% of study participants could have avoided chemotherapy if treated according to genomic risk versus the traditional clinicopathologic assessment of recurrence by the Adjuvant! Online program (215).

The Symphony trial: Using Symphony in Treatment Decisions Concerning Adjuvant Systemic Therapy (Symphony), NCT02209857 will measure and compare the proportion of patients receiving adjuvant chemotherapy in the group of patients receiving MammaPrint and the group that does not receive MammaPrint.

Commonly Used Adjuvant Chemotherapy Regimens

To understand the current use of adjuvant chemotherapy, one needs to appreciate the history and multiple trials conducted to prove the therapies' benefit. Meta-analyses showed that standard CMF compared to standard four cycles of doxorubicin and cyclophosphamide (AC) were equivalent (RR 0.98, SE 0.05, $2P = .67$) and that anthracycline-based regimens with substantially higher cumulative dose of anthracycline than standard four doses of AC (eg, CAF or CEF) were superior to standard CMF (RR 0.78, SE 0.06, $2P = .0004$). Trials versus no chemotherapy also suggested higher mortality reductions with CAF (RR 0.64, $2P < .0001$) than with standard 4AC (RR 0.78, $2P = .01$) or standard CMF (RR 0.76, $2P < .0001$) (228). We include a brief synopsis of the history and trials that led to a transition from first to third generation regimens frequently used in the United States. In all EBCTCG chemotherapy meta-analyses involving taxane- or anthracycline-based regimens, proportional risk reductions were not affected by age, LN status, tumor size or differentiation, ER expression, or tamoxifen use. Addition of four cycles of a taxane to a fixed anthracycline regimen, reduced BC mortality (RR 0.86, two-sided significance [2P] = .0005) (228). While third generation regimens are more effective, they can have a high side-effect profile—with the small but present risk of late-onset complications of myelodysplastic syndrome, secondary leukemia, and heart failure. Therefore, for lower risk disease, a second generation regimen such as TC may be appropriate. For patients who are elderly, have multiple comorbidities, and who are frail, but still need adjuvant chemotherapy, even a first generation regimen such as CMF may still be an option. Commonly used contemporary chemotherapy regimens and dosing schedules are listed in Tables 5.9 and 5.10.

FIRST GENERATION—CMF AND AC

Cyclophosphamide, methotrexate, and 5-fluorouracil (CMF). In 1973 cyclo-phosphamide, methotrexate, and 5-fluorouracil (CMF) was one of the first com-bination adjuvant chemotherapy regimens tested in a prospective clinical trial for the treatment of BC. This trial randomized women with LN+ BC after radical mastectomy to 12 cycles of CMF, administered every 28 days versus no additional treatment.

Results: Improved DFS (HR 0.71; $P = .005$) and OS (HR 0.79; $P = .04$) for CMF was observered as compared to the control population (229). A subsequent study found that 6 cycles of adjuvant CMF was as effective as 12 cycles of adjuvant CMF (230).

NSABP-B-15—doxorubicin and cyclophosphamide (AC): Around the same time the CMF regimen was developed, researchers found that doxorubicin was highly active in the treatment of metastatic BC (231,232). The NSABP B-15 trial was a trial randomizing women with LN+ BC to doxorubicin and cyclophospha-mide (AC) every 3 weeks for 4 cycles given over 12 weeks versus CMF given for 6 cycles over 24 weeks.

Results: The 3-year DFS (62% vs. 63%; $P = .5$) and OS rates (83% vs. 82%; $P = .8$) were similar for AC compared to CMF (233).

Table 5.9 Examples of Commonly Used Adjuvant Chemotherapy Regimens	
Generation	**Regimen**
First	Cyclophosphamide, methotrexate, 5-fluorouracil (CMF) Doxorubicin and cyclophosphamide (AC) 5-fluorouracil, epirubicin, and cyclophosphamide (FEC50)
Second	Fluorouracil, cyclophosphamide, and epirubicin (FEC100) Cyclophosphamide, doxorubicin, and 5-fluorouracil (CAF or FAC) Sequential doxorubicin/cyclophosphamide followed by paclitaxel (AC-T) Sequential epirubicin followed by CMF Docetaxel plus cyclophosphamide (TC)
Third	Docetaxel, doxorubicin, and cyclophosphamide (TAC) Sequential FEC-taxane therapy Dose dense sequential doxorubicin/cyclophosphamide paclitaxel (dose dense AC-T)

Table 5.10 Common Regimen Details

Generation	Regimen	Drug	Dose and route	Days	Cycle length	Number of cycles	Key toxicities
Third	DD-AC + weekly paclitaxel	Doxorubicin	60 mg/m^2 IV	Day 1	Every 14 days	4	– High risk for emesis and for febrile neutropenia – Risk for cardiotoxicity, allergic reaction, and peripheral neuropathy
		Cyclophosphamide	600 mg/m^2 IV	Day 1			
		Paclitaxel	80 mg/m^2 IV	Weekly	Every 7 days	12	
Third	DD-AC + DD paclitaxel	Doxorubicin	60 mg/m^2 IV	Day 1	Every 14 days	4	– High risk for emesis for febrile neutropenia – Risk for cardiotoxicity – Paclitaxel has high risk for allergic reaction and peripheral neuropathy
		Cyclophosphamide	600 mg/m^2 IV	Day 1			
		Paclitaxel	175 mg/m^2 IV	Every 2 weeks	Every 14 days	6	
Third	TAC	Docetaxel	75 mg/m^2 IV	Day 1	Every 21 days	6	– High risk for emesis and febrile neutropenia – Risk for cardiotoxicity, allergic reaction, fluid retention, and peripheral neuropathy
		Doxorubicin	50 mg/m^2 IV	Day 1			
		Cyclophosphamide	500 mg/m^2	Day 1			
Second	TC	Docetaxel	75 mg/m^2 IV	Day 1	Every 21 days	4	– Moderate risk emesis – Intermediate febrile neutropenia – High risk for allergic reaction
		Cyclophosphamide	600 mg/m^2 IV	Day 1			

(continued)

Table 5.10 Common Regimen Details (*continued*)

Generation	Regimen	Drug	Dose and route	Days	Cycle length	Number of cycles	Key toxicities
First	CMF	Cyclophosphamide	600 mg/m^2 IV or 100 mg/m^2 orally on days 1–14	Days 1 and 8	Every 28 days	6	– Moderate risk for emesis – Low risk for febrile neutropenia – Adjust renal function methotrexate if CrCl <50 – Adjust cyclophosphamide bili >3
		Methotrexate	40 mg/m^2 IV	Days 1 and 8			
		5-fluorouracil	600 mg/m^2 IV	Days 1 and 8			
First	AC	Doxorubicin	60 mg/m^2 IV	Day 1	Every 21 days	4	– High-risk emesis – Doxorubicin cardiomyopathy
		Cyclophosphamide	600 mg/m^2 IV	Day 1			

SECOND GENERATION—ADDITION OF TAXANE

CALGB 9344—sequential doxorubicin/cyclophosphamide followed by paclitaxel (AC-T): In the 1990s, taxanes were developed and shown to have efficacy in the treatment of BC (234,235). However, concurrent administration of paclitaxel with doxorubicin, another highly active cytotoxic agent for metastatic BC, was associated with substantial cardiotoxicity due to paclitaxel resulting in greater doxorubicin exposure (236).

The CALGB 9344 study was therefore developed to evaluate the benefit of paclitaxel when given following completion of AC in LN+ operable BC. The study employed a 2 × 2 factorial design to evaluate escalating doses of doxorubicin in combination with cyclophosphamide every 21 days for four cycles, given alone or followed sequentially by four cycles of paclitaxel.

Results: The study found that the addition of four cycles of paclitaxel after four cycles of AC was associated with improved DFS (HR 0.83; P = .0023) and OS (HR 0.82; P = .006) compared to AC alone (235). The study also found that the escalation of doxorubicin dose had no effect on outcomes (235).

US Oncology Research Trial 9735—Docetaxel and cyclophosphamide (TC): In an effort to find a nonanthracycline-based BC chemotherapy regimen, the U.S. Oncology Research phase III trial evaluated the efficacy of docetaxel and cyclophosphamide (TC) compared to doxorubicin and cyclophosphamide (AC) in the treatment of patients with operable BC. Patients were assigned to four 3-week cycles of AC or TC.

Results: TC was associated with significantly improved DFS (HR 0.74; P = .033) and OS (HR 0.69; P = .032) compared to AC. However, the study did not have sufficient power to show superiority of one regimen over the other (237).

THIRD GENERATION—TRIPLETS AND DOSE DENSE

BCIRG 001 (TAC vs. FAC): The BCIRG 0001 trial compared six cycles of docetaxel, doxorubicin, and cyclophosphamide (TAC) with cyclophosphamide, doxorubicin, and 5-fluorouracil (FAC) every 3 weeks as adjuvant treatment for women with operable, LN+ BC (238).

Results: At 10-year follow-up, there were improvements in DFS at 62% (95% CI 58%–65%) for the TAC group versus 55% (95% CI 51%–59%) for the FAC group (HR 0.80; P = .0043) (239); 10-year OS was also improved, from 69% in the FAC group to 76% in the TAC group (HR 0.74; P = .002). It is notable TAC was associated with more toxicity (239,240).

BCIRG 005 trial (TAC vs. AC followed by T): In this study TAC × 6 cycles every 3 weeks was compared to 4 cycles of AC every 3 weeks followed by 4 cycles of docetaxel every 3 weeks in women with LN+, HER2-negative operable BC.

Results: 5-year DFS rates (HR 1.0; P = .98) and OS rates were equal (HR 0.91; P = .37) between treatment arms (241). However, the treatment toxicity profile differed. TAC was associated with more febrile neutropenia and thrombocytopenia, and AC-T was associated with more sensory neuropathy, nail changes, and myalgia (241).

CALGB 9741 (Dose dense A-C-T): "Dose density" is the concept of administering chemotherapy at more frequent intervals to reduce time for cancer cells to repair (242). CALGB 9741 assessed the impact of dose density (2 weeks vs. 3 weeks) and treatment sequence (concurrent vs. sequential) using A, C, and T in patients with LN+ operable BC. Patients were randomized to receive sequential A × 4 (doses) → T × 4 → C × 4 every 3 wk, or sequential A × 4 → T × 4 → C × 4 every 2 wk with filgrastim, or concurrent AC × 4 → T × 4 every 3 wk, or concurrent AC × 4 → T × 4 every 2 wk with filgrastim.

Results: At 36 months there was no difference in either DFS or OS between the concurrent and sequential schedule (243). However, the dose dense regimen improved DFS (HR 0.74; P = .01) and OS (HR 0.69; P = .04) (243). The dose dense chemotherapy arms had higher rates of nonhematological adverse events compared to the every 3 weeks chemotherapy arms (243).

Taxane Schedule—Weekly Paclitaxel

Eastern Cooperative Oncology Group (ECOG) E1199 NCT00004125: This trial was designed to compare the efficacy (DFS primary end point) of paclitaxel with that of docetaxel and to compare the standard taxane schedule (every 3 weeks) with a weekly schedule. Almost 5,000 women with axillary LN+ or high-risk, LN– operable BC were randomized to 1 of 4 treatment arms, AC every 3 weeks followed by weekly or every 3 weeks paclitaxel or docetaxel.

Results: The estimated 5-year OS rates were 86.5% (paclitaxel every 3 wk × 4 cycles), 89.7% (paclitaxel × 12 wk), 87.3% (docetaxel every 3 wk × 4 cycles), and 86.2% (docetaxel × 12 wk) (244). As compared with the group receiving paclitaxel every 3 wk, OS was significantly better in the group receiving weekly paclitaxel (odds ratio, 1.32; P = .01), but not in the groups receiving docetaxel every 3 wk (odds ratio, 1.13; P = .25) or weekly docetaxel (odds ratio, 1.02; P = .80). Treatment with AC followed by weekly paclitaxel × 12 wk was associated with improved DFS and OS compared to treatment with AC followed by paclitaxel given every 3 wk × 4 cycles with a 32% reduction in death with weekly paclitaxel (244). In addition, the investigators found no evidence that women with ER/PR+, HER2-negative BC derived less benefit than those with BC ER/PR+ or positive for HER2 (244).

SWOG S0221—Dosing of the taxane portion was a phase III open label 2 × 2 factorial design for women with LN+ or high-risk LN– operable BC. The trial aimed to compare the use of dose dense AC (as previously described) for 6 cycles versus weekly doxorubicin (24 mg/m²) + oral daily cyclophosphamide 60 mg/m² for 15 weeks. The second evaluation was paclitaxel at 80 mg/m² IV weekly for 12 wk versus paclitaxel 175 mg/m² IV every 14 days for 6 cycles. Growth factor support was used. The study was amended eventually to only include AC every 2 wk for 4-cycle arm.

Results: The study found no difference in outcomes comparing weekly paclitaxel (12 wk) to biweekly paclitaxel (6 cycles) at a higher dose (245). However, toxicities differed between the two paclitaxel regimens. Weekly paclitaxel was associated with more hematologic toxicity (leukopenia and neutropenia), while there was a higher incidence of peripheral neuropathy, allergic reactions, and musculoskeletal pain toxicity with the biweekly higher dose paclitaxel schedule (245).

Chemotherapy and Trastuzumab for HER2-Positive Disease

HER2 overexpression in BC is a poor prognostic indicator, but is also predictive for the benefit of anti-HER2 therapy. On November 16, 2006, the FDA granted approval to trastuzumab (Herceptin) as part of a treatment regimen containing doxorubicin, cyclophosphamide, and paclitaxel for the adjuvant treatment of women with LN+, HER2-overexpressing BC. The approval was based on evidence of a significant prolongation in DFS in women receiving trastuzumab + chemotherapy compared to those receiving chemotherapy alone (246). Serial monitoring of cardiac function (low-normal left ventricular ejection fraction [LVEF]) approximately every 3 months is recommended as 2% of patients in trastuzumab + chemotherapy (anthracycline based) and 0.4% in the chemotherapy alone group experienced clinically symptomatic cardiomyopathy.

SMALL HER2+ POSITIVE TUMORS

A retrospective review by Gonzalez at MD Anderson Cancer Center included 965 T1a and T1b (<10 mm) tumors not treated with chemotherapy, 77% ER/PR+, 13% triple negative, and 10% HER2+.

Results: In this review, the 5-year RFS was 77% for the HER2+ cohort versus 94% in the HER2− ($P < .001$) (247); distant RFS was 86% in the HER2+ versus 97% in the HER2− group ($P < .001$) (247). A validation cohort was analyzed at two other institutions that reproduced similar data with a 5-year RFS of 87% versus 97%, but did not reach statistical significance.

Another study evaluating patients with LN−, HER2+ tumors measuring less than 2 cm found that the 10-year rate of RFS was 68.4% for patients with HER2+ untreated disease and 81.8% for patients with HER2− untreated disease (248).

These studies show that the risk of recurrence for patients with small HER2+ tumors remains higher than their HER2− counterparts. The advent of the monoclonal antibody trastuzumab allows for targeted therapy against HER2. A meta-analysis of eight trials including 12,000 patients comparing chemotherapy + trastuzumab to chemotherapy alone demonstrated an HR of 0.6 for DFS favoring the addition of trastuzumab (95% CIs [0.50, 0.71]) (249).

> ➤ Based on these findings, we recommend chemotherapy + trastuzumab for any patient with tumors greater than 1 cm and consideration of chemotherapy + trastuzumab in those with tumors <1 cm as per guidelines in Table 5.5.

Dosing and Common side effects of the anti-HER2 regimens are in Table 5.11.

Length of anti-HER2 adjuvant therapy: Two major studies were completed evaluating the ideal duration of adjuvant trastuzumab therapy.

The **Herceptin Adjuvant (HERA) trial** was an international, multicenter, randomized trial that compared 1 or 2 years of trastuzumab given every 3 weeks with observation in patients with HER2+, operable BC who had completed local–regional therapy and at least 4 cycles of neoadjuvant or adjuvant chemotherapy.

Results: The unadjusted hazard ratio (HR) for an event in the trastuzumab group, as compared to the observation group, was 0.64; $P < .0001$, which corresponds to an absolute DFS benefit of 6.3% (80.6% vs. 74.3%) at 3 years (250). At 8 years of follow-up, there was no DFS or OS difference between the 1 and 2 years' adjuvant trastuzumab duration arms (251).

The **Protocol for Herceptin as Adjuvant Therapy with Reduced Exposure (PHARE) trial** evaluated 6 months versus 1 year of trastuzumab addition to standard chemotherapy in patients with operable HER2+ BC; 3,380 patients were randomized.

Results: The 2-year DFS was shorter in the 6-month arm (91% vs. 94%) (252). The HR for death was elevated at 1.46 (95% CIs [1.06, +2.01]) and there were more

Table 5.11 HER2-Positive Disease

Regimen	Drug	Dose and route	Days	Cycle length	Number of cycles	Key toxicities
DD-AC-TH	Doxorubicin	60 mg/m² IV	Day 1	14 days*	Cycles 1–4	– High risk for emesis and febrile neutropenia, for DD-AC-GCSF prophylaxis is required – Risk for cardiotoxicity, allergic reaction, and peripheral sensory neuropathy – Check LVEF before AC and before trastuzumab
	Cyclophosphamide	600 mg/m² IV	Day 1			
	Paclitaxel	80 mg/m² IV	Weekly	7 days	12 weeks	
	Trastuzumab	4 mg/m² IV (loading dose)	With first dose of paclitaxel	Once	1	
	Trastuzumab	2 mg/kg IV Many will change to 6 mg/kg every 3 weeks after paclitaxel completed	Weekly	7 days 21 days	Completion of 1 year	
TCH	Docetaxel	75 mg/m² IV	Day 1	21 days	Cycles 1–6	– High-risk emesis – Intermediate febrile neutropenia-peripheral sensory neuropathy, renal dysfunction – Check LVEF before treatment and every 3 months while on trastuzumab due to risk of cardiotoxicity
	Carboplatin	AUC 6	Day 1			
	Trastuzumab	8 mg/kg IV (loading dose)	Day 1 of cycle 1	Once	Cycle 1	
	Trastuzumab	6 mg/kg IV	Day 1	21 days	Following cycle 1 for completion of 1 year (counting from first dose of trastuzumab)	

(continued)

Table 5.11 HER2-Positive Disease (*continued*)

Regimen	Drug	Dose and route	Days	Cycle length	Number of cycles	Key toxicities
Paclitaxel + Trastuzumab	Paclitaxel	80 mg/m^2 IV	Weekly	7 days	Cycles 1–12	Risk infusion reaction, sensory neuropathy Check LVEF before trastuzumab and every 3 months due to risk of cardiomyopathy
	Trastuzumab	4 mg/kg IV (loading dose)	Day 1 of cycle 1	Once	Cycle 1 (with first dose of paclitaxel)	
	Trastuzumab	6 mg/kg IV	Day 1	21 days	Following cycle 1 for completion of 1 year	

*The N9831/NSABPB-31 AC was q 3 not q 2 weeks, but the DD AC was adopted given better efficacy.
AUC, area under the curve.

distant recurrences; HR 1.33 (95% CIs [1.04, +1.71]) (252). The multivariate analysis in the control group identified a relationship between shorter metastasis free survival (MFS) and tumor size (>2 cm, HR = 1.78, 95% CIs [1.19, 2.66]; $P < .005$) and nodal involvement (1–3 involved nodes: HR = 2.25, 95% CIs [1.37, 3.70]; >3 involved nodes: HR = 5.89, 95% CIs [3.65, 9.51]; $P < .01$) (253). At 42.5 months of median follow-up, 6 months of trastuzumab was noninferior to 12 months, thus confirming that 1-year duration should still remain the standard.

> ➤ Based on the HERA and PHARE studies, 1 year of adjuvant trastuzumab has become standard in the adjuvant setting.

Additionally, the HERA trial also confirmed the benefit of anti-HER2 therapy when given every 3 weeks after adjuvant chemotherapy is completed. Therefore, in cases where the HER2+ status is not known until after adjuvant chemotherapy is completed, we recommend 1 year of adjuvant trastuzumab therapy.

HER2-Positive Chemotherapy Regimens

Anthracyclines: The NSABP and the North Central Cancer Treatment Group (NCCTG) designed similar trials evaluating the addition of trastuzumab to anthracycline- and taxane-based chemotherapy. Given that both trastuzumab and anthracyclines have cardiac toxicity, the AC was given first every 3 weeks × 4 cycles and then trastuzumab given weekly was combined with the paclitaxel × 4 cycles every 3 weeks or given sequentially after paclitaxel and continued to complete 1 year of therapy. The **NSABP B-31 and NCCTG N9831** included women with LN+ and high-risk LN− (defined as ER+/PR+ tumors >2 cm in diameter or ER−/PR−tumors >1 cm in diameter) operable BC.

Results: The data from these studies were combined and showed that following the four cycles of AC, 1 year of trastuzumab given concurrently with paclitaxel significantly reduced the risk of recurrence and extended OS in all planned subgroups. Adding trastuzumab to chemotherapy led to a 37% relative improvement in OS (HR, 0.63; $P < .001$) with a 10-year OS rate of 75.2% to 84% and DFS improved 40% (HR, 0.60; $P < .001$) with a 10-year DFS rate of 62.2% to 73.7% (254).

Nonanthracycline Regimen—TCH: Many patients are not candidates for anthracycline-based chemotherapy or are concerned about the long-term side effects of therapy. The **Breast Cancer International Research Group BCIRG-006** performed a three-arm trial comparing anthracycline + cyclophosphamide + taxane + trastuzumab (ACTH), the nonanthracycline regimen of docetaxel + carboplatin + trastuzumab (TCH), and anthracycline + cyclophosphamide + taxane (ACT). Patients with HER2+ disease were eligible for this trial if they had LN+, or high-risk LN− operable BC.

Results: At a median follow-up of 5.5 years, the trastuzumab treated arms had statistically significantly improved ACTH versus TCH versus ACT—DFS (84% vs. 81% vs. 75%) and OS (92% vs. 91% vs. 87%), respectively (255). The differences in DFS and OS between ACTH and TCH were not statistically significant (255). At the final analysis, 10-year DFS was 74.6% with AC-TH ($P < .0001$), 73% with TCH ($P = .0011$), and 67.9% with AC-T. OS at 10 years was 85.9%, 83.3% and 78.7% respectively (256). Compared to a anthracycline-based regimen, TCH resulted in less congestive heart failure (0.4% vs. 2%) and subclinical loss of left ventricular ejection fraction (9% vs. 18%) (256). As in Table 5.5, given the long-term side-effect profile of anthracyclines, we recommend consideration of TCH as the preferred regimen. In patients with Stage II and III disease, the addition of pertuzumab (discussed in the following) may be considered. This is not an approved FDA indication, however, the NCCN notes consideration and we offer in high risk patients after discussion of the indications.

Nonanthracycline—Adjuvant Paclitaxel Trastuzumab (APT) trial: The earlier regimens of AC followed by TH and TCH are associated with significant toxicities. For patients with small HER2+ tumors, the absolute benefit of such a regimen is less than those with larger LN+ tumors. Weekly paclitaxel is known to be a very tolerable regimen with significantly fewer side effects. APT investigated the effect of adjuvant weekly paclitaxel × 12 weeks and Herceptin for 1 year in patients with early-stage (<3 cm, LN−) HER2+ BC. This trial was a nonrandomized single-arm phase II study.

Results: With a median follow-up of 4 years, the 3-year survival from invasive disease was 98.7% (95% CIs [97.6, 99.8]). The treatment was well tolerated with 6% of patients withdrawing for adverse events (257). Although not a randomized phase III trial, this data is convincing and we feel it is reasonable to consider **weekly paclitaxel with trastuzumab as per the APT trial for patients with small LN− HER2+ BC.**

Other HER2 Agents in the Adjuvant Setting

Pertuzumab is a humanized monoclonal antibody that targets domain II on the HER2 molecule and blocks ligand-dependent heterodimerization of the HER2 with other HER2 family members needed to activate the downstream cell proliferation signaling. In addition, evidence suggests that pertuzumab mediates antibody-dependent cell-mediated cytotoxicity. In 2013 pertuzumab was given accelerated FDA approval in the neoadjuvant setting for HER2+ BC which is LN+ or with tumor >2 cm in diameter (258). However, if a patient does not receive neoadjuvant therapy and is found to have stage 2 or 3 BC at pathologic review, adjuvant trastuzumab and pertuzumab can be considered (NCCN guidelines).

Currently, the Breast International Group is evaluating the addition of pertuzumab to trastuzumab and standard chemotherapy in the adjuvant setting in the phase III **APHINITY trial—NCT01358877.** Accrual was completed in 2013 of 4,800 patients with preliminary results expected in the near future.

Lapatinib (Tykerb) is a tyrosine kinase inhibitor approved in combination with capecitabine in the metastatic setting.

- **Tykerb Evaluation After Chemotherapy (TEACH)** evaluated lapatinib efficacy in the adjuvant setting. Following chemotherapy, lapatinib alone did not improve mortality or recurrence (259).
- **Adjuvant Lapatinib and/or Trastuzumab Treatment Options (ALTTO)** trial with a median follow-up of 4.5 years showed a 16% reduction in the DFS observed with lapatinib + trastuzumab compared to trastuzumab alone (HR, 0.84; 95% CIs [0.7, 1.02]; P = .048), and a nonsignificant 4% reduction was observed with trastuzumab followed by lapatinib compared to trastuzumab alone (HR, 0.96; P = .61) (260). Lapatinib treated patients experienced more

diarrhea, cutaneous rash, and hepatic toxicity compared to trastuzumab-treated patients. The incidence of cardiac toxicity was low in all treatment arms. Given the substantial side effects and the minimal nonsignificant increase in DFS, 1 year of trastuzumab alone remains the standard of care.

Neratinib is another tyrosine kinase inhibitor. The **ExteNET trial** was a double-blind, placebo-controlled, phase III trial of neratinib versus placebo after adjuvant treatment with trastuzumab in women with early-stage, HER2+ BC. The primary end point of the trial was invasive DFS. Neratinib resulted in a 2% absolute reduction and 33% reduction of risk of invasive disease recurrence or death versus placebo (HR = 0.67; P = .009) with a 2-year DFS rate of 93.9% in the neratinib arm and 91.6% in the placebo arm (261). As of 2016, neratinib has not been FDA approved for any use in the treatment of HER2+ BC.

> ## ➤ MANAGEMENT PEARLS FOR HER2-POSITIVE DISEASE
>
> 1. Given that both anthracycline and nonanthracycline regimens combined with 1 year of trastuzumab have similar efficacy but differ in toxicity profiles, we recommend the nonanthracycline regimen (TCH).
> 2. One year of therapy with trastuzumab every 3 weeks is the standard of care.
> 3. We consider single agent paclitaxel weekly for 12 weeks with 1 year of trastuzumab for patients with small LN–, HER2+ tumors.
> 4. Although it is preferable to give trastuzumab concurrently with nonanthracycline-based regimens or concurrently with a taxane after anthracycline-based regimens, it is acceptable to complete 1 year of adjuvant trastuzumab after all chemotherapy is completed.
> 5. Dosing and schedules are in Table 5.11.

Triple Negative Breast Cancer (TNBC)

Tumors <0.5 cm, no lymph node involvement: There is inadequate data to make general recommendations regarding adjuvant chemotherapy in patients with very small TNBC tumors (<0.5 cm). The NCCN guidelines do not recommend adjuvant chemotherapy for TNBC tumors less than 0.5 cm. In contrast to the NCCN guidelines, the St. Gallen 2013 chemotherapy guidelines recommend chemotherapy for all invasive TNBC regardless of size (small BC). Many practitioners treat very small TNBC based on studies showing patients with small TNBC have poorer overall outcomes compared to their ER/PR+ counterparts (262–264).

In a retrospective analysis of 1,691 women with T1mic, a, b N0 BC, patients with TNBC phenotype had an increased risk of local–regional relapse (HR 3.58, 95% CIs [1.4, 9.13]) and BC-related event (HR 2.18, 95% CIs [1.04, –4.57]) compared to luminal A subtypes (263). Another study of 1,012 patients with chemotherapy naïve T1a, b N0 BC demonstrated women with TNBC had almost 3 times worse RFS and over 2 times worse distant RFS as compared to women with ER/PR+ disease (264).

Tumors ≥0.5 cm or with lymph node involvement: Studies have suggested that there is a larger benefit to adjuvant chemotherapy among patients with TNBC. One such study was an analysis of three randomized trials involving over 6,000 women with LN+ BC, where researchers evaluated risk of recurrence and OS between women with ER+ BC and women with ER− BC. The study found that at 5 years following adjuvant chemotherapy, women with ER− versus ER+ BC had a larger reduction in risk of recurrence (55% [95% CI, 37%–68%] vs. 26% [95% CI, 4%–48%]) respectively, resulting in a higher absolute improvement in DFS (23% vs. 7%) from the addition of chemotherapy (265). Women with ER− versus ER+ BC at 5 years also had a larger reduction in the risk of death (55% [95% CI, 38%–69%] vs. 23% [95% CI, 17%–49%]), resulting in a larger benefit in OS (17% vs. 4%) (265). Based on these findings, adjuvant chemotherapy is recommended for women with T ≥ 0.5 cm or LN+ positive TNBC. NCCN guidelines recommend considering adjuvant therapy for TNBC tumors 0.5 to 1 cm and gives category 1 recommendation to adjuvant therapy for all tumors greater than 1 cm or LN+.

Important Ongoing Adjuvant Clinical Trials

ER/PR+ HER2−

PENELOPE-B NCT01864746: Given the trend for worse outcomes with residual disease after neoadjuvant therapy, PENELOPE-B is a large phase III clinical trial for ER+ patients who receive neoadjuvant therapy and have residual disease at surgery. Patients are randomized to adjuvant therapy to palbociclib (CDK 4–6 inhibitor) versus standard hormone adjuvant therapy. 1,100 patients are planned for accrual with a primary completion date in 2020.

    S1207 NCT01674140: Phase III randomized, placebo-controlled clinical trial evaluating the use of adjuvant endocrine therapy +/− 1 year of everolimus in patients with high-risk, hormone-receptor-positive and HER2/neu negative breast cancer.

TNBC

Given the high risk of recurrence for TNBC, additional effective adjuvant treatments are an unmet need. Platinums and poly adenosine diphosphate ribose [ADP]-ribose polymerase (PARP) inhibitors are promising targets.

    NRG-R003—NCT02488967 is a large phase III trial aiming to accrue 990 patients with operable BC and randomize to dose dense doxorubicin + cyclophosphamide followed by weekly paclitaxel plus or minus carboplatin. The primary end point is invasive DFS. A similar approach is being evaluated in the neoadjuvant setting with increased pathologic complete responses (pCRs) being observed.

    NSABP B55—NCT02032823: OlympiA study is evaluating olaparib versus placebo adjuvant therapy for 2 years after standard adjuvant chemotherapy in patients with *BRCA* mutation. Patients with *germline BRCA1/2* mutations and high-risk HER2-negative primary breast cancer who have completed definitive local treatment and neoadjuvant or adjuvant chemotherapy are eligible.

    NCT02593227—Folate Receptor Alpha Peptide Vaccine with granulocyte macrophage colony stimulating factor (GM-CSF) in patients with triple negative breast cancer. This phase II trial evaluates the safety and immunogenicity of two doses of the folate receptor alpha (FRα) peptide vaccine mixed with GM-CSF as a vaccine adjuvant, with or without immune priming with cyclophosphamide, as a consolidation therapy after neoadjuvant or adjuvant treatment of patients with stage IIb–III TNBC.

HER2+

Ado-trastuzumab emtansine (Kadcyla) is a rationally designed antibody drug conjugate (ADC) developed that pairs trastuzumab with a microtubule-based chemotherapy connected by a linker molecule. The chemotherapy is not active until endocytosed in HER2+ cells. Ado-trastuzumab emtansine gained FDA approval in the metastatic BC setting for second-line therapy in the EMILIA study in 2013. Two large phase III trials and one phase II adjuvant trial with ado-trastuzumab emtansine are currently accruing.

KATHERINE NCT01772472 study evaluates adjuvant ado-trastuzumab emtansine compared to standard trastuzumab in patients with residual disease following neoadjuvant chemotherapy (NACT).

KAITLIN NCT01966471 study evaluates the combination of ado-trastuzumab emtansine + pertuzumab compared to trastuzumab + pertuzumab + taxane following anthracycline chemotherapy. Eligible participants include LN+ (pN $\geq$ 1), or lymph node negative disease (pN0) with pathologic tumor size >2.0 cm.

NCT02414646 Adjuvant Ado-Trastuzumab Emtansine (T-DM1) for Older Patients With Human Epidermal Growth Factor Receptor 2 (HER2)-Positive stage 1–3 Breast Cancer. Patients receive trastuzumab emtansine intravenously over 30 to 90 minutes on day 1 every 21 days for 17 courses in the absence of disease progression or unacceptable toxicity. Primary objective is invasive disease free survival.

NEOADJUVANT TREATMENT APPROACHES

Neoadjuvant Chemotherapy

NACT is the practice of administering chemotherapy to patients prior to surgical resection. In the 1990s, multiple studies evaluated the safety of neoadjuvant therapy. The **NSABP B-18** (AC × 4 cycles pre- or postsurgery) and **NSABP B-27** (benefit of adding docetaxel to AC pre- or postsurgery) and **EORTC trial 10902** (FEC × 4 cycles pre- or postsurgery) were some of the larger prospective clinical trials that found no significant difference in DFS or OS based on preoperative versus postoperative timing of systemic chemotherapy (266,267). The benefits of NACT therapy included the shrinkage of tumor to allow breast conservation, real-time appraisal of response, and prognostic significance. The NACT approach enables significant scientific research.

Patients with locally advanced breast cancer (LABC) or inflammatory BC (Figures 5.13 and 5.14) who are unresectable can be converted to operative candidates by using NACT. Even patients with resectable stage II or III BC may benefit from NACT as they can convert from a mastectomy to breast conservation. In addition, patients with medical contraindications to surgery at the time of diagnosis (such as pregnancy, recent pulmonary embolism, or recent myocardial infarction) may benefit from NACT or neoadjuvant hormonal therapy as a bridge to surgery.

In general, tumors with a higher proliferative index (Ki-67) respond better to NACT. One analysis of over 6,300 tumors showed pathologic complete response (pCR) using NACT in breast and lymph nodes in 31% to 36% basal (triple negative),

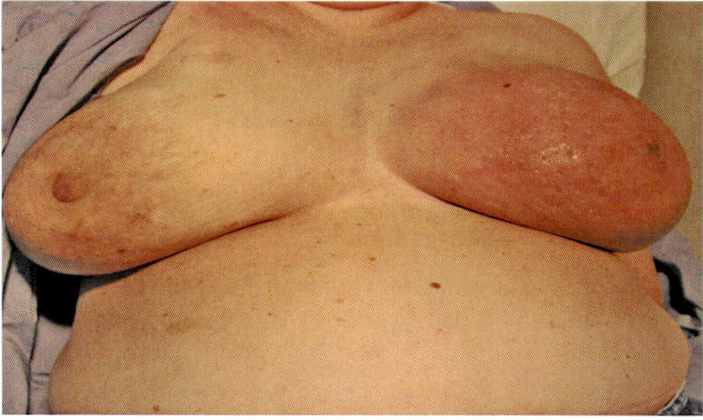

Figure 5.13 Left breast inflammatory breast carcinoma, erythema, peau d'orange changes of the skin, inverted nipple.

32% to 51% HER2-positive, 11% to 32% luminal B, and 6% to 9% luminal A tumors (268). The **I-SPY 1 trial** found a 45% pCR in the ER/PR– HER2+ subset, 35% in triple negative, and 9% in the ER/PR+ HER2– (269). The pCR rates have increased to over 60% in ER/PR– HER2+ BC with the use of pertuzumab and trastuzumab in addition to standard chemotherapy (269). While luminal A tumors may have low pCR to NACT, they may respond well to neoadjuvant hormonal therapy (NAHT), which is discussed later in this chapter.

The association between pCR and outcomes from BC has been a source of interest. The U.S. FDA conducted a meta-analysis known as Collaborative Trials in Neoadjuvant Breast Cancer (CTNeoBC). The goals of the analysis were to establish the relationship between pCR, EFS, and OS and determine the tumor subtypes in which pCR correlates with long-term outcome. **In HER2+ and TNBC, pCR is a prognostic marker of survival in BC patients** (270).

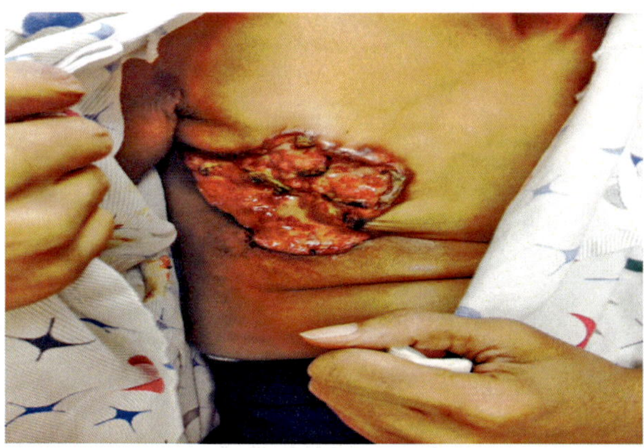

Figure 5.14 Locally advanced breast cancer—large right breast ulceration.

CTNeoBC identified 12 large neoadjuvant studies (>200 participants) that when combined had 11,955 patients. The study found that pCR in both the breast and lymph nodes correlated most with improved EFS and OS. Patients who experienced a pCR had EFS improvement with HR 0.48 (95% CIs [0.43, 0.54]) and improvement in OS with HR 0.36 (95% CIs [0.31, 0.42]) (270). This result was stronger in triple negative patients (EFS: HR 0.24, 95% CIs [0.18, 0.33]; OS: HR 0.16, 95% CIs [0.11, 0.25]) and HER2+, ER/PR− patients (EFS: HR = 0.15, 95% CIs [0.09, 0.27]; OS: HR 0.08, 95% CIs [0.03, 0.22]) (270). However, the analysis failed to find on a trial level an association between increases in frequency of pCR and EFS (R^2 = 0.03, 95% CIs [0.00, 0.25]) and OS (R^2 = 0.24, 0.00–0.70) (270).

NACT by Receptor Status

ER/PR+ HER2− BC AND NACT

As mentioned previously, patients with ER+ HER2− BC are less likely to have a clinical or pCR to NACT. However, in patients with unresectable tumors and inflammatory BC or those with locally advanced disease, particularly those with tumors that may respond to NACT (high grade, high Oncotype DX or MammaPrint), NACT may be considered to downsize the tumor. The CTNeoBC found a 7.5% pCR in grade 1 or 2 ER+ tumors and 16.2% pCR in grade 3 ER+ tumors. For long-term outcomes, the attainment of a pCR in the grade 1 or 2 had an HR for OS of 0.47, but this was not statistically significant (270). A pCR in Grade 3 ER+ HER2− was associated with improved OS with an HR of 0.29 (0.13–0.65) (270).

> ➤ For patients with ER/PR+ HER2− tumors who are candidates for neoadjuvant therapy, we recommend a discussion of the low likelihood of complete response, but potential benefit of downsizing and better surgical outcomes. We monitor these patients carefully for response. We typically use a third generation combination chemotherapy regimen that includes an anthracycline and taxane.

TRIPLE NEGATIVE BREAST CANCER AND NEOADJUVANT CHEMOTHERAPY

Patients with TNBC have been shown to have a pCR rate ranging from 31% to 45% with NACT (268,269,271). With such a high pCR, NACT is routinely considered in patients with stage 1 through 3 BC. As already stated, the pCR is prognostic in TNBC with residual disease portending a worse prognosis (269). The CTNeoBC found OS to be significantly improved with an HR of 0.16 (95% CIs [0.11, 0.25]) with attainment of a pCR in the breast and nodes (270).

Patients with TNBC who have more than minimal residual disease at surgery have a higher risk of early distant disease recurrence. Therefore, the opportunity to achieve higher pCR suggests that long-term benefits may be seen. Several studies suggest that the addition of carboplatin to the weekly taxane portion of ddAC with weekly paclitaxel can result in higher pCR (up to 54%) and improve candidacy for BCS compared to standard therapy (anthracycline and taxane based) (268). Carboplatin may be dosed at an AUC of 6 every 3 weeks or AUC 1.5 weekly.

CALGB 40603 and GeparSixto data showed improved EFS with carboplatin (CALBG 40603) and DFS (GeparSixto) with carboplatin (272,273).

In **CALGB 40603**, the 3-year EFS was 86% for patients achieving pCR in the breast/axilla, versus 62% for those who did not ($P < .0001$). The 3-year OS rates were 93% and 73%, respectively ($P < .0001$) (274).

In **GeparSixto** TNBC subgroup, pCR increased from 37% to 53% with carboplatin ($P = .005$) and DFS was 85.8% with carboplatin and 76.1% without (HR = 0.56; $P = .0350$). Compared to standard chemotherapy, patients who received carboplatin had higher rates of grade 3 to 4 neutropenia and delayed treatment due to treatment-related toxicities (273).

> ➤ We recommend considering clinical trial participation with the addition of carboplatin for TNBC patients eligible for neoadjuvant therapy. In the absence of a clinical trial, the data using carboplatin suggests it can be administered in a well-informed, TNBC patient.

HER2- OVEREXPRESSED BREAST CANCER AND NEOADJUVANT CHEMOTHERAPY

Patients with HER2+ BC have the highest rate of pCR to NACT, particularly the HR– HER2+ subset (270,275,276). The pCR increases significantly when treatment includes a HER2-directed agent. The Investigation of Serial Studies to Predict Your Therapeutic Response with Imaging and Molecular Analysis (I-SPY 1) trial evaluated 221 patients with tumors ≥3 cm who received NACT (doxorubicin and cyclophosphamide plus paclitaxel). The pCR using NACT in patients with HER2+ disease was 39% without trastuzumab and 60% with chemotherapy and trastuzumab, as compared to 18% for individuals with HER2– BC (269).

The **NeO Adjuvant Herceptin (NOAH) study** showed improved pCR with the addition of trastuzumab from 19% to 38% (277). In patients who achieved a pCR, improvements in EFS HR 0.64 (95% CIs [0.44, 0.93]) and OS HR 0.66 (95% CIs [0.43, 1.01]) were observed (278). Therefore, targeted treatment against HER2 is recommended as part of NACT for HER2+ patients.

Lapatinib, the small molecule tyrosine kinase inhibitor approved in the metastatic setting for HER2+ BC in combination with capecitabine, has been tested in the neoadjuvant setting. It has been found to be less effective than trastuzumab (279–281).

In **GeparQuinto**, patients receiving epirubicin + cyclophosphamide were randomized to treatment with docetaxel + either trastuzumab or lapatinib. The trastuzumab arm had a higher rate of pCR compared to lapatinib (OR 0.68, 95% CIs [0.47, 0.97]; 30% vs. 23%) (279). In the lapatinib arm there were more adverse events with 33% discontinuing therapy compared to 14% in the trastuzumab arm.

Lapatinib and trastuzumab combination therapy was evaluated in **NEO-ALLTO, Cher lob, and NSABP-B41.** These studies showed increased pCR ranging between 47% and 62% with combination therapy (280–282). In NEOALLTO, while the combination of trastuzumab and lapatinib did increase pCR, EFS, and OS were not increased as a whole (280). Patients who achieved a pCR did have increased EFS at 3 years HR 0.38 (95% CIs [0.22, 0.63]) (280). However, given the more severe side-effect profile (diarrhea, rash, liver abnormalities, neutropenia) for lapatinib, lack of long-term data on EFS and OS, and approval of pertuzumab, combination lapatinib and trastuzumab did not become a standard of care.

Pertuzumab is a monoclonal antibody that binds to a different domain than trastuzumab on the HER2 molecule and prevents the dimerization needed for cell signaling and proliferation. Pertuzumab is used in combination with trastuzumab and received FDA approval in the metastatic setting and gained accelerated FDA approval in the neoadjuvant setting based on a set of phase II trials: NEOSPHERE and TRYEPHENA.

In **Neoadjuvant Study of Pertuzumab + Herceptin in an Early Regimen Evaluation (NEOSPHERE)**, patients were randomized to receive four neoadjuvant cycles of either trastuzumab + docetaxel (group A), pertuzumab + trastuzumab + docetaxel (group B), pertuzumab + trastuzumab (group C), or pertuzumab + docetaxel (group D).

Results: Patients receiving pertuzumab + trastuzumab + docetaxel had a significantly improved pCR rate at 45.8% (95% CIs [36.1, 55.7]) compared to those given trastuzumab + docetaxel 29.0% (95% CIs [20.6, 38.5]; P = .0141) (275). Patients who received pertuzumab + docetaxel had a pCR of 24.0% (95% CIs [15.8, 33.7]) and those who received the two antibodies alone had a pCR of 16.8% (95% CIs [10.3, 25.3]) (275). The addition of pertuzumab was well tolerated with mild increases in rash, diarrhea, and mucosal inflammation.

Trastuzumab + Pertuzumab in Neoadjuvant HER2-Positive Breast Cancer (*TRYEPHENA*) randomized patients to treatment with trastuzumab + pertuzumab with concurrent docetaxel + carboplatin (TCHP), trastuzumab + pertuzumab with concurrent FEC (fluorouracil, epirubicin, cyclophosphamide), or FEC followed by trastuzumab + pertuzumab.

Results: The primary end point of the trial was cardiac toxicity and a secondary end point was pCR. The TCHP regimen was found to have the lowest decreased ejection fraction rate at 2.6% and the highest pCR at 63.6% (95% CIs [51, 74]) (276).

TDM1—ado-trastuzumab emtansine (Kadcyla): This Antibody Drug Conjugate (ADC) is approved as second-line therapy in HER2+ MBC. It has been evaluated in the neoadjuvant setting in the **ADAPT trial** NCT01745965. Participating patients with ER/PR+ HER2+ BC were randomized to receive either ado-trastuzumab emtansine, ado-trastuzumab emtansine + hormone therapy, or trastuzumab + hormone therapy. This treatment was administered in four cycles and followed by surgery + 1-year treatment of the standard adjuvant chemotherapy + trastuzumab.

Results: After four cycles (12 weeks) of treatment, a pCR in breast and lymph nodes was seen in 40.5% with ado-trastuzumab emtansine alone, 45.8% with ado-trastuzumab emtansine + hormone therapy, and 6.7% with trastuzumab + hormone therapy (P < 0.001 for both ado-trastuzumab emtansine groups vs. trastuzumab) (283). Although interesting, currently this approach cannot be recommended for routine use in the neoadjuvant setting.

> ➤ Based on the data of NEOSPHERE and TRYEPHENA, the FDA approved pertuzumab for stage II (>2 cm or LN+) and stage III HER2+ BC in the neoadjuvant setting.

> ➤ Given the high pCR seen to date, we recommend the TCHP regimen for HER2+ BC patients treated with NACT; alternatively, THP can be offered to older patients or patients with poor PS or comorbidities.

In Tables 5.12 and 5.13 we summarize commonly used chemotherapy +/− HER2 therapy regimens.

NEOADJUVANT HORMONAL THERAPY (NAHT)

Early studies of NAHT focused on the use of tamoxifen as the primary treatment for elderly women with ER/PR+ LABC who were not medically fit for chemotherapy or surgery. Subsequently, randomized trials were conducted to assess the role of neoadjuvant tamoxifen compared to surgery or tamoxifen compared to surgery + tamoxifen in the neoadjuvant setting. These studies demonstrated that surgery is necessary for optimal local control, whereas tamoxifen lowered the risk of metastases (284–287). A meta-analysis of six studies comparing primary surgery with NAHT using tamoxifen in women over the age of 70 showed no statistically significant difference in OS between the two treatment arms (HR: 0.98; $P = .9$) (288). NAHT alone is ineffective in achieving a cure and should be reserved for women who are unfit or refuse surgery (289,290).

Neoadjuvant hormonal versus chemotherapy: Limited data exist from clinical trials evaluating the use of NAHT versus NACT. Semiglazov and colleagues compared neoadjuvant therapy with AIs to chemotherapy in 239 postmenopausal women with untreated invasive ER/PR+ BC.

Results: There was no significant difference between the two arms in terms of overall response, pCR, or disease progression (291). The breast conservation rate was higher in the AI group at 33% compared to 24% in the chemotherapy arm (291).

The Grupo Español de Investigación del Cáncer de Mama (GEICAM) trial randomized 95 patients with ER/PR+ BC to NACT or exemestane. This study differed from the Semiglazov trial in that more than 50% of patients were premenopausal. Premenopausal women assigned to chemotherapy had a higher response rate. However, in postmenopausal women the response rates were comparable between chemotherapy and hormone therapy.

Results: Although not statistically significant, more patients assigned to the AI arm (56% vs. 47%) were able to undergo BCS (292).

Choice of NAHT

As shown in multiple trials in the adjuvant setting, third generation AIs are superior to tamoxifen. Several neoadjuvant hormonal therapy trials were conducted to compare the efficacy of tamoxifen with a third generation AI.

Table 5.12 NACT Regimen Details HER2-Negative Neoadjuvant Regimens (for Timing and Dosing, see Table 5.10)
Dose dense doxorubicin and cyclophosphamide, followed by paclitaxel weekly or biweekly (DDAC-T)
Doxorubicin, cyclophosphamide, and docetaxel (TAC)
Dose dense doxorubicin and cyclophosphamide, followed by paclitaxel weekly (DDAC-T) +/− carboplatin at AUC 6 every 3 weeks or 1.5 weekly during the paclitaxel (for TNBC)
Docetaxel and cyclophosphamide (TC) for patients who cannot tolerate anthracycline

Table 5.13 HER2-Positive Neoadjuvant Regimens

Regimen	Drug	Dose and route	Days	Cycle length	Number of cycles	Key toxicities
TCHP	Docetaxel	75 mg/m^2 IV	Day 1	21 days	Cycles 1–6	High risk for emesis High risk for allergic reaction and fluid retention Carboplatin-taste changes, electrolyte loss, function-monitor LVEF every 3 months-Trastuzumab/pertuzumab-decrease EF, rash, infusion reactions Monitor hepatic function (may need to dose modify if bili >1.3, ALT >2.5 ULN)
	Carboplatin	AUC 6	Day 1			
	Trastuzumab	8 mg/kg IV	Day 1 of cycle 1 (loading dose)	Once	Cycle 1	
	Pertuzumab	840 mg IV	Day 1 of cycle 1 (loading dose)	Once	Cycle 1	
	Trastuzumab	6 mg/kg IV	Day 1	21 days	Cycle 2–6	
	Pertuzumab	420 mg IV	Day 1	21 days	Cycle 2–6	
	Trastuzumab	6 mg/kg IV	Day 1	21 days	Following cycle 6 for completion of 1 year (counting from first dose of trastuzumab)	

(continued)

Table 5.13 HER2-Positive Neoadjuvant Regimens (*continued*)

Regimen	Drug	Dose and route	Days	Cycle length	Number of cycles	Key toxicities
THP3-FEC	Pertuzumab	840 mg IV	Day 1 of cycle 1 (loading dose)	Once	Cycle 1	Fluid retention, allergic reactions, cardiotoxicity
	Trastuzumab	8 mg/kg IV	Day 1 of cycle 1 (loading dose)	Once	Cycle 1	
	Docetaxel	75–100 mg/m^2 IV	Day 1	21 days	Cycle 1–4	
	Pertuzumab	420 mg IV	Day 1	21 days	Cycle 2–4	
	Trastuzumab	6 mg/kg IV	Day 1	21 days	Cycle 2–4	
				Surgery		
	Fluorouracil	600 mg/m^2 IV	Day 1	21 days	Cycles 1–3 postsurgery	
	Epirubicin	90 mg/m^2 IV	Day 1	21 days	Cycles 1–3 postsurgery	
	Cyclophosphamide	600 mg/m^2 IV	Day 1	21 days	Cycles 1–3 postsurgery	
	Trastuzumab	6 mg/kg IV	Day 1	21 days	10 cycles after FEC	

The P024 trial randomized 337 women with ER/PR+ BC to treatment with letrozole or tamoxifen followed by surgery. Compared to tamoxifen, letrozole resulted in a significantly higher overall response rate and higher rate of BCS (293).

The IMPACT trial randomized 330 postmenopausal women with ER/PR+ BC to anastrozole, tamoxifen, or the combination for 12 weeks prior to surgery. There was no significant difference in response rates between patients receiving tamoxifen, anastrozole, or the combination (294). However, in the biomarker analysis, the change in the Ki-67 proliferative index was more significant in the anastrozole arm. There was also a trend toward an improved rate of BCS in patients who received anastrozole, but the difference was not statistically significant (294,295).

The PROACT trial randomized 451 postmenopausal women with ER/PR+ BC to 3 months of neoadjuvant anastrozole or tamoxifen. This study differed in that it permitted concomitant chemotherapy at the investigator's discretion (29% of patients on anastrozole vs. 32% on tamoxifen). There was no significant difference in overall response between the two arms. However, in those patients who received HT alone, BCS was possible in 43% of patients in the anastrozole arm compared to 31% in the tamoxifen arm (296).

A meta-analysis of these trials supported the notion that AIs resulted in higher BCS rates than tamoxifen (297).

Choice of AI: There is no preferred agent among the AIs based on current evidence.

ACOSOG Z1031 trial randomized 277 postmenopausal women with stage 2 or 3 ER/PR+ BC with high ER expression (Allred score 6–8) to treatment with exemestane, letrozole, or anastrozole prior to surgery (298). There were no observed differences in clinical response rates, surgical outcomes, or changes in Ki-67.

Duration of NAHT: Current evidence supports the use of NAHT for at least 3 to 4 months in most patients. However, if the tumor is responding to NAHT and there is no evidence of progression, it is acceptable to continue therapy for 6 months or longer with appropriate monitoring. In most studies investigating NAHT, patients were treated for 3 to 4 months prior to surgery. However, not all patients will have maximal response at 3 to 4 months as demonstrated in a study by Llombart-Cussac and colleagues (299). In a study by Dixon et al, 32 women were treated with letrozole for a minimum of 4 months. Those who responded were allowed to continue letrozole for a maximum of 8 months and were shown to have increased rates of BCS, 69.8% at 3 months versus 83.5% after prolonged treatment (300).

NAHT Patient Selection and Assessment of Response: ER-positivity is the most important eligibility criteria for NAHT. **The P024 and IMPACT** trials both demonstrated higher response rates in patients with higher ER expression (294,295,301). The ACOSOG Z1031 trial demonstrated that patients with luminal A tumors by PAM50 analysis or a Ki-67 ≤10% achieved better response rates, although response rates were also good in patients with luminal B tumors (298). Other genomic tests, such as the 21-gene RS, may also be useful in selecting patients for NAHT.

In regard to response, a change in Ki-67 after short-term exposure to NAHT has been utilized to evaluate the efficacy of treatment. Dowsett et al demonstrated that a reduction in Ki-67 expression level after initiation of NAHT treatment was more strongly associated with RFS (log-rank $P = .008$) than baseline Ki-67 level (log-rank $P = .07$) (295). The prognostic significance of posttreatment Ki-67 levels on RFS was also demonstrated for patients treated in the P024 trial (301). A change in the Ki-67 proliferative index after short-term hormone therapy provides prognostic information on a long-term outcome. This may help to select patients whose tumors are exquisitely sensitive to estrogen deprivation who may be considered for treatment with hormone therapy alone.

The Preoperative Endocrine Prognostic Index (PEPI score) was developed from the analysis of tumors from patients treated in the P024 trial and includes posttreatment ER status, Ki-67 proliferative index, tumor size, and nodal status. The total PEPI score assigned to each patient is the sum of the risk points derived from the residual pT stage, pN stage, Ki-67 level, and ER status of the surgical specimen. Those patients with a PEPI score of 0 after NAHT have a very low risk of recurrence and may be considered for adjuvant endocrine therapy alone; those patients with a high PEPI score ≥ 4 should be considered for more aggressive adjuvant therapy (302).

It is expected that pretreatment genomic sequencing of the tumor will play a critical role in identifying patients who will benefit most from neoadjuvant therapy. Several studies are under way, including the MNT1 trial to test the ability of genomic assays such as MammaPrint to predict response to neoadjuvant therapy.

Surgical Management of Breast Cancer Patients After Neoadjuvant Therapy (NST)

As mentioned earlier, there are several potential benefits to administering systemic therapy prior to surgery. First, neoadjuvant systemic therapy (NST) may **convert patients with inoperable tumors to operative candidates**. Second, patients may be eligible for **less extensive or more cosmetically favorable** operations after neoadjuvant therapy including BCS, skin-sparing or nipple-sparing mastectomy, and less extensive axillary surgery. Finally, response to NST provides important **prognostic information,** which may help to guide recommendations for additional treatment. Management of the breast and axillary lymph nodes in patients undergoing NST depends on the initial staging and the distribution of cancer in the breast prior to the neoadjuvant therapy. In patients with MF or MC disease, NST may not alter the surgical plan and mastectomy may still be recommended after neoadjuvant treatment.

The **NSABP B-18 trial** randomized patients to preoperative or postoperative AC. This study showed an increase in BCS rates in patients treated with NST, particularly those patients with tumors >5 cm at diagnosis. The overall BCS rate was 67% in patients who received NST (303).

The **ACOSOG Z1031 trial,** which compared three AIs—letrozole, anastrozole, and exemestane—in the neoadjuvant setting, also demonstrated significant improvements in surgical outcomes. Over 50% of patients who were only considered eligible for mastectomy at the start of treatment were able to undergo BCS, and 83% of patients who were marginal candidates for BCS at the start of treatment were able to have BCS (298).

Inflammatory Breast Cancer (IBC):

> For patients with IBC at diagnosis, the recommendation is to proceed with a multimodality treatment approach which includes NACT, followed by modified radical mastectomy and adjuvant RT (304–309).

These patients are not considered candidates for BCS or limited axillary lymph node procedures. In addition, immediate reconstruction is not considered in these patients due to the high risk of LR.

MANAGEMENT OF THE AXILLARY LYMPH NODES

Assessment of the axillary lymph nodes prior to NST is usually performed by clinical examination of the axilla and axillary US. Suspicious lymph nodes by clinical exam or imaging should be sampled by CNB or fine needle aspiration (FNA) prior to initiation of systemic therapy to establish a pretreatment nodal status.

Clinically negative lymph nodes prior to NST: In patients with clinically negative lymph nodes at diagnosis, SLNB may be performed after NST. It is recommended that both radiotracer and blue dye be utilized in this setting since this increases SLN identification rates. Numerous studies have evaluated SLN identification rates and FNRs after NST (310–314). One of the largest studies reported results from the NSABP B-27 trial in which multiple participating surgeons performed SLNB prior to the required ALND. This study showed an SLN identification rate of 84.8% and an FNR of 10.7% (310). The success rate of SLNB was improved with the use of radiotracer. A second large study from MD Anderson Cancer Center of 575 clinically node-negative patients who received NST followed by surgery reported a SLN identification rate of 97.4% and an FNR of 5.9% (312). The FNRs reported in both of these studies are similar to those commonly accepted for SLNB at the time of primary surgical resection (91,315,316).

> In patients with clinically negative lymph nodes undergoing neoadjuvant systemic therapy (NST), we recommend SLNB using a combination of radiotracer and blue dye at the time of surgery.

CLINICALLY POSITIVE LYMPH NODES PRIOR TO NST

In patients with clinically positive lymph nodes at diagnosis, ALND after NST has been considered the standard approach. However, pCR rates in the breast and axillary lymph nodes have increased significantly in patients receiving NST with the use of third generation chemotherapy agents and targeted therapy. NST down-stages axillary lymph nodes in 30% to 40% of patients with potentially higher percentages in triple negative and HER2+ patients. Avoiding ALND in these patients would significantly decrease surgical morbidity. Multiple small studies have examined whether SLNB alone may be an accurate predictor of axillary lymph node status after NST (317–320). These studies have reported a wide range of FNRs (5%–35%) using SLNB in node-positive patients who convert to clinically node negative after NST.

The **ACOSOG Z1071** study investigated the FNR of SLNB after NST in patients with clinically positive nodes at diagnosis (321). The goal was to attain an FNR ≤ 10%. This study included patients with T0-4 N1-2 disease; however, the primary analysis was performed for patients with clinical N1 (cN1) disease. SLNB was attempted in all patients followed by ALND. At least one SLN was identified in 92.9% of patients with cN1 disease. The FNR of SLNB in patients with cN1 disease who had at least 2 SLNs removed was 12.6%, so the trial did not meet the FNR threshold. However, it was noted that when ≥3 SLNs were removed, the FNR decreased to <10% (9.1%).

The **SENTINA trial** also examined the use of SLNB after NST in patients with clinically positive nodes prior to treatment (314). In this trial, a cohort of patients with cN1 disease who converted to clinical node negative after treatment underwent SLNB and ALND. The SLN identification rate in this group was 80.1% and the FNR was 14.2%. The FNR rate was decreased to less than 10% when a greater number of SLNs were removed and with the use of radiocolloid and blue dye for lymphatic mapping.

Multiple centers are investigating the use of clip placement in biopsied axillary lymph nodes prior to NST to allow for targeted axillary dissection at the time of surgery (322,323). A recent publication demonstrated that the clipped node predicted the status of the axillary lymph node basin in almost all patients with residual nodal disease with an FNR of 4.2% (323). The clipped node was not retrieved as an SLN in 23% of the cases. However, in patients who had SLNB combined with removal of the clipped node followed by ALND, the FNR was decreased to 2.0%. Therefore, this appears to be a promising approach for management of the axillary lymph nodes in patients with clinically positive nodes prior to NST who convert to clinically node negative.

> ➤ In patients with clinically positive nodes undergoing NST, we recommend axillary US and lymph node core biopsy with clip placement prior to treatment. After therapy, the axilla is reevaluated by imaging and clinical exam. Based on response to treatment, select patients may be considered for SLNB. In order to achieve an acceptable FNR, SLN mapping is performed with radiotracer and blue dye and the clipped lymph node is also localized so that it can be removed during surgery.

Radiation Following Neoadjuvant Therapy

The use of NST has also led to multiple questions regarding RT since historically local–regional treatment was based on clinical and pathologic factors from upfront surgery. Clinicians now face questions including proper pathologic assessment, axillary surgical assessment (SLNB, ALND), type and timing of reconstruction, and, for radiation oncologists, the use and design of radiation (ie, which nodal stations to radiate).

Local–Regional Relapse Risk Factors Following a Mastectomy

Given that there are currently no randomized data regarding radiation after NAC (324,325), radiation oncologists face difficult clinical decisions regarding the local–regional treatment in these patients who undergo a mastectomy. Thus, pathological response as well as risk factors predictive of LRR are helpful in making this decision.

Multiple MDACC Retrospective Experiences evaluating risk factors predictive of LRR following NAC who were treated surgically with a mastectomy have been published. Buchholz et al (326) evaluated LRR in 150 patients with NAC compared to 1,031 with adjuvant chemotherapy; no patients received radiation. They found the 5-year LRR was significantly higher in the NAC group (27% vs. 15%) at all tumor sizes. LRR did not differ by the number of lymph nodes except for ≥4 lymph nodes (NAC 53% vs. 23%). When looking at both tumor size and number of positive lymph nodes, LRR was significantly higher in the NAC group in patients with pT2 pN1-3+. Clinical stage IIIB, four or more pathologic positive nodes, and no tamoxifen use were significant risk factors for LRR. Evaluating the 150 patients who received NAC, an LRR of 19% was found following a pCR versus 28% following a partial response. Therefore, one can argue that achievement of pCR does not necessarily negate the need for PMRT. Another retrospective experience from MDACC by Huang et al (327) compared the outcomes of 542 patients treated with NAC, mastectomy, and PMRT to 134 patients treated with NAC and mastectomy and found an overall significant reduction in LRR from 22% to 11% with the use of PMRT. When looking at stage III–IV patients who achieved pCR, they found a significant difference in 10-year LRR of 3% with PMRT versus 33% without PMRT. On multivariate analysis, significant poor prognostic factors for cancer-specific survival included lack of radiation, clinical stage IIIB to stage IV disease, residual pathological tumor involvement after chemotherapy, four or more positive nodes, minimal or worse clinical response to NACT, fewer than 10 axillary nodes sampled, no tamoxifen, and ER disease.

These studies illustrate that while LRR is lower with pCR, it is still substantial and the decision to give adjuvant radiation needs to incorporate pretreatment clinical factors such as stage and age. Garg et al (328) focused on patients with age less than 35 years old presenting with stage II–III disease and found a 5-year LRR of 12% with PMRT versus 37% without PMRT, implying that age is also an important factor. Similarly, Shim et al (329) evaluated 151 stage II–III patients treated with NAC and mastectomy and achieved pCR and found that age <40 years old was a significant prognostic factor for DFS. McGuire et al (330) reviewed 106 patients with stage II–III patients and found that while the LRR reduction with the use of PMRT was not significant in stage II patients, it was significant in stage III patients (7% vs. 33%), implying that PMRT should be used in clinical stage III patients despite pCR but there may be no benefit in stage II patients. In addition, patients with initial cT3N1 disease who received NACT were found to substantially benefit from radiation even if they had a pCR in the axilla. This series (331) demonstrated a substantial benefit even though there was bias to radiate patients who were younger and those with less than a pCR in the lymph nodes.

A reanalysis of the prospective NSABP B18 and B27 trials (332) reviewed the LRR outcomes of 3,088 patients who underwent mastectomy (no radiation) with nodal staging by clinical exam only. It is important to note that 90% of patients were stage I-II and 30% presented with nodal disease; thus, the results are more applicable to early-stage patients. Multivariate analysis showed that ypN+ was the most significant predictor of LRR (HR 4.48) followed by residual breast disease (HR 2.21), clinical node positive prior to NAC (HR 1.53), and pre-NAC tumor size >5 cm (HR 1.58). Compared to ypN– patients with breast pCR, patients with ypN+ disease had higher LRR regardless of tumor size or clinical node status. Finally, the authors found that all patients with 1 to 3 pathological positive nodes had LRR rates greater than 10%.

Thus, while residual nodal disease is indeed a driver for LRR, clinicians need to consider a combination of factors including residual primary disease, clinical stage, pretreatment clinical nodal status, receptor subtype, grade, and age. There are current NAC trials including NSABP B-51 and A011202 that will help to address this issue. In the meantime, patients with an estimated LRR risk of at least 10% warrant discussion on the use of adjuvant radiation. Stage I–II patients with pCR, especially older patients, low grade, and/or ER+ receptor status, will likely not benefit from PMRT. Patients with residual nodal or primary disease regardless of stage and stage III patients regardless of response warrant radiation. The intermediate group should be discussed in a multidisciplinary setting or should be sent to a radiation oncologist for consult and discussion.

Clinical Trials for Radiation After NAC

There are many areas of concern in the application of RT in NAC patients. **Current NCCN guidelines advocate PMRT following NAC for advanced BC.** Two currently accruing trials are addressing the role of radiation in NAC patients.

NSABP B-51/RTOG 1304 (NCT01872975) is a phase III multicenter trial looking specifically at cT1-T3 N1 (by FNA or core biopsy) patients who undergo NACT and then surgery (BCS or mastectomy) and must achieve pN0 (ypN0(i+) or ypN0 (mol+) are still eligible) either by SLNB +/− ALND or ALND. SLNB can be performed alone provided at least two SLNs are removed; at least three SLNs and use of dual tracer are recommended but not mandated. Mastectomy patients are then randomized to receive comprehensive nodal and chest wall RT or no radiation. BCS patients are randomized to standard whole breast RT with no nodal radiation or comprehensive nodal and breast RT. Internal mammary nodes are included in nodal RT. The primary end point is invasive BC recurrence-free interval with goal accrual of 1,636 patients. All patients will receive additional systemic therapy as planned.

Alliance 012202 trial (NCT01901094) is also evaluating patients with cT1-T3 N1 (by FNA or core biopsy) who undergo NAC with follow-up negative axilla by physical exam and then surgery with SLNB. The trial pertains to those patients whose SLNB is positive either intraoperatively or on final pathology. Patients are then randomized to ALND + nodal RT (without RT to dissected axilla) or axillary + nodal RT (no ALND). If the SLNB is not able to be performed or is negative on final pathology, then the patient is not eligible for the trial.

While we await the final accrual and results of the two previous trials, clinicians still need to make informed decisions for their current patients. As with upfront surgery, while axillary status is an important consideration in determining local–regional treatment, other important clinical and pathologic factors need to be taken into consideration as discussed earlier.

REFERENCES

Epidemiology/General Characteristics

1. Siegel RL, Miller KD, Jemal A. Cancer statistics, 2016. *CA Cancer J Clin.* 2016;66(1):7–30.
2. McCormack VA, dos Santos Silva I. Breast density and parenchymal patterns as markers of breast cancer risk: a meta-analysis. *Cancer Epidemiol Biomarkers Prev.* 2006;15(6):1159–1169.
3. Boyd NF, Guo H, Martin LJ, et al. Mammographic density and the risk and detection of breast cancer. *N Engl J Med.* 2007;356(3):227–236.
4. Hartmann LC, Radisky DC, Frost MH, et al. Understanding the premalignant potential of atypical hyperplasia through its natural history: a longitudinal cohort study. *Cancer Prev Res (Phila).* 2014;7(2):211–217.
5. Chuba PJ, Hamre MR, Yap J, et al. Bilateral risk for subsequent breast cancer after lobular carcinoma-in-situ: analysis of surveillance, epidemiology, and end results data. *J Clin Oncol.* 2005 20;23(24):5534–5541.
6. Page DL, Kidd TE, Dupont WD, et al. Lobular neoplasia of the breast: higher risk for subsequent invasive cancer predicted by more extensive disease. *Hum Pathol.* 1991;22(12):1232–1239.
7. Li CI, Malone KE, Saltzman BS, Daling JR. Risk of invasive breast carcinoma among women diagnosed with ductal carcinoma in situ and lobular carcinoma in situ, 1988–2001. *Cancer.* 2006;106(10):2104–2112.
8. Narod SA, Iqbal J, Giannakeas V, et al. Breast cancer mortality after a diagnosis of ductal carcinoma in situ. *JAMA Oncol.* 2015;1(7):888–896.
9. Nichols HB, Berrington de Gonzalez A, Lacey JV, Jr, et al. Declining incidence of contralateral breast cancer in the United States from 1975 to 2006. *J Clin Oncol.* 2011;29(12):1564–1569.
10. Colditz GA, Willett WC, Hunter DJ, et al. Family history, age, and risk of breast cancer: prospective data from the Nurses' Health Study. *JAMA.* 1993;270(3):338–343.
11. Collaborative Group on Hormonal Factors in Breast Cancer. Familial breast cancer: collaborative reanalysis of individual data from 52 epidemiological studies including 58,209 women with breast cancer and 101,986 women without the disease. *Lancet.* 2001; 358(9291):1389–1399.
12. Ritte R, Lukanova A, Tjønneland A, et al. Height, age at menarche and risk of hormone receptor-positive and -negative breast cancer: A cohort study. *Int J Cancer.* 2013; 132(11):2619–2629.
13. Rosner B, Colditz GA, Willett WC. Reproductive risk factors in a prospective study of breast cancer: the Nurses' Health Study. *Am J Epidemiol.* 1994;139(8):819–835.
14. Colditz GA, Rosner B. Cumulative risk of breast cancer to age 70 years according to risk factor status: data from the Nurses' Health Study. *Am J Epidemiol.* 2000;152(10):950–964.
15. Chlebowski RT, Hendrix SL, Langer RD, et al. Influence of estrogen plus progestin on breast cancer and mammography in healthy postmenopausal women: the Women's Health Initiative Randomized Trial. *JAMA.* 2003;289(24):3243–3253.
16. Bagnardi V, Rota M, Botteri E, et al. Light alcohol drinking and cancer: a meta-analysis. *Ann Oncol.* 2013;24(2):301–308.
17. Han X, Stevens J, Truesdale KP, et al. Body mass index at early adulthood, subsequent weight change and cancer incidence and mortality. *Int J Cancer.* 2014;135(12):2900–2909.
18. Gunter MJ, Hoover DR, Yu H, et al. Insulin, insulin-like growth factor-I, and risk of breast cancer in postmenopausal women. *J Natl Cancer Inst.* 2009;101(1):48–60.

19. Hormones TE, Group BCC. Insulin-like growth factor 1 (IGF1), IGF binding protein 3 (IGFBP3), and breast cancer risk: pooled individual data analysis of 17 prospective studies. *Lancet Oncol.* 2010;11(6):530–542.

20. van den Brandt PA, Spiegelman D, Yaun SS, et al. Pooled analysis of prospective cohort studies on height, weight, and breast cancer risk. *Am J Epidemiol.* 2000;152(6):514–527.

21. Guibout C, Adjadj E, Rubino C, et al. Malignant breast tumors after radiotherapy for a first cancer during childhood. *J Clin Oncol.* 2005;23(1):197–204.

22. Horwich A, Swerdlow A. Second primary breast cancer after Hodgkin's disease. *Br J Cancer.* 2004;90(2):294–298.

23. Lynch BM, Friedenreich CM, Winkler EA, et al. Associations of objectively assessed physical activity and sedentary time with biomarkers of breast cancer risk in post-menopausal women: findings from NHANES (2003–2006). *Breast Cancer Res Treat.* 2011;130(1):183–194.

24. Stuebe AM, Willett WC, Xue F, Michels KB. Lactation and incidence of premenopausal breast cancer: a longitudinal study. *Arch Intern Med.* 2009;169(15):1364–1371.

25. Tryggvadottir L, Tulinius H, Eyfjord JE, Sigurvinsson T. Breastfeeding and reduced risk of breast cancer in an Icelandic cohort study. *Am J Epidemiol.* 2001;154(1):37–42.

26. Mathis KL, Hoskin TL, Boughey JC, et al. Palpable presentation of breast cancer persists in the era of screening mammography. *J Am Coll Surg.* 2010;210(3):314–318.

27. Ma I, Dueck A, Gray R, et al. Clinical and self breast examination remain important in the era of modern screening. *Anna Surg Oncol.* 2012;19(5):1484–1490.

28. Smith RL, Pruthi S, Fitzpatrick LA. Evaluation and management of breast pain. *Mayo Clin Proc.* 2004;79:353–372.

29. Kennecke H, Yerushalmi R, Woods R, et al. Metastatic behavior of breast cancer subtypes. *J Clin Oncol.* 2010;28(20):3271–3277.

30. Schnipper LE, Smith TJ, Raghavan D, et al. American Society of Clinical Oncology identifies five key opportunities to improve care and reduce costs: the top five list for oncology. *J Clin Oncol.* 2012;30(14):1715–1724.

31. Edge S, Byrd DR, Compton CC, et al. *AJCC Cancer Staging Handbook: From the AJCC Cancer Staging Manual.* 7th ed. New York, NY: Springer Science + Business Media; 2010.

Pathology

32. Say CC, Donegan WL. Invasive carcinoma of the breast: prognostic significance of tumor size and involved axillary lymph nodes. *Cancer.* 1974;34(2):468–471.

33. Carter CL, Allen C, Henson DE. Relation of tumor size, lymph node status, and survival in 24,740 breast cancer cases. *Cancer.* 1989;63(1):181–187.

34. Mayer EL, Dominici LS. Breast cancer axillary staging: much ado about micrometastatic disease. *J Clin Oncol.* 2015;33(10):1095–1097.

35. Houvenaeghel G, Classe J, Garbay J, et al. Prognostic value of isolated tumor cells and micrometastases of lymph nodes in early-stage breast cancer: a French sentinel node multicenter cohort study. *Breast.* 2014;23(5):561–566.

36. Borst MJ, Ingold JA. Metastatic patterns of invasive lobular versus invasive ductal carcinoma of the breast. *Surgery.* 1993;114(4):637–641; discussion 641–642.

37. Li C, Uribe D, Daling J. Clinical characteristics of different histologic types of breast cancer. *Br J Cancer.* 2005;93(9):1046–1052.

38. Arpino G, Bardou VJ, Clark GM, Elledge RM. Infiltrating lobular carcinoma of the breast: tumor characteristics and clinical outcome. *Breast Cancer Res.* 2004;6(3):R149–R156.

39. Mai KT, Yazdi HM, Isotalo PA. Resection margin status in lumpectomy specimens of infiltrating lobular carcinoma. *Breast Cancer Res Treat.* 2000;60(1):29–33.

40. Rakha EA, van Deurzen CH, Paish EC, et al. Pleomorphic lobular carcinoma of the breast: is it a prognostically significant pathological subtype independent of histological grade? *Mod Pathol.* 2013;26(4):496–501.

41. Pedersen L, Holck S, Schiødt T, et al. Medullary carcinoma of the breast, prognostic importance of characteristic histopathological features evaluated in a multivariate Cox analysis. *Eur J Cancer.* 1994;30(12):1792–1797.

42. Huober J, Gelber S, Goldhirsch A, et al. Prognosis of medullary breast cancer: analysis of 13 International Breast Cancer Study Group (IBCSG) trials. *Ann Oncol.* 2012; 23(11):2843–2851.

43. Vo T, Xing Y, Meric-Bernstam F, et al. Long-term outcomes in patients with mucinous, medullary, tubular, and invasive ductal carcinomas after lumpectomy. *Am J Surg.* 2007;194(4):527–531.

44. Walsh MM, Bleiweiss IJ. Invasive micropapillary carcinoma of the breast: eighty cases of an underrecognized entity. *Hum Pathol.* 2001;32(6):583–589.

45. Pinder S, Murray S, Ellis I, et al. The importance of the histologic grade of invasive breast carcinoma and response to chemotherapy. *Cancer.* 1998;83(8):1529–1539.

46. Hoda S, Brogi E, Koener F, Rosen P. *Rosen's Breast Pathology.* 4th ed. Philadelphia, PA: Lippincott Williams and Wilkins; 2014.

47. Hammond MEH, Hayes DF, Wolff AC, et al. American Society of Clinical Oncology/ College of American Pathologists guideline recommendations for immunohistochemical testing of estrogen and progesterone receptors in breast cancer. *J Oncol Pract.* 2010;6(4):195–197.

48. Wolff AC, Hammond ME, Hicks DG, et al. Recommendations for human epidermal growth factor receptor 2 testing in breast cancer: American Society of Clinical Oncology/ College of American Pathologists clinical practice guideline update. *J Clin Oncol.* 2013;31(31):3997–4013.

49. Inwald E, Klinkhammer-Schalke M, Hofstädter F, et al. Ki-67 is a prognostic parameter in breast cancer patients: results of a large population-based cohort of a cancer registry. *Breast Cancer Res Treat.* 2013;139(2):539–552.

50. Georgiannos SN, Chin Aleong J, Goode AW, Sheaff M. Secondary neoplasms of the breast. *Cancer.* 2001;92(9):2259–2266.

51. Hajdu SI, Urban JA. Cancers metastatic to the breast. *Cancer.* 1972;29(6):1691–1696.

52. Bacchi CE, Wludarski SC, Ambaye AB, et al. Metastatic melanoma presenting as an isolated breast tumor: a study of 20 cases with emphasis on several primary mimickers. *Arch Pathol Lab Med.* 2013;137(1):41–49.

53. DeLair DF, Corben AD, Catalano JP, et al. Non-mammary metastases to the breast and axilla: a study of 85 cases. *Mod Pathol.* 2013;26(3):343–349.

54. Hejmadi R, Day L, Young J. Extramammary metastatic neoplasms in the breast: a cytomorphological study of 11 cases. *Cytopathology.* 2003;14(4):191–194.

55. Kothadia JP, Arju R, Kaminski M, et al. Metastatic colonic adenocarcinoma in breast: report of two cases and review of the literature. *Case Rep Oncol Med.* 2015;2015:1–6. doi:10.1155/2015/458423

56. Shen Y, Sui Y, Zhang X, et al. Ipsilateral breast metastasis from a pulmonary adenocarcinoma: a case report and a focused review of the literature. *Int J Clin Exp Pathol.* 2015;8(8):9647–9654.

57. Lee AH. The histological diagnosis of metastases to the breast from extramammary malignancies. *J Clin Pathol.* 2007;60(12):1333–1341.

58. David O, Gattuso P, Razan W, et al. Unusual cases of metastases to the breast. *Acta Cytol.* 2002;46(2):377–385.

59. Rodríguez-Gil Y, Pérez-Barrios A, Alberti-Masgrau N, et al. Fine-needle aspiration cytology diagnosis of metastatic nonhaematological neoplasms of the breast: a series of seven cases. *Diagn Cytopathol.* 2012;40(4):297–304.

60. Wood B, Sterrett G, Frost F, Swarbrick N. Diagnosis of extramammary malignancy metastatic to the breast by fine needle biopsy. *Pathology.* 2008;40(4):345–351.

Surgery

61. Sakorafas G, Safioleas M. Breast cancer surgery: an historical narrative. Part II. 18th and 19th centuries. *Eur J Cancer Care (Engl).* 2010;19(1):6–29.

62. Sakorafas G, Safioleas M. Breast cancer surgery: an historical narrative. Part III. From the sunset of the 19th to the dawn of the 21st century. *Eur J Cancer Care (Engl).* 2010;19(2):145–166.

63. Fisher B, Anderson S, Bryant J, et al. Twenty-year follow-up of a randomized trial comparing total mastectomy, lumpectomy, and lumpectomy plus irradiation for the treatment of invasive breast cancer. *N Engl J Med.* 2002;347(16):1233–1241.

64. Veronesi U, Cascinelli N, Mariani L, et al. Twenty-year follow-up of a randomized study comparing breast-conserving surgery with radical mastectomy for early breast cancer. *N Engl J Med.* 2002;347(16):1227–1232.

65. Poggi MM, Danforth DN, Sciuto LC, et al. Eighteen-year results in the treatment of early breast carcinoma with mastectomy versus breast conservation therapy. *Cancer.* 2003;98(4):697–702.

66. Arriagada R, Le MG, Rochard F, Contesso G. Conservative treatment versus mastectomy in early breast cancer: patterns of failure with 15 years of follow-up data. Institut Gustave-Roussy Breast Cancer Group. *J Clin Oncol.* 1996;14(5):1558–1564.

67. van Dongen JA, Voogd AC, Fentiman IS, et al. Long-term results of a randomized trial comparing breast-conserving therapy with mastectomy: European Organization for Research and Treatment of Cancer 10801 trial. *J Natl Cancer Inst.* 2000;92(14):1143–1150.

68. Blichert-Toft M, Rose C, Andersen JA, et al. Danish randomized trial comparing breast conservation therapy with mastectomy: six years of life-table analysis. Danish Breast Cancer Cooperative Group. *J Natl Cancer Inst Monogr.* 1992;(11):19–25.

69. Houssami N, Macaskill P, Marinovich ML, Morrow M. The association of surgical margins and local recurrence in women with early-stage invasive breast cancer treated with breast-conserving therapy: a meta-analysis. *Ann Surg Oncol.* 2014;21(3):717–730.

70. Moran MS, Schnitt SJ, Giuliano AE, et al. Society of Surgical Oncology–American Society for Radiation Oncology consensus guideline on margins for breast-conserving surgery with whole-breast irradiation in stages I and II invasive breast cancer. *Int J Radiat Oncol Biol Phys.* 2014;88(3):553–564.

71. Gentilini O, Botteri E, Rotmensz N, et al. Conservative surgery in patients with multifocal/multicentric breast cancer. *Breast Cancer Res Treat.* 2009;113(3):577–583.

72. Medina-Franco H, Vasconez LO, Fix RJ, et al. Factors associated with local recurrence after skin-sparing mastectomy and immediate breast reconstruction for invasive breast cancer. *Ann Surg.* 2002;235(6):814–819.

73. Carlson GW, Styblo TM, Lyles RH, et al. Local recurrence after skin-sparing mastectomy: tumor biology or surgical conservatism? *Ann Surg Oncol.* 2003;10(2):108–112.

74. Spiegel AJ, Butler CE. Recurrence following treatment of ductal carcinoma in situ with skin-sparing mastectomy and immediate breast reconstruction. *Plast Reconstr Surg.* 2003;111(2):706–711.

75. Greenway RM, Schlossberg L, Dooley WC. Fifteen-year series of skin-sparing mastectomy for stage 0 to 2 breast cancer. *Am J Surg.* 2005;190(6):933–938.

76. Yi M, Kronowitz SJ, Meric-Bernstam F, et al. Local, regional, and systemic recurrence rates in patients undergoing skin-sparing mastectomy compared with conventional mastectomy. *Cancer.* 2011;117(5):916–924.

77. Romics L, Chew B, Weiler-Mithoff E, et al. Ten-year follow-up of skin-sparing mastectomy followed by immediate breast reconstruction. *Br J Surg.* 2012;99(6):799–806.

78. Foster RD, Esserman LJ, Anthony JP, et al. Skin-sparing mastectomy and immediate breast reconstruction: a prospective cohort study for the treatment of advanced stages of breast carcinoma. *Ann Surg Oncol.* 2002;9(5):462–466.

79. Downes KJ, Glatt BS, Kanchwala SK, et al. Skin-sparing mastectomy and immediate reconstruction is an acceptable treatment option for patients with high-risk breast carcinoma. *Cancer.* 2005;103(5):906–913.

80. Prabhu R, Godette K, Carlson G, et al. The impact of skin-sparing mastectomy with immediate reconstruction in patients with stage III breast cancer treated with neoadjuvant chemotherapy and postmastectomy radiation. *Int J Radiat Oncol Biol Phys.* 2012;82(4):e587–e593.

81. de Alcantara Filho P, Capko D, Barry JM, et al. Nipple-sparing mastectomy for breast cancer and risk-reducing surgery: the Memorial Sloan-Kettering Cancer Center experience. *Ann Surg Oncol.* 2011;18(11):3117–3122.

82. Jensen JA, Orringer JS, Giuliano AE. Nipple-sparing mastectomy in 99 patients with a mean follow-up of 5 years. *Ann Surg Oncol.* 2011;18(6):1665–1670.

83. Peled AW, Foster RD, Garwood ER, et al. The effects of acellular dermal matrix in expander-implant breast reconstruction after total skin-sparing mastectomy: results of a prospective practice improvement study. *Plast Reconstr Surg.* 2012;129(6):901e–908e.

84. Weidong L, Shuling W, Xiaojing G, et al. Nipple involvement in breast cancer: retrospective analysis of 2323 consecutive mastectomy specimens. *Int J Surg Pathol.* 2011; 19(3):328–334.

85. Giuliano AE, Kirgan DM, Guenther JM, Morton DL. Lymphatic mapping and sentinel lymphadenectomy for breast cancer. *Ann Surg.* 1994;220(3):391–398; discussion 398–401.

86. Giuliano AE, Dale PS, Turner RR, et al. Improved axillary staging of breast cancer with sentinel lymphadenectomy. *Ann Surg.* 1995;222(3):394–399; discussion 399–401.

87. Krag D, Weaver D, Ashikaga T, et al. The sentinel node in breast cancer—a multicenter validation study. *N Engl J Med.* 1998;339(14):941–946.

88. Wong SL, Edwards MJ, Chao C, et al. Sentinel lymph node biopsy for breast cancer: impact of the number of sentinel nodes removed on the false-negative rate. *J Am Coll Surg.* 2001;192(6):684–689.

89. Chagpar A, Martin RC III, Chao C, et al. Validation of subareolar and periareolar injection techniques for breast sentinel lymph node biopsy. *Ann Surg.* 2004;139(6):614–620.

90. McMasters KM, Wong SL, Martin RC, et al. Dermal injection of radioactive colloid is superior to peritumoral injection for breast cancer sentinel lymph node biopsy: results of a multiinstitutional study. *Ann Surg.* 2001;233(5):676–687.

91. Krag DN, Anderson SJ, Julian TB, et al. Sentinel-lymph-node resection compared with conventional axillary-lymph-node dissection in clinically node-negative patients with breast cancer: overall survival findings from the NSABP B-32 randomised phase 3 trial. *Lancet Oncol.* 2010;11(10):927–933.

92. Giuliano AE, McCall L, Beitsch P, et al. Locoregional recurrence after sentinel lymph node dissection with or without axillary dissection in patients with sentinel lymph node metastases: the American College of Surgeons Oncology Group Z0011 randomized trial. *Ann Surg.* 2010;252(3):426–432; discussion 432–433.

93. Giuliano AE, Hunt KK, Ballman KV, et al. Axillary dissection vs no axillary dissection in women with invasive breast cancer and sentinel node metastasis: a randomized clinical trial. *JAMA.* 2011;305(6):569–575.

94. Galimberti V, Cole BF, Zurrida S, et al. Axillary dissection versus no axillary dissection in patients with sentinel-node micrometastases (IBCSG 23–01): a phase 3 randomised controlled trial. *Lancet Oncol.* 2013;14(4):297–305.

95. Donker M, van Tienhoven G, Straver ME, et al. Radiotherapy or surgery of the axilla after a positive sentinel node in breast cancer (EORTC 10981-22023 AMAROS): a randomised, multicentre, open-label, phase 3 non-inferiority trial. *Lancet Oncol.* 2014;15(12):1303–1310.

Radiation Therapy in the Adjuvant Setting Following Surgery

96. Marks LB, Prosnitz LR. Reducing local therapy in patients responding to preoperative systemic therapy: are we outsmarting ourselves? *J Clin Oncol.* 2014;32(6):491–493.

Radiation Therapy as an Adjuvant to BCS for Early-Stage BC

97. NIH consensus conference. Treatment of early-stage breast cancer. *JAMA.* 1991;265(3): 391–395.

98. Fisher B, Jeong JH, Anderson S, et al. Twenty-five-year follow-up of a randomized trial comparing radical mastectomy, total mastectomy, and total mastectomy followed by irradiation. *N Engl J Med.* 2002;347(8):567–575.

99. Clarke M, Collins R, Darby S, et al. Effects of radiotherapy and of differences in the extent of surgery for early breast cancer on local recurrence and 15-year survival: an overview of the randomised trials. *Lancet.* 2005;366(9503):2087–2106.

100. Early Breast Cancer Trialists' Collaborative Group; Darby S, McGale P, Correa C, et al. Effect of radiotherapy after breast-conserving surgery on 10-year recurrence and 15-year breast cancer death: meta-analysis of individual patient data for 10,801 women in 17 randomised trials. *Lancet.* 2011;378(9804):1707–1716. doi:10.1016/S0140-6736(11)61629-2

101. Fisher B, Bryant J, Dignam JJ, et al. Tamoxifen, radiation therapy, or both for prevention of ipsilateral breast tumor recurrence after lumpectomy in women with invasive breast cancers of one centimeter or less. *J Clin Oncol.* 2002;20(20):4141–4149.

102. Hughes KS, Schnaper LA, Berry D, et al. Lumpectomy plus tamoxifen with or without irradiation in women 70 years of age or older with early breast cancer. *N Engl J Med.* 2004;351(10):971–977.

103. Hughes KS, Schnaper LA, Bellon JR, et al. Lumpectomy plus tamoxifen with or without irradiation in women age 70 years or older with early breast cancer: long-term follow-up of CALGB 9343. *J Clin Oncol.* 2013;31(19):2382–2387.

104. Kunkler IH, Williams LJ, Jack WJ, et al. Breast-conserving surgery with or without irradiation in women aged 65 years or older with early breast cancer (PRIME II): a randomised controlled trial. *Lancet Oncol.* 2015;16(3):266–273.

105. Tanguturi SK, Lyatskaya Y, Chen Y, et al. Prospective assessment of deep inspiration breath-hold using 3-dimensional surface tracking for irradiation of left-sided breast cancer. *Pract Radiat Oncol.* 2015;5(6):358–365. doi:10.1016/j.prro.2015.06.002

106. Krengli M, Masini L, Caltavuturo T, et al. Prone versus supine position for adjuvant breast radiotherapy: a prospective study in patients with pendulous breasts. *Radiat Oncol.* 2013;8;8:232. doi:10.1186/1748-717X-8-232

107. Veldeman L, Schiettecatte K, De Sutter C, et al. The 2-year cosmetic outcome of a randomized trial comparing prone and supine whole-breast irradiation in large-breasted women. *Int J Radiat Oncol Biol Phys.* 2016;95:1210–1217. doi:10.1016/j.ijrobp.2016.03.003

108. Donovan E, Bleakley N, Denholm E, et al. Randomised trial of standard 2D radiotherapy (RT) versus intensity modulated radiotherapy (IMRT) in patients prescribed breast radiotherapy. *Radiother Oncol.* 2007;82:254–264.

109. Pignol J, Olivotto I, Rakovitch E, et al. A multicenter randomized trial of breast intensity-modulated radiation therapy to reduce acute radiation dermatitis. *J Clin Oncol.* 2008;26:2085–2092.

110. Freedman G, Li T, Nicolaou N, Anderson P. Breast intensity modulated radiation therapy reduces time spent with acute dermatitis for women of all breast sizes during radiation. *Int J Radiat Oncol Biol Phys.* 2009;74:689–694.

111. McDonald MW, Godette KD, Butker EK, et al. Long-term outcomes of IMRT for breast cancer: a single-institution cohort analysis. *Int J Radiat Oncol Biol Phys.* 2008;72:1031–1040.

112. Harsolia A, Kestin L, Grills I, et al. Intensity-modulated radiotherapy results in significant decrease in clinical toxicities compared with conventional wedge-based breast radiotherapy. *Int J Radiat Oncol Biol Phys.* 2007;68:1375–1380.

113. Murphy C, Anderson PR, Li T, et al. Impact of the radiation boost on outcomes after breast-conserving surgery and radiation. *Int J Radiat Oncol Biol Phys.* 2011;81(1):69–76. doi:10.1016/j.ijrobp.2010.04.067

114. Rosen PP, Fracchia AA, Urban JA, et al. "Residual" mammary carcinoma following simulated partial mastectomy. *Cancer.* 1975;35(3):739–747.

115. Bentzen SM, Agrawal RK, Aird EG, et al. The UK Standardisation of Breast Radiotherapy (START) Trial A of radiotherapy hypofractionation for treatment of early breast cancer: a randomised trial. *Lancet Oncol.* 2008;9(4):331–341.

116. Bentzen SM, Agrawal RK, Aird EG, et al. The UK Standardisation of Breast Radiotherapy (START) Trial B of radiotherapy hypofractionation for treatment of early breast cancer: a randomised trial. *Lancet.* 2008;371(9618):1098–1107.

117. Owen JR, Ashton A, Bliss JM, et al. Effect of radiotherapy fraction size on tumour control in patients with early-stage breast cancer after local tumour excision: long-term results of a randomised trial. *Lancet Oncol.* 2006;7(6):467–471.

118. Whelan T, MacKenzie R, Julian J, et al. Randomized trial of breast irradiation schedules after lumpectomy for women with lymph node-negative breast cancer. *J Natl Cancer Inst.* 2002;94(15):1143–1150.

119. Whelan TJ, Pignol JP, Julian J, et al. Long-term results of a randomized trial of accelerated hypofractionated whole breast irradiation following breast conserving surgery in women with node-negative breast cancer. *Int J Radiat Oncol Biol Phys.* 2008;72(suppl):A60, S28.

120. Yarnold J, Ashton A, Bliss J, et al. Fractionation sensitivity and dose response of late adverse effects in the breast after radiotherapy for early breast cancer: long-term results of a randomised trial. *Radiother Oncol.* 2005;75(1):9–17.

121. Whelan TJ, Pignol JP, Levine MN, et al. Long-term results of hypofractionated radiation therapy for breast cancer. *N Engl J Med.* 2010;362(6):513–520.

122. Haviland JS, Owen JR, Dewar JA, et al. The UK Standardisation of Breast Radiotherapy (START) trials of radiotherapy hypofractionation for treatment of early breast cancer: 10-year follow-up results of two randomised controlled trials. *Lancet Oncol.* 2013;14(11):1086–1094.

123. Shaitelman SF, Schlembach PJ, Arzu I, et al. Acute and short-term toxic effects of conventionally fractionated vs hypofractionated whole-breast irradiation: a randomized clinical trial. *JAMA Oncol.* 2015;1(7):931–941.

124. Jagsi R, Griffith KA, Boike TP, et al. Differences in the acute toxic effects of breast radiotherapy by fractionation schedule: comparative analysis of physician-assessed and patient-reported outcomes in a large multicenter cohort. *JAMA Oncol.* 2015;1(7):918–930.

125. Smith BD, Bentzen SM, Correa CR, et al. Fractionation for whole breast irradiation: an American Society for Radiation Oncology (ASTRO) evidence-based guideline. *Int J Radiat Oncol Biol Phys.* 2011;81(1):59–68.

126. Clark RM, Whelan T, Levine M, et al. Randomized clinical trial of breast irradiation following lumpectomy and axillary dissection for node-negative breast cancer: an update. Ontario Clinical Oncology Group. *J Natl Cancer Inst.* 1996;88(22):1659–1664.

127. Holli K, Saaristo R, Isola J, et al. Lumpectomy with or without postoperative radiotherapy for breast cancer with favourable prognostic features: results of a randomized study. *Br J Cancer.* 2001;84(2):164–169.

128. Liljegren G, Holmberg L, Bergh J, et al. 10-year results after sector resection with or without postoperative radiotherapy for stage I breast cancer: a randomized trial. *J Clin Oncol.* 1999;17(8):2326–2333.

129. Romestaing P, Lehingue Y, Carrie C, et al. Role of a 10-Gy boost in the conservative treatment of early breast cancer: results of a randomized clinical trial in Lyon, France. *J Clin Oncol.* 1997;15(3):963–968.

130. Bartelink H, Horiot JC, Poortmans P, et al. Recurrence rates after treatment of breast cancer with standard radiotherapy with or without additional radiation. *N Engl J Med.* 2001;345(19):1378–1387.

131. Poortmans PM, Collette L, Bartelink H, et al. The addition of a boost dose on the primary tumour bed after lumpectomy in breast conserving treatment for breast cancer. A summary of the results of EORTC 22881-10882 "boost versus no boost" trial. *Cancer Radiother.* 2008;12(6–7):565–570.

132. Bartelink H, Horiot JC, Poortmans PM, et al. Impact of a higher radiation dose on local control and survival in breast-conserving therapy of early breast cancer: 10-year results of the randomized boost versus no boost EORTC 22881-10882 trial. *J Clin Oncol.* 2007;25(22):3259–3265.

133. Nattinger AB, Kneusel RT, Hoffmann RG, Gilligan MA. Relationship of distance from a radiotherapy facility and initial breast cancer treatment. *J Natl Cancer Inst.* 2001;93:1344–1346.

134. Nattinger AB, Hoffmann RG, Kneusel RT, Schapira MM. Relation between appropriateness of primary therapy for early-stage breast carcinoma and increased use of breast-conserving surgery. *Lancet.* 2000;356:1148–1153.

135. Strnad V, Ott OJ, Hildebrandt G, et al. 5-year results of accelerated partial breast irradiation using sole interstitial multicatheter brachytherapy versus whole-breast irradiation with boost after breast-conserving surgery for low-risk invasive and in-situ carcinoma of the female breast: a randomised, phase 3, non-inferiority trial. *Lancet.* 2016;387(10015):229–238. doi:10.1016/S0140-6736(15)00471-7

136. Vaidya JS, Joseph DJ, Tobias JS, et al. Targeted intraoperative radiotherapy versus whole breast radiotherapy for breast cancer (TARGIT-A trial): an international, prospective, randomised, non-inferiority phase 3 trial. *Lancet.* 2010;376:91–102.

137. Orecchia R. ELIOT trials in Milan: results. *Radiother Oncol.* 2012;103:S4.

138. Olivotto IA, Whelan TJ, Parpia S, et al. Interim cosmetic and toxicity results from RAPID: a randomized trial of accelerated partial breast irradiation using three-dimensional conformal external beam radiation therapy. *J Clin Oncol.* 2013;31:4038–4045.

139. Leonard KL, Hepel JT, Hiatt JR, et al. The effect of dose-volume parameters and interfraction interval on cosmetic outcome and toxicity after 3-dimensional conformal accelerated partial breast irradiation. *Int J Radiat Oncol Biol Phys.* 2013;85:623–629.

140. Hepel JT, Tokita M, MacAusland SG, et al. Toxicity of three-dimensional conformal radiotherapy for accelerated partial breast irradiation. *Int J Radiat Oncol Biol Phys.* 2009;75:1290–1296.

141. Smith GL, Xu Y, Buchholz TA, et al. Association between treatment with brachytherapy vs whole-breast irradiation and subsequent mastectomy, complications, and survival among older women with invasive breast cancer. *JAMA.* 2012;307(17):1827–1837. doi:10.1001/jama.2012.3481

142. Smith BD, Arthur DW, Buchholz TA, et al. Accelerated partial breast irradiation consensus statement from the American Society for Radiation Oncology (ASTRO). *Int J Radiat Oncol Biol Phys.* 2009;74(4):987–1001.

143. Shaitelman SF, Vicini FA, Beitsch P, et al. Five-year outcome of patients classified using the American Society for Radiation Oncology consensus statement guidelines for the application of accelerated partial breast irradiation: an analysis of patients treated on the American Society of Breast Surgeons MammoSite Registry Trial. *Cancer.* 2010;116(20):4677–4685. doi:10.1002/cncr.25383

144. Vicini F, Shah C, Ben Wilkinson J, et al. Should ductal carcinoma-in-situ (DCIS) be removed from the ASTRO consensus panel cautionary group for off-protocol use of accelerated partial breast irradiation (APBI)? A pooled analysis of outcomes for 300 patients with DCIS treated with APBI. *Ann Surg Oncol.* 2013;20(4):1275–1281. doi:10.1245/s10434-012-2694-7

145. Julian TB, Costantino JP, Vicini FA, et al. Early toxicity results with 3-d conformal external beam therapy (CEBT) from the NSABP B-39/RTOG 0413 Accelerated Partial Breast Irradiation (APBI) Trial [abstract]. *Int J Radiat Oncol Biol Phys.* 2011; 81(suppl 2):S7.

146. Yu CX, Shao X, Zhang J, et al. GammaPod—a new device dedicated for stereotactic radiotherapy of breast cancer. *Med Phys.* 2013;40:051703.

147. Ödén J, Toma-Dasu I, Yu CX, et al. Dosimetric comparison between intra-cavitary breast brachytherapy techniques for accelerated partial breast irradiation and a novel stereotactic radiotherapy device for breast cancer: GammaPod™. *Phys Med Biol.* 2013;58:4409–4421.

148. Mutaf YD, Yu C, Nichols EN, et al. Localization accuracy of a novel prone breast stereotactic immobilization. *Med Phys.* 2013;40:93. doi:10.1118/1.4813969

149. Snider III JW, Mutaf Y, Hall A, et al. Dosimetric improvements based on vacuum assisted breast immobilization utilized with a novel breast stereotactic radiation therapy (BSRT) device. 2015;93(3)(suppl):E53.

150. Nichols EM, Dhople AA, Mohiuddin MM, et al. Comparative analysis of the post-lumpectomy target volume versus the use of pre-lumpectomy tumor volume for early stage breast cancer: implications for the future. *Int J Radiat Oncol Biol Phys.* 2010;77:197–202.

151. Nichols EM, Feigenberg SJ, Marter K, et al. Preoperative radiation therapy significantly increases patient eligibility for accelerated partial breast irradiation using 3D-conformal radiotherapy. *Am J Clin Oncol.* 2013;36:232–238.

152. Overgaard M, Hansen PS, Overgaard J, et al. Postoperative radiotherapy in high-risk premenopausal women with breast cancer who receive adjuvant chemotherapy. Danish Breast Cancer Cooperative Group 82b Trial. *N Engl J Med.* 1997;337(14):949–955.

153. Overgaard M, Jensen MB, Overgaard J, et al. Postoperative radiotherapy in high-risk postmenopausal breast-cancer patients given adjuvant tamoxifen: Danish Breast Cancer Cooperative Group DBCG 82c randomised trial. *Lancet.* 1999;353(9165):1641–1648.

154. Ragaz J, Olivotto IA, Spinelli JJ, et al. Locoregional radiation therapy in patients with high-risk breast cancer receiving adjuvant chemotherapy: 20-year results of the British Columbia randomized trial. *J Natl Cancer Inst.* 2005;97(2):116–126.

155. Recht A, Edge SB, Solin LJ, et al. Postmastectomy radiotherapy: clinical practice guidelines of the American Society of Clinical Oncology. *J Clin Oncol.* 2001;19(5):1539–1569.

156. Olson JA, Jr, McCall LM, Beitsch P, et al. Impact of immediate versus delayed axillary node dissection on surgical outcomes in breast cancer patients with positive sentinel nodes: results from American College of Surgeons Oncology Group Trials Z0010 and Z0011. *J Clin Oncol.* 2008;26(21):3530–3535.

157. Jagsi R, Chadha M, Moni J, et al. Radiation field design in the ACOSOG Z0011 (Alliance) Trial. *J Clin Oncol.* 2014;32(32):3600–3606.

158. Poortmans PM, Collette S, Kirkove C, et al. Internal mammary and medial supraclavicular irradiation in breast cancer. *N Engl J Med.* 2015;373(4):317–327.

159. Whelan TJ, Olivotto IA, Parulekar WR, et al. Regional nodal irradiation in early-stage breast cancer. *N Engl J Med.* 2015;373(4):307–316.

160. Thorsen LB, Offersen BV, Dano H, et al. DBCG-IMN: a population-based cohort study on the effect of internal mammary node irradiation in early node-positive breast cancer. *J Clin Oncol.* 2016;34(4):314–320. doi:10.1200/JCO.2015.63.6456

161. Darby SC, Ewertz M, McGale P, et al. Risk of ischemic heart disease in women after radiotherapy for breast cancer. *N Engl J Med.* 2013;368(11):987–998.

162. Early Breast Cancer Trialists' Collaborative Group; McGale P, Taylor C, Correa C, et al. Effect of radiotherapy after mastectomy and axillary surgery on 10-year recurrence and 20-year breast cancer mortality: meta-analysis of individual patient data for 8135 women in 22 randomised trials. *Lancet.* 2014;383(9935):2127–2135. doi:10.1016/S0140-6736(14)60488-8

163. Floyd SR, Taghian AG. Post-mastectomy radiation in large node-negative breast tumors: does size really matter? *Radiother Oncol.* 2009;91(1):33–37. doi:10.1016/j.radonc.2008.09.015

164. Johnson ME, Handorf EA, Martin JM, Hayes SB. Postmastectomy radiation therapy for T3N0: a SEER analysis. *Cancer.* 2014;120(22):3569–3574. doi:10.1002/cncr.28865

165. Kyndi M, Sørensen FB, Knudsen H, et al. Estrogen receptor, progesterone receptor, HER-2, and response to postmastectomy radiotherapy in high-risk breast cancer: the Danish Breast Cancer Cooperative Group. *J Clin Oncol.* 2008;26(9):1419–1426. doi:10.1200/JCO.2007.14.5565

166. Wallgren A, Bonetti M, Gelber RD, et al. Risk factors for locoregional recurrence among breast cancer patients: results from International Breast Cancer Study Group Trials I through VII. *J Clin Oncol.* 2003;21(7):1205–1213.

167. Jagsi R, Abrahamse P, Morrow M, et al. Patterns and correlates of adjuvant radiotherapy receipt after lumpectomy and after mastectomy for breast cancer. *J Clin Oncol.* 2010;28(14):2396–2403. doi:10.1200/JCO.2009.26.8433

168. Kyndi M, Overgaard M, Nielsen HM, et al. High local recurrence risk is not associated with large survival reduction after postmastectomy radiotherapy in high-risk breast cancer: a subgroup analysis of DBCG 82 b&c. *Radiother Oncol.* 2009;90(1):74–79. doi:10.1016/j.radonc.2008.04.014

169. Truong PT, Sadek BT, Lesperance MF, et al. Is biological subtype prognostic of locoregional recurrence risk in women with pT1-2N0 breast cancer treated with mastectomy? *Int J Radiat Oncol Biol Phys.* 2014;88(1):57–64. doi:10.1016/j.ijrobp.2013.09.024

170. Karlsson P, Cole BF, Chua BH, et al. Patterns and risk factors for locoregional failures after mastectomy for breast cancer: an International Breast Cancer Study Group report. *Ann Oncol.* 2012;23(11):2852–2858. doi:10.1093/annonc/mds118

171. Freedman GM, Fowble BL, Hanlon AL, et al. A close or positive margin after mastectomy is not an indication for chest wall irradiation except in women aged fifty or younger. *Int J Radiat Oncol Biol Phys.* 1998;41(3):599–605.

172. Childs SK, Chen YH, Duggan MM, et al. Surgical margins and the risk of local-regional recurrence after mastectomy without radiation therapy. *Int J Radiat Oncol Biol Phys.* 2012;84(5):1133–1138. doi:10.1016/j.ijrobp.2012.02.048

173. Katz A, Strom EA, Buchholz TA, et al. The influence of pathologic tumor characteristics on locoregional recurrence rates following mastectomy. *Int J Radiat Oncol Biol Phys.* 2001;50(3):735–742.

Systemic Adjuvant Therapy

174. Anampa J, Makower D, Sparano JA. Progress in adjuvant chemotherapy for breast cancer: an overview. *BMC Med.* 2015;13:195.

175. Brown-Glaberman U, Dayao Z, Royce M. HER2-targeted therapy for early-stage breast cancer: a comprehensive review. *Oncology (Williston Park).* 2014;28(4):281–289.

176. Isakoff S. Triple-negative breast cancer: role of specific chemotherapy agents. *Cancer J.* 2010;16(1):53–61.

177. Loprinzi CL, Thomé SD. Understanding the utility of adjuvant systemic therapy for primary breast cancer. *J Clin Oncol.* 2001;19(4):972–979.

178. Miller E, Lee HJ, Lulla A, et al. Current treatment of early breast cancer: adjuvant and neoadjuvant therapy [version 1; referees: 2 approved]. *F1000Res.* 2014;3:198.

179. Early Breast Cancer Trialists' Collaborative Group. Comparisons between different polychemotherapy regimens for early breast cancer: meta-analyses of long-term outcome among 100 000 women in 123 randomised trials. *Lancet.* 2012;379(9814):432–444.

180. Early Breast Cancer Trialists' Collaborative Group. Effects of chemotherapy and hormonal therapy for early breast cancer on recurrence and 15-year survival: an overview of the randomised trials. *Lancet.* 2005;365(9472):1687–1717.

181. Coates AS, Winer EP, Goldhirsch A, et al. Tailoring therapies—improving the management of early breast cancer: St Gallen International Expert Consensus on the Primary Therapy of Early Breast Cancer 2015. *Ann Oncol.* 2015;26(8):1533–1546.

182. Fornier MN, Modi S, Panageas KS, et al. Incidence of chemotherapy-induced, long-term amenorrhea in patients with breast carcinoma age 40 years and younger after adjuvant anthracycline and taxane. *Cancer* [Internet]. 2005;104(8):1575–1579. doi:10.1002/cncr.21385

183. Goss PE, Strasser K. Aromatase inhibitors in the treatment and prevention of breast cancer. *J Clin Oncol.* 2001;19(3):881–894.

184. Lønning PE, Lien EA. Mechanisms of action of endocrine treatment in breast cancer. *Crit Rev Oncol.* 1995;21(1):158–193.

185. DeVita VTL, Theodore S, Rosenberg SA. *DeVita, Hellman, and Rosenberg's Cancer: Principles & Practice of Oncology.* Ninth, North American Edition. 2011.

186. Early Breast Cancer Trialists' Collaborative Group. Relevance of breast cancer hormone receptors and other factors to the efficacy of adjuvant tamoxifen: patient-level meta-analysis of randomised trials. *Lancet.* 2011;378(9793):771–784.

187. Fisher B, Dignam J, Bryant J, et al. Five versus more than five years of tamoxifen therapy for breast cancer patients with negative lymph nodes and estrogen receptor-positive tumors. *J Natl Cancer Inst.* 1996;88(21):1529–1542.

188. Fisher B, Dignam J, Bryant J, Wolmark N. Five versus more than five years of tamoxifen for lymph node-negative breast cancer: updated findings from the National Surgical Adjuvant Breast and Bowel Project B-14 randomized trial. *J Natl Cancer Inst.* 2001;93(9):684–690.

189. Davies C, Pan H, Godwin J, et al. Long-term effects of continuing adjuvant tamoxifen to 10 years versus stopping at 5 years after diagnosis of oestrogen receptor-positive breast cancer: ATLAS, a randomised trial. *Lancet.* 2013;381(9869):805–816.

190. Gray RG, Rea D, Handley K, et al. aTTom: Long-term effects of continuing adjuvant tamoxifen to 10 years versus stopping at 5 years in 6,953 women with early breast cancer. *J Clin Oncol.* 2013;31(18)(suppl):Abstract 5.

191. Early Breast Cancer Trialists' Collaborative Group. Aromatase inhibitors versus tamoxifen in early breast cancer: patient-level meta-analysis of the randomised trials. *Lancet.* 2015;386(10001):1341–1352.

192. Baum M, Budzar A, Cuzick J, et al. ATAC Trialists' Group. Anastrozole alone or in combination with tamoxifen versus tamoxifen alone for adjuvant treatment of postmenopausal women with early breast cancer: first results of the ATAC randomised trial. *Lancet.* 2002;359(9324):2131–2139.

193. Cuzick J, Sestak I, Baum M, et al. Effect of anastrozole and tamoxifen as adjuvant treatment for early-stage breast cancer: 10-year analysis of the ATAC trial. *Lancet Oncol.* 2010;11(12):1135–1141.

194. Breast International Group (BIG) 1-98 Collaborative Group; Thurlimann B, Keshaviah A, Coates AS, et al. A comparison of letrozole and tamoxifen in postmenopausal women with early breast cancer. *N Engl J Med.* 2005;353(26):2747–2757.

195. BIG 1-98 Collaborative Group; Mouridsen H, Giobbie-Hurder A, Goldhirsch A, et al. Letrozole therapy alone or in sequence with tamoxifen in women with breast cancer. *N Engl J Med.* 2009;361(8):766–776.

196. Van de Velde CJ, Rea D, Seynaeve C, et al. Adjuvant tamoxifen and exemestane in early breast cancer (TEAM): a randomised phase 3 trial. *Lancet.* 2011;377(9762):321–331.

197. Coombes RC, Hall E, Gibson LJ, et al. A randomized trial of exemestane after two to three years of tamoxifen therapy in postmenopausal women with primary breast cancer. *N Engl J Med.* 2004;350(11):1081–1092.

198. Coombes R, Kilburn L, Snowdon C, et al. Survival and safety of exemestane versus tamoxifen after 2–3 years' tamoxifen treatment (Intergroup Exemestane Study): a randomised controlled trial. *Lancet.* 2007;369(9561):559–570.

199. Goss PE, Ingle JN, Martino S, et al. Randomized trial of letrozole following tamoxifen as extended adjuvant therapy in receptor-positive breast cancer: updated findings from NCIC CTG MA.17. *J Natl Cancer Inst.* 2005;97(17):1262–1271.

200. Goss PE, Ingle JN, Martino S, et al. Efficacy of letrozole extended adjuvant therapy according to estrogen receptor and progesterone receptor status of the primary tumor: National Cancer Institute of Canada Clinical Trials Group MA.17. *J Clin Oncol.* 2007;25(15):2006–2011.

201. Jin H, Tu D, Zhao N, et al. Longer-term outcomes of letrozole versus placebo after 5 years of tamoxifen in the NCIC CTG MA.17 trial: analyses adjusting for treatment crossover. *J Clin Oncol.* 2012;30(7):718–721.

202. Goss PE, Ingle JN, Pater JL, et al. Late extended adjuvant treatment with letrozole improves outcome in women with early-stage breast cancer who complete 5 years of tamoxifen. *J Clin Oncol.* 2008;26(12):1948–1955.

203. Mamounas EP, Jeong JH, Wickerham DL, et al. Benefit from exemestane as extended adjuvant therapy after 5 years of adjuvant tamoxifen: intention-to-treat analysis of the National Surgical Adjuvant Breast and Bowel Project B-33 trial. *J Clin Oncol.* 2008;26(12):1965–1971.

204. Goss PE, Ingle JN, Pritchard KI, et al. Extending Aromatase-Inhibitor Adjuvant Therapy to 10 Years. *N Engl J Med.* 2016;375:209–219. doi:10.1056/NEJMoa1604700

205. Goss PE, Ingle JN, Pritchard KI, et al. Exemestane versus anastrozole in postmenopausal women with early breast cancer: NCIC CTG MA.27—a randomized controlled phase III trial. *J Clin Oncol.* 2013;31(11):1398–1404.

206. O'Shaughnessy J, Yardley D, Burris H, et al. Abstract PD2-01: randomized phase 3 trial of adjuvant letrozole versus anastrozole in postmenopausal patients with hormone receptor positive, node positive early breast cancer: Final efficacy and safety results of the femara versus anastrozole clinical evaluation (Face) trial. *Cancer Res.* 2016; 76(4)(suppl):PD2,01-PD2-01.

207. Francis PA, Regan MM, Fleming GF, et al. Adjuvant ovarian suppression in premenopausal breast cancer. *N Engl J Med.* 2015;372(5):436–446.

208. Pagani O, Regan MM, Walley BA, et al. Adjuvant exemestane with ovarian suppression in premenopausal breast cancer. *N Engl J Med.* 2014;371(2):107–118.

209. Kaufmann M, Jonat W, Hilfrich J, et al. Improved overall survival in postmenopausal women with early breast cancer after anastrozole initiated after treatment with tamoxifen compared with continued tamoxifen: the ARNO 95 Study. *J Clin Oncol.* 2007;25(19):2664–2670.

210. Jakesz R, Gnant M, Griel R, et al. Tamoxifen and anastrozole as a sequencing strategy in postmenopausal women with hormone-responsive early breast cancer: updated data from the Austrian breast and colorectal cancer study group trial 8. *Cancer Res.* 2009;69(2)(suppl):14.

211. Boccardo F, Rubagotti A, Puntoni M, et al. Switching to anastrozole versus continued tamoxifen treatment of early breast cancer: preliminary results of the Italian Tamoxifen Anastrozole Trial. *J Clin Oncol.* 2005;23(22):5138–5147.

212. Jakesz R, Jonat W, Gnant M, et al. Switching of postmenopausal women with endocrine-responsive early breast cancer to anastrozole after 2 years' adjuvant tamoxifen: combined results of ABCSG trial 8 and ARNO 95 trial. *Lancet.* 2005;366(9484): 455–462.

213. Jakesz R, Greil R, Gnant M, et al. Extended adjuvant therapy with anastrozole among postmenopausal breast cancer patients: results from the randomized Austrian Breast and Colorectal Cancer Study Group Trial 6a. *J Natl Cancer Inst.* 2007;99(24):1845–1853.

214. Saphner T, Tormey DC, Gray R. Annual hazard rates of recurrence for breast cancer after primary therapy. *J Clin Oncol.* 1996;14(10):2738–2746.

215. Piccart M, Rutgers E, van' t Veer L, et al. Primary analysis of the EORTC 10041/ BIG 3-04 MINDACT study: a prospective, randomized study evaluating the clinical utility of the 70-gene signature (MammaPrint) combined with common clinical-pathological criteria for selection of patients for adjuvant chemotherapy in breast cancer with 0 to 3 positive nodes [abstract]. In: Proceedings of the 107th Annual Meeting of the American Association for Cancer Research; April 16–20, 2016; New Orleans, LA. Philadelphia, PA: AACR; *Cancer Res.* 2016;76(14)(suppl):Abstract nr CT039.

216. Sparano JA, Gray RJ, Makower DF, et al. Prospective validation of a 21-gene expression assay in breast cancer. *N Engl J Med.* 2015;373(21):2005–2014.

217. Fan C, Oh DS, Wessels L, et al. Concordance among gene-expression–based predictors for breast cancer. *N Engl J Med.* 2006;355(6):560–569.

218. Paik S, Tang G, Shak S, et al. Gene expression and benefit of chemotherapy in women with node-negative, estrogen receptor–positive breast cancer. *J Clin Oncol.* 2006;24(23): 3726–3734.

219. Paik S, Shak S, Tang G, et al. A multigene assay to predict recurrence of tamoxifen-treated, node-negative breast cancer. *N Engl J Med.* 2004;351(27):2817–2826.

220. Goldstein LJ, Gray R, Badve S, et al. Prognostic utility of the 21-gene assay in hormone receptor-positive operable breast cancer compared with classical clinicopathologic features. *J Clin Oncol.* 2008;26(25):4063–4071.

221. Albain KS, Barlow WE, Shak S, et al. Prognostic and predictive value of the 21-gene recurrence score assay in postmenopausal women with node-positive, oestrogen-receptor-positive breast cancer on chemotherapy: a retrospective analysis of a randomised trial. *Lancet Oncol.* 2010;11(1):55–65.

222. National Cancer Institute. Hormone therapy with or without combination chemotherapy in treating women who have undergone surgery for node-negative breast cancer (The TAILORx Trial). *ClinicalTrials.gov* [Internet]. Bethesda, MD: National Library of Medicine (US); 2000. https://clinicaltrials.gov/show/NCT00310180

223. Van De Vijver MJ, He YD, van't Veer LJ, et al. A gene-expression signature as a predictor of survival in breast cancer. *N Engl J Med.* 2002;347(25):1999–2009.

224. Delahaye LJM, Wehkamp D, Floore AN, et al. Performance characteristics of the MammaPrint breast cancer diagnostic gene signature. *Personalized Medicine.* http://www.agendia.com/performance-characteristics-of-the-mammaprint-breast-cancer-diagnostic-gene-signature

225. Drukker CA, Bueno-de-Mesquita J, Retèl VP, et al. A prospective evaluation of a breast cancer prognosis signature in the observational RASTER study. *Int J Cancer.* 2013;133(4):929–936.

226. Buyse M, Loi S, van't Veer L, et al. Validation and clinical utility of a 70-gene prognostic signature for women with node-negative breast cancer. *J Natl Cancer Inst.* 2006;98(17): 1183–1192.

227. Cardoso F, van't Veer LJ, Bogaerts J, et al. 70-gene signature as an aid to treatment decisions in early-stage breast cancer. *N Engl J Med.* 2016;375(8):717–729.

228. Early Breast Cancer Trialists' Collaborative Group; Peto R, Davies C, Godwin J, et al. Comparisons between different polychemotherapy regimens for early breast cancer: meta-analyses of long-term outcome among 100,000 women in 123 randomised trials. *Lancet.* 2012;379(9814):432–444. http://dx.doi.org/10.1016/s0140-6736(11)61625-5

229. Bonadonna G, Brusamolino E, Valagussa P, et al. Combination chemotherapy as an adjuvant treatment in operable breast cancer. *N Engl J Med.* 1976;294(8):405–410.

230. Tancini G, Bonadonna G, Valagussa P, et al. Adjuvant CMF in breast cancer: comparative 5-year results of 12 versus 6 cycles. *J Clin Oncol.* 1983;1(1):2–10.

231. Tan C, Etcubanas E, Wollner N, et al. Adriamycin? An antitumor antibiotic in the treatment of neoplastic diseases. *Cancer.* 1973;32(1):9–17.

232. Brambilla C, Valagussa P, Bonadonna G. Sequential combination chemotherapy in advanced breast cancer. *Cancer Chemother Pharmacol.* 1978;1(1):35–39.

233. Fisher B, Brown AM, Dimitrov NV, et al. Two months of doxorubicin-cyclophosphamide with and without interval reinduction therapy compared with 6 months of cyclophosphamide, methotrexate, and fluorouracil in positive-node breast cancer patients with tamoxifen-nonresponsive tumors: results from the National Surgical Adjuvant Breast and Bowel Project B-15. *J Clin Oncol.* 1990;8(9):1483–1496.

234. Wani M, Taylor H, Wall M, et al. Plant antitumor agents. VI. The isolation and structure of taxol, a novel antileukemic and antitumor agent from Taxus brevifolia. *J Am Chem Soc.* 1971;96:2325–2327.

235. Henderson IC, Berry DA, Demetri GD, et al. Improved outcomes from adding sequential paclitaxel but not from escalating doxorubicin dose in an adjuvant chemotherapy regimen for patients with node-positive primary breast cancer. *J Clin Oncol.* 2003;21(6):976–983.

236. Sparano J. Doxorubicin/taxane combinations: cardiac toxicity and pharmacokinetics. *Semin Oncol.* 1999;26(3):14–19.

237. Jones S, Holmes FA, O'Shaughnessy J, et al. Docetaxel with cyclophosphamide is associated with an overall survival benefit compared with doxorubicin and cyclophosphamide: 7-year follow-up of US oncology research trial 9735. *J Clin Oncol.* 2009;27(8):1177–1183.

238. Martin M, Pienkowski T, Mackey J, et al. Adjuvant docetaxel for node-positive breast cancer. *N Engl J Med.* 2005;352(22):2302–2313.

239. Mackey JR, Martin M, et al. Adjuvant docetaxel, doxorubicin, and cyclophosphamide in node-positive breast cancer: 10-year follow-up of the phase 3 randomised BCIRG 001 trial. *Lancet Oncol.* 2013;14(1):72–80.

240. Nabholtz J, Pienkowski T, Mackey J, et al. Phase III trial comparing TAC (docetaxel, doxorubicin, cyclophosphamide) with FAC (5-fluorouracil, doxorubicin, cyclophosphamide) in the adjuvant treatment of node positive breast cancer (BC) patients: interim analysis of the BCIRG 001 study. *Proc Am Soc Clin Oncol.* 2002;21:141.

241. Eiermann W, Pienkowski T, Crown J, et al. Phase III study of doxorubicin/cyclophosphamide with concomitant versus sequential docetaxel as adjuvant treatment in patients with human epidermal growth factor receptor 2–normal, node-positive breast cancer: BCIRG-005 trial. *J Clin Oncol.* 2011;29(29):3877–3884.

242. Norton L. Adjuvant breast cancer therapy: current status and future strategies—growth kinetics and the improved drug therapy of breast cancer. *Semin Oncol.* 1999;26(1):1–4.

243. Citron ML, Berry DA, Cirrincione C, et al. Randomized trial of dose-dense versus conventionally scheduled and sequential versus concurrent combination chemotherapy as postoperative adjuvant treatment of node-positive primary breast cancer: First report of intergroup trial C9741/cancer and leukemia Group B trial 9741. *J Clin Oncol.* 2003;21(8):1431–1439.

244. Sparano JA, Wang M, Martino S, et al. Weekly paclitaxel in the adjuvant treatment of breast cancer. *N Engl J Med.* 2008;358(16):1663–1671.

245. Budd GT, Barlow WE, Moore HCF, et al. SWOG S0221: a Phase III trial comparing chemotherapy schedules in high-risk early-stage breast cancer. *J Clin Oncol.* 2015;33(1):58–64.

246. Herceptin [package insert]. San Franscisco, CA: Genetech; 2016.

247. Gonzalez-Angulo AM, Litton JK, Broglio KR, et al. High risk of recurrence for patients with breast cancer who have human epidermal growth factor receptor 2–positive, node-negative tumors 1 cm or smaller. *J Clin Oncol.* 2009;27(34):5700–5706.

248. Chia S, Norris B, Speers C, et al. Human epidermal growth factor receptor 2 overexpression as a prognostic factor in a large tissue microarray series of node-negative breast cancers. *J Clin Oncol.* 2008;26(35):5697–5704.

249. Moja L, Tagliabue L, Balduzzi S, et al. Trastuzumab containing regimens for early breast cancer. *Cochrane Database Syst Rev.* 2012;(4):CD006243.

250. Smith I, Procter M, Gelber RD, et al. 2-year follow-up of trastuzumab after adjuvant chemotherapy in HER2-positive breast cancer: a randomised controlled trial. *Lancet.* 2007;369(9555):29–36.

251. Goldhirsch A, Gelber RD, Piccart-Gebhart MJ, et al. 2 years versus 1 year of adjuvant trastuzumab for HER2-positive breast cancer (HERA): an open-label, randomised controlled trial. *Lancet.* 2013;382(9897):1021–1028.

252. Pivot X, Romieu G, Debled M, et al. 6 months versus 12 months of adjuvant trastuzumab for patients with HER2-positive early breast cancer (PHARE): a randomised phase 3 trial. *Lancet Oncol.* 2013;14(8):741–748.

253. Kramar A, Bachelot T, Madrange N, et al. Trastuzumab duration effects within patient prognostic subgroups in the PHARE trial. *Ann Oncol* [Internet]. 2014;25(8):1563–1570. doi:10.1093/annonc/mdu177

254. Perez EA, Romond EH, Suman VJ, et al. Trastuzumab plus adjuvant chemotherapy for human epidermal growth factor receptor 2-positive breast cancer: planned joint analysis of overall survival from NSABP B-31 and NCCTG N9831. *J Clin Oncol.* 2014;32(33):3744–3752.

255. Slamon D, Eiermann W, Robert N, et al. Adjuvant trastuzumab in HER2-positive breast cancer. *N Engl J Med.* 2011;365(14):1273–1283.

256. Slamon DJ, Eiermann W, Robert NJ, et al. Ten-year follow-up of BCIRG-006 comparing doxorubicin plus cyclophosphamide followed by docetaxel with doxorubicin plus cyclophosphamide followed by docetaxel and trastuzumab with docetaxel, carboplatin and trastuzumab in HER2-positive early breast cancer patients. 2015 San Antonio Breast Cancer Symposium. December 11, 2015; Abstract S5–04.

257. Tolaney SM, Barry WT, Dang CT, et al. Adjuvant paclitaxel and trastuzumab for node-negative, HER2-positive breast cancer. *N Engl J Med.* 2015;372(2):134–141.

258. Perjeta Prescribing Highlights [package insert]. San Francisco, CA: Genetech; 2016.

259. Goss PE, Smith IE, O'Shaughnessy J, et al. Adjuvant lapatinib for women with early-stage HER2-positive breast cancer: a randomised, controlled, phase 3 trial. *Lancet Oncol.* 2013;14(1):88–96.

260. Piccart-Gebhart M, Holmes E, Baselga J, et al. Adjuvant lapatinib and trastuzumab for early human epidermal growth factor receptor 2-positive breast cancer: results from the randomized Phase III adjuvant lapatinib and/or trastuzumab treatment optimization trial. *J Clin Oncol.* 2016;34(10):1034–1042.

261. Chan A, Delaloge S, Holmes FA, et al. Neratinib after adjuvant chemotherapy and trastuzumab in HER2-positive early breast cancer: Primary analysis at 2 years of a phase 3, randomized, placebo-controlled trial (ExteNET). *J Clin Oncol.* 2015;33:508.

262. Tryfonidis K, Zardavas D, Cardoso F. Small breast cancers: when and how to treat. *Cancer Treat Rev.* 2014;40(10):1129–1136.

263. Cancello G, Maisonneuve P, Rotmensz N, et al. Prognosis in women with small (T1mic,T1a,T1b) node-negative operable breast cancer by immunohistochemically selected subtypes. *Breast Cancer Res Treat.* 2011;127(3):713–720.

264. Theriault RL, Litton JK, Mittendorf EA, et al. Age and survival estimates in patients who have node-negative t1ab breast cancer by breast cancer subtype. *Clin Breast Cancer.* 2011;11(5):325–331.

265. Berry D, Cirrincione C, Henderson C, et al. Estrogen-receptor status and outcomes of modern chemotherapy for patients with node-positive breast cancer. *JAMA.* 2006;295(14):1658–1667.

Neoadjuvant Treatment Approaches

266. Wolmark N, Wang J, Mamounas E, et al. Preoperative chemotherapy in patients with operable breast cancer: nine-year results from National Surgical Adjuvant Breast and Bowel Project B-18. *J Natl Cancer Inst Monogr.* 2001;30:96–102.

267. van der Hage JA, van de Velde CJ, Julien JP, et al. Preoperative chemotherapy in primary operable breast cancer: results from the European Organization for Research and Treatment of Cancer trial 10902. *J Clin Oncol.* 2001;19(22):4224–4237.

268. von Minckwitz G, Untch M, Blohmer J, et al. Definition and impact of pathologic complete response on prognosis after neoadjuvant chemotherapy in various intrinsic breast cancer subtypes. *J Clin Oncol.* 2012;30(15):1796–1804.

269. Esserman LJ, Berry DA, DeMichele A, et al. Pathologic complete response predicts recurrence-free survival more effectively by cancer subset: results from the I-SPY 1 TRIAL—CALGB 150007/150012, ACRIN 6657. *J Clin Oncol.* 2012;30(26):3242–3249.

270. Cortazar P, Zhang L, Untch M, et al. Pathological complete response and long-term clinical benefit in breast cancer: the CTNeoBC pooled analysis. *Lancet.* 2014;384(9938):164–172.

271. Rouzier R, Perou CM, Symmans WF, et al. Breast cancer molecular subtypes respond differently to preoperative chemotherapy. *Clin Cancer Res.* 2005;11(16):5678–5685.

272. Sikov W, Berry D, Perou C, et al. Event-free and overall survival following neoadjuvant weekly paclitaxel and dose-dense AC/carboplatin and/or bevacizumab in triple-negative breast cancer: outcomes from CALGB 40603 (Alliance). *San Antonio Breast Cancer Symposium.* December 8–12, 2015; San Antonio, TX. doi:10.1158/1538-7445. SABCS15-S2-05

273. von Minckwitz G, Schneeweiss A, Loibl S, et al. Neoadjuvant carboplatin in patients with triple-negative and HER2-positive early breast cancer (GeparSixto; GBG 66): a randomised phase 2 trial. *Lancet Oncol.* 2014;15(7):747–756.

274. Sikov WM, Berry DA, Perou CM, et al. Impact of the addition of carboplatin and/or bevacizumab to neoadjuvant once-per-week paclitaxel followed by dose-dense doxorubicin and cyclophosphamide on pathologic complete response rates in stage II to III triple-negative breast cancer: CALGB 40603 (Alliance). *J Clin Oncol.* 2015;33(1):13–21.

275. Gianni L, Pienkowski T, Im Y, et al. Efficacy and safety of neoadjuvant pertuzumab and trastuzumab in women with locally advanced, inflammatory, or early HER2-positive breast cancer (NeoSphere): a randomised multicentre, open-label, phase 2 trial. *Lancet Oncology.* 2012;13(1):25–32.

276. Schneeweiss A, Chia S, Hickish T, et al. Pertuzumab plus trastuzumab in combination with standard neoadjuvant anthracycline-containing and anthracycline-free chemotherapy regimens in patients with HER2-positive early breast cancer: a randomized phase II cardiac safety study (TRYPHAENA). *Ann Oncol.* 2013;24(9):2278–2284.

277. Gianni L, Eiermann W, Semiglazov V, et al. Neoadjuvant chemotherapy with trastuzumab followed by adjuvant trastuzumab versus neoadjuvant chemotherapy alone, in patients with HER2-positive locally advanced breast cancer (the NOAH trial): a randomised controlled superiority trial with a parallel HER2-negative cohort. *Lancet.* 2010;375(9712):377–384.

278. Gianni L, Eiermann W, Semiglazov V, et al. Neoadjuvant and adjuvant trastuzumab in patients with HER2-positive locally advanced breast cancer (NOAH): follow-up of a randomised controlled superiority trial with a parallel HER2-negative cohort. *Lancet Oncol.* 2014;15(6):640–647.

279. Untch M, Loibl S, Bischoff J, et al. Lapatinib versus trastuzumab in combination with neoadjuvant anthracycline-taxane-based chemotherapy (GeparQuinto, GBG 44): a randomised phase 3 trial. *Lancet Oncol.* 2012;13(2):135–144.

280. Baselga J, Bradbury I, Eidtmann H, et al. Lapatinib with trastuzumab for HER2-positive early breast cancer (NeoALTTO): a randomised, open-label, multicentre, phase 3 trial. *Lancet.* 2012;379(9816):633–640.

281. Guarneri V, Frassoldati A, Bottini A, et al. Preoperative chemotherapy plus trastuzumab, lapatinib, or both in human epidermal growth factor receptor 2-positive operable breast cancer: results of the randomized phase II CHER-LOB study. *J Clin Oncol.* 2012;30(16):1989–1995.

282. Robidoux A, Tang G, Rastogi P, et al. Lapatinib as a component of neoadjuvant therapy for HER2-positive operable breast cancer (NSABP protocol B-41): an open-label, randomised phase 3 trial. *Lancet Oncol.* 2013;14(12):1183–1192.

283. Harbeck N, Gluz O, Christgen M, et al. Efficacy of 12-weeks of neoadjuvant TDM1 with or without endocrine therapy in HER2-positive hormone-receptor-positive early breast cancer: WSG-ADAPT HER2 /HR phase II trial. *J Clin Oncol.* 2015;33:506.

284. Gazet J, Ford H, Bland J, et al. Prospective randomised trial of tamoxifen versus surgery in elderly patients with breast cancer. *Lancet.* 1988;331(8587):679–681.

285. Robertson J, Ellis I, Elston C, Blamey R. Mastectomy or tamoxifen as initial therapy for operable breast cancer in elderly patients: 5-year follow-up. *Eur J Cancer.* 1992;28(4):908–910.

286. Mustacchi G, Milani S, Pluchinotta A, et al. Tamoxifen or surgery plus tamoxifen as primary treatment for elderly patients with operable breast cancer: The G.R.E.T.A. Trial. Group for Research on Endocrine Therapy in the Elderly. *Anticancer Res.* 1994;14(5B):2197–2200.

287. Bates T, Riley D, Houghton J, et al. Breast cancer in elderly women: a Cancer Research Campaign trial comparing treatment with tamoxifen and optimal surgery with tamoxifen alone. *Br J Surg.* 1991;78(5):591–594.

288. Hind D, Wyld L, Beverley C, Reed MW. Surgery versus primary endocrine therapy for operable primary breast cancer in elderly women (70 years plus). *Cochrane Database Syst Rev.* 2006;1(1).

289. Bergman L, Van Dongen J, Van Ooijen B, Van Leeuwen F. Should tamoxifen be a primary treatment choice for elderly breast cancer patients with locoregional disease? *Breast Cancer Res Treat.* 1995;34(1):77–83.

290. Preece PE, Wood RA, Mackie CR, Cuschieri A. Tamoxifen as initial sole treatment of localised breast cancer in elderly women: a pilot study. *Br Med J (Clin Res Ed).* 1982;284(6319):869–870.

291. Semiglazov VF, Semiglazov VV, Dashyan GA, et al. Phase 2 randomized trial of primary endocrine therapy versus chemotherapy in postmenopausal patients with estrogen receptor-positive breast cancer. *Cancer.* 2007;110(2):244–254.

292. Alba E, Calvo L, Albanell J, et al. Chemotherapy (CT) versus hormone therapy (HT) as neoadjuvant treatment in luminal breast cancer: a multicenter, randomized phase II study (GEICAM/2006-03). *Ann Oncol.* 2012; doi:10.1093/annonc/mds132

293. Eiermann W, Paepke S, Appfelstaedt J, et al. Preoperative treatment of postmenopausal breast cancer patients with letrozole: a randomized double-blind multicenter study. *Ann Oncol.* 2001;12(11):1527–1532.

294. Smith IE, Dowsett M, Ebbs SR, et al. Neoadjuvant treatment of postmenopausal breast cancer with anastrozole, tamoxifen, or both in combination: the Immediate Preoperative Anastrozole, Tamoxifen, or Combined with Tamoxifen (IMPACT) multicenter double-blind randomized trial. *J Clin Oncol.* 2005;23(22):5108–5116.

295. Dowsett M, Smith IE, Ebbs SR, et al. Prognostic value of Ki67 expression after short-term presurgical endocrine therapy for primary breast cancer. *J Natl Cancer Inst.* 2007;99(2):167–170.

296. Cataliotti L, Buzdar AU, Noguchi S, et al. Comparison of anastrozole versus tamoxifen as preoperative therapy in postmenopausal women with hormone receptor-positive breast cancer. *Cancer.* 2006;106(10):2095–2103.

297. Seo JH, Kim YH, Kim JS. Meta-analysis of pre-operative aromatase inhibitor versus tamoxifen in postmenopausal woman with hormone receptor-positive breast cancer. *Cancer Chemother Pharmacol.* 2009;63(2):261–266.

298. Ellis MJ, Suman VJ, Hoog J, et al. Randomized phase II neoadjuvant comparison between letrozole, anastrozole, and exemestane for postmenopausal women with estrogen receptor-rich stage 2 to 3 breast cancer: clinical and biomarker outcomes and predictive value of the baseline PAM50-based intrinsic subtype—ACOSOG Z1031. *J Clin Oncol.* 2011;29(17):2342–2349.

299. Llombart-Cussac A, Guerrero Á, Galán A, et al. Phase II trial with letrozole to maximum response as primary systemic therapy in postmenopausal patients with ER/PgR [+] operable breast cancer. *Clin Transl Oncol.* 2012;14(2):125–131.

300. Dixon JM, Renshaw L, Macaskill EJ, et al. Increase in response rate by prolonged treatment with neoadjuvant letrozole. *Breast Cancer Res Treat.* 2009;113(1):145–151.

301. Ellis MJ, Ma C. Letrozole in the neoadjuvant setting: the P024 trial. *Breast Cancer Res Treat.* 2007;105(1):33–43.

302. Ellis MJ, Tao Y, Luo J, et al. Outcome prediction for estrogen receptor-positive breast cancer based on postneoadjuvant endocrine therapy tumor characteristics. *J Natl Cancer Inst.* 2008;100(19):1380–1388.

303. Fisher B, Bryant J, Wolmark N, et al. Effect of preoperative chemotherapy on the outcome of women with operable breast cancer. *J Clin Oncol.* 1998;16(8):2672–2685.

304. Ueno NT, Buzdar AU, Singletary SE, et al. Combined-modality treatment of inflammatory breast carcinoma: twenty years of experience at M. D. Anderson Cancer Center. *Cancer Chemother Pharmacol.* 1997;40(4):321–329.

305. Cristofanilli M, Buzdar AU, Sneige N, et al. Paclitaxel in the multimodality treatment for inflammatory breast carcinoma. *Cancer.* 2001;92(7):1775–1782.

306. Harris EE, Schultz D, Bertsch H, et al. Ten-year outcome after combined modality therapy for inflammatory breast cancer. *Int J Radiat Oncol Biol Phys.* 2003;55(5):1200–1208.

307. Baldini E, Gardin G, Evagelista G, et al. Long-term results of combined-modality therapy for inflammatory breast carcinoma. *Clin Breast Cancer.* 2004;5(5):358–363.

308. Cristofanilli M, Gonzalez-Angulo AM, Buzdar AU, et al. Paclitaxel improves the prognosis in estrogen receptor negative inflammatory breast cancer: the M. D. Anderson Cancer Center experience. *Clin Breast Cancer.* 2004;4(6):415–419.

309. Hennessy BT, Gonzalez-Angulo AM, Hortobagyi GN, et al. Disease-free and overall survival after pathologic complete disease remission of cytologically proven inflammatory breast carcinoma axillary lymph node metastases after primary systemic chemotherapy. *Cancer.* 2006;106(5):1000–1006.

310. Mamounas EP, Brown A, Anderson S, et al. Sentinel node biopsy after neoadjuvant chemotherapy in breast cancer: results from National Surgical Adjuvant Breast and Bowel Project Protocol B-27. *J Clin Oncol.* 2005;23(12):2694–2702.

311. Rastogi P, Anderson SJ, Bear HD, et al. Preoperative chemotherapy: updates of National Surgical Adjuvant Breast and Bowel Project Protocols B-18 and B-27. *J Clin Oncol.* 2008;26(5):778–785.

312. Hunt KK, Yi M, Mittendorf EA, et al. Sentinel lymph node surgery after neoadjuvant chemotherapy is accurate and reduces the need for axillary dissection in breast cancer patients. *Ann Surg.* 2009;250(4):558–566.

313. Takahashi M, Jinno H, Hayashida T, et al. Correlation between clinical nodal status and sentinel lymph node biopsy false negative rate after neoadjuvant chemotherapy. *World J Surg.* 2012;36(12):2847–2852.

314. Kuehn T, Bauerfeind I, Fehm T, et al. Sentinel-lymph-node biopsy in patients with breast cancer before and after neoadjuvant chemotherapy (SENTINA): a prospective, multicentre cohort study. *Lancet Oncol.* 2013;14(7):609–618.

315. Kuehn T, Vogl FD, Helms G, et al. Sentinel-node biopsy for axillary staging in breast cancer: results from a large prospective German multi-institutional trial. *Eur J Surg Oncol.* 2004;30(3):252–259.

316. Kim T, Giuliano AE, Lyman GH. Lymphatic mapping and sentinel lymph node biopsy in early-stage breast carcinoma: a metaanalysis. *Cancer.* 2006;106(1):4–16.

317. Le Bouedec G, Geissler B, Gimbergues P, et al. Sentinel lymph node biopsy for breast cancer after neoadjuvant chemotherapy: influence of nodal status before treatment. *Bull Cancer.* 2006;93(4):415–419.

318. Lee S, Kim EY, Kang SH, et al. Sentinel node identification rate, but not accuracy, is significantly decreased after pre-operative chemotherapy in axillary node-positive breast cancer patients. *Breast Cancer Res Treat.* 2007;102(3):283–288.

319. Newman EA, Sabel MS, Nees AV, et al. Sentinel lymph node biopsy performed after neoadjuvant chemotherapy is accurate in patients with documented node-positive breast cancer at presentation. *Ann Surg Oncol.* 2007;14(10):2946–2952.

320. Shen J, Gilcrease MZ, Babiera GV, et al. Feasibility and accuracy of sentinel lymph node biopsy after preoperative chemotherapy in breast cancer patients with documented axillary metastases. *Cancer.* 2007;109(7):1255–1263.

321. Boughey JC, Suman VJ, Mittendorf EA, et al. Sentinel lymph node surgery after neoadjuvant chemotherapy in patients with node-positive breast cancer: the ACOSOG Z1071 (Alliance) clinical trial. *JAMA.* 2013;310(14):1455–1461.

322. Boughey JC, Ballman KV, Le-Petross HT, et al. Identification and resection of clipped node decreases the false-negative rate of sentinel lymph node surgery in patients presenting with node-positive breast cancer (T0-T4, N1-N2) who receive neoadjuvant chemotherapy: results from ACOSOG Z1071 (Alliance). *Ann Surg.* 2016 Apr;263(4):802–807. doi:10.1097/SLA.0000000000001375

323. Caudle AS, Yang WT, Krishnamurthy S, et al. Improved axillary evaluation following neoadjuvant therapy for patients with node-positive breast cancer using selective evaluation of clipped nodes: implementation of targeted axillary dissection. *J Clin Oncol.* 2016 Apr;34(10):1072–1078. doi:10.1200/JCO.2015.64.0094

324. Buchholz TA, Lehman CD, Harris JR, et al. Statement of the science concerning locoregional treatments after preoperative chemotherapy for breast cancer: a National Cancer Institute conference. *J Clin Oncol.* 2008;26(5):791–797. doi:10.1200/JCO.2007.15.0326

325. Garg AK, Buchholz TA. Influence of neoadjuvant chemotherapy on radiotherapy for breast cancer. *Ann Surg Oncol.* 2015;22(5):1434–1440. doi:10.1245/s10434-015-4402-x

326. Buchholz TA, Katz A, Strom EA, et al. Pathologic tumor size and lymph node status predict for different rates of locoregional recurrence after mastectomy for breast cancer patients treated with neoadjuvant versus adjuvant chemotherapy. *Int J Radiat Oncol Biol Phys.* 2002;53(4):880–888.

327. Huang EH, Strom EA, Perkins GH, et al. Comparison of risk of local-regional recurrence after mastectomy or breast conservation therapy for patients treated with neoadjuvant chemotherapy and radiation stratified according to a prognostic index score. *Int J Radiat Oncol Biol Phys.* 2006;66(2):352–357.

328. Garg AK, Oh JL, Oswald MJ, et al. Effect of postmastectomy radiotherapy in patients <35 years old with stage II-III breast cancer treated with doxorubicin-based neoadjuvant chemotherapy and mastectomy. *Int J Radiat Oncol Biol Phys.* 2007;69(5):1478–1483.

329. Shim SJ, Park W, Huh SJ, et al. The role of postmastectomy radiation therapy after neoadjuvant chemotherapy in clinical stage II-III breast cancer patients with pN0: a multicenter, retrospective study (KROG 12-05). *Int J Radiat Oncol Biol Phys.* 2014;88(1):65–72. doi:10.1016/j.ijrobp.2013.09.021

330. McGuire SE, Gonzalez-Angulo AM, Huang EH, et al. Postmastectomy radiation improves the outcome of patients with locally advanced breast cancer who achieve a pathologic complete response to neoadjuvant chemotherapy. *Int J Radiat Oncol Biol Phys.* 2007;68(4):1004–1009.

331. Nagar H, Mittendorf EA, Strom EA, et al. Local-regional recurrence with and without radiation therapy after neoadjuvant chemotherapy and mastectomy for clinically staged T3N0 breast cancer. *Int J Radiat Oncol Biol Phys.* 2011;81(3):782–787. doi:10.1016/j.ijrobp.2010.06.027

332. Mamounas EP, Anderson SJ, Dignam JJ, et al. Predictors of locoregional recurrence after neoadjuvant chemotherapy: results from combined analysis of National Surgical Adjuvant Breast and Bowel Project B-18 and B-27. *J Clin Oncol.* 2012;30(32):3960–3966. doi:10.1200/JCO.2011.40.8369

6 Metastatic Breast Cancer

Katherine H. R. Tkaczuk, Paula Rosenblatt, Angela DeRidder, Syed S. Mahmood, Reshma L. Mahtani, Geetha Pukazhendhi, Susan B. Kesmodel, Jason Molitoris, and Randi Cohen

Despite an increase in detection of early-stage breast cancer over the past 30 years, approximately 5% to 10% of patients diagnosed with breast cancer present with de novo metastatic disease; in addition, up to 30% of lymph node (LN)-negative and 70% of LN-positive patients will eventually develop metastases (1,2). The primary goals of systemic treatment for MBC are palliation of symptoms, maintenance and improvement in quality of life, and prolongation of survival. These goals must be balanced against toxicities associated with treatment.

The 5-year survival of MBC has increased from 5% to 10% in 1990 to 26% presently based on Surveillance, Epidemiology, and End Results (SEER) data (3,4). In a series from MD Anderson, the median overall survival (OS) for patients with de novo stage IV and relapsed disease was 39.2 and 27.2 months, respectively ($P < .0001$) (5). Improved survival among patients with recurrent or newly diagnosed metastatic disease has been attributed to more aggressive management and the availability of effective therapeutics (6,7).

This chapter reviews the initial assessment and management of MBC. We review hormonal therapy (HT), combination hormonal and targeted therapy, single agent chemotherapy, and combination chemotherapy. Finally, while systemic therapy is the mainstay of treatment for MBC, there are certain situations in which radiation and surgery may play prominently in management for palliation of symptoms, maintenance and improvement in quality of life, and prolongation of survival. These situations are discussed at the end of the chapter.

INITIAL ASSESSMENT

At the diagnosis of metastatic disease, initial assessment should include:

- **Tissue diagnosis of invasive breast cancer with markers (estrogen receptor [ER], progesterone receptor [PR], and HER2) is mandatory before systemic therapy is considered.** We prefer to rebiopsy metastatic sites before final recommendations are made as a change in receptor status can alter treatment decisions in 20% of cases (8).
- **History and physical exam.** MBC patients who are being considered for systemic chemotherapy should be carefully evaluated in terms of clinical symptoms, physical exam (PE), and social support. The PE should include assessment of vital signs, performance status (PS), and comprehensive clinical exam. These assessments should continue with each prechemotherapy

exam. Low PS is a predictor of poor survival, increased toxicity, and decreased chemotherapy response (9).

- **Laboratories.** Routine prechemotherapy labs should include a complete blood count (CBC) and comprehensive metabolic panel (CMP). Tumor markers (CA 15-3, 27.29) and circulating tumor cells (CTCs) can be considered but should never be used as a sole assessment of response to therapy. CTCs have prognostic significance (10).
- **Imaging.** We recommend baseline staging within 4 weeks of initiation of new systemic therapy and we do not routinely stage the central nervous system (CNS) unless there are specific symptoms to suggest CNS involvement. We recommend to stage with contrast-enhanced CTs of chest/abdomen/pelvis + bone scan or fludeoxyglucose (FDG) PET with diagnostic CTs initially.
- **Genomic tumor tissue testing.** Genomic tumor tissue testing looks to identify what may account for the differences in response to treatment and to guide use of therapies that target the tumor's specific genes, proteins, or the tissue environment that contributes to growth and survival. At present, treatments using these approaches are still considered investigational and are being examined in multiple ongoing clinical trials (NCI-MATCH/EAY131 Trial, NCT02465060). We do not routinely send genomic analysis of tumor for newly diagnosed metastatic patients.

Choice of Therapy

The choice of treatment for MBC is influenced by several factors including hormone receptors, estrogen-ER, progesterone-PR (ER/PR) and HER2-neu status, presence of symptoms from disease, presence of visceral crisis, PS, prior receipt of adjuvant treatments, number of prior treatments for metastatic disease and presence of residual side effects of therapy, response to prior treatments, duration of response, time to treatment failure/progression, and comorbidities (11). As the goal of treatment for MBC is quality of life, if a patient is eligible for HT, this is chosen as first-line treatment. Earlier studies have shown response to HT to be a predictive factor for rate and duration of response to chemotherapy (12). Patients with symptomatic visceral disease (liver, lymphangitic lung, bone marrow) involvement should be considered for upfront chemotherapy regardless of ER/PR status, as chemotherapy is more likely to offer rapid relief of symptoms. Single agent and combination therapies are discussed in the following.

Follow-Up

Close follow-up is important in all patients with MBC. Patients receiving hormonal/endocrine therapy (HT) will be seen monthly and then visits spaced depending on the pace of their disease. Our approach is to see our MBC patients on chemotherapy approximately every 2 to 4 weeks depending on the treatment and schedule. We do not see our weekly chemotherapy patients every week, unless toxicities are reported, and nursing visits are done in between MD visits. We feel that this schedule of follow-up allows adequate clinical assessments and assessment of toxicity to therapy. A thorough history with assessment for changes in PS, weight loss, fatigue, gastrointestinal symptoms, neuropathy, depression, and distress should be performed at each visit. A complete PE with specific documentation of abnormalities should be completed and labs should be monitored for cytopenias, kidney function, and liver function.

Assessment of Response to Therapy

- *Imaging* should be completed **every two to four cycles of chemotherapy in the absence of clinical symptoms and signs of progression.** We adhere to the **RECIST 1.1 criteria for assessment of response** and changing therapies (13). We do not recommend routine imaging with PET/CT scans. While we often obtain a baseline PET/CT to determine the location of metastatic lesions, **we typically restage and follow disease status with contrast-enhanced CTs and bone scans.**
- *Tumor markers (CA15-3 or CA 27.29)* are optional in follow-up of patients with MBC. We do not recommend any changes to systemic therapy solely based on rising or declining levels of these tumor markers. If tumor markers were not initially elevated, we do not continue to check routinely.
- *CTC* enumeration is not routine in our assessment of response to therapy. We do utilize CTCs for the purpose of assessment of tissue markers (ER, HER2), in particular when tumor tissue may not be available, not accessible for biopsy, or in cases of bone only disease when there is a concern about reliability of the immunohistochemical (IHC) stains for ER or HER2 after bone decalcification.

DURATION OF THERAPY

The optimal duration of systemic chemotherapy is unknown and must be individualized. Benefit of therapy must be balanced against the toxicities and effects on quality of life. Patients with ER/PR+ disease can be switched to maintenance HT, while patients with HER2+ disease can continue with anti-HER2 therapies +/− HTs without chemotherapy after best response is achieved with chemotherapy. Patients with triple-negative breast cancer may come off palliative chemotherapy and take a "chemotherapy holiday" at the time best response is achieved and monitored closely for increased burden of disease and new symptoms. Clinical trials should be considered and discussed with patients early in the treatment of MBC.

HORMONE THERAPY FOR METASTATIC BREAST CANCER

Indications for Endocrine (Hormonal) Therapy in MBC

Initial assessment of the patient with ER/PR+ MBC is crucial in determining the optimal treatment strategy. The landscape of hormonal treatment is vast and includes ovarian suppression, selective estrogen receptor modulators (SERMs), selective estrogen receptor degrader (SERD), aromatase inhibitors (AI), mammalian target of rapamycin (mTOR) inhibitors, and cyclin-dependent kinase (CDK) 4/6 inhibitors. Choosing the optimum strategy takes into account menopausal status, location and extent of disease, and history of prior adjuvant HT. In the latter case, the duration of disease-free or treatment-free interval is relevant and may influence the choice of the next hormonal agents or transition to chemotherapy, as possible resistance mechanisms or primary or secondary hormone insensitivity need to be considered if the patient is not responding to HT.

The former approach that all visceral disease in MBC requires upfront chemotherapy treatment is no longer supported for clinical practice unless the disease burden is large, causing symptoms, rapidly progressing, or there is evidence of end-organ dysfunction (visceral crisis due to extensive involvement of

the liver, lymphangitic lung involvement, or bone marrow involvement with cytopenias) where immediate response is required.

A high-quality systematic review in 2003 assessing randomized clinical trials compared frontline HT to chemotherapy and showed no difference in OS (hazard ratio [HR] 0.94; $P = .5$), albeit a statistical significance for overall response rate (ORR) (relative risk 1.25; $P = .04$) did favor chemotherapy, while treatment-related toxicities were notably increased in the chemotherapy arms (14). **Furthermore, there is no benefit from combining HT with chemotherapy in ER/PR+ HER2-negative MBC (15,16).**

ER or PR Positivity and Response to Therapy

ER and/or PR prognostic and predictive values have been demonstrated in the metastatic setting. The presence and degree of tissue ER/PR expression strongly predicts response to hormonal treatments, with responses seen in approximately 60% of patients with both ER+ and PR+ tumors, versus 30% in patients with either ER+ or PR+ status alone, versus fewer than 10% of women with receptor negative (ER–/PR–) disease (17,18). Patients with both ER+ and PR+ MBC have been shown to have a more favorable prognosis with longer OS than their counterpart single ER or PR+ tumors. This was assessed in an analysis of three phase III trials of AIs according to ER and PR status, showing that although there were no differences in clinical benefit, the median OS of women with ER+/PR+ tumors was significantly longer than those with single ER or PR+ tumors (800 vs. 600 days, $P = .01$) (19). Additionally in women with ER+ tumors, the median OS of those with tumors that were also PR+ was significantly longer than those that were PR– (800 vs. 625 days, $P = .02$) (19).

DURATION OF HORMONAL THERAPY

Tumor response assessments while on HT should be similar to other therapies. However, ER/PR+ disease is more often associated with bone only disease, which is not considered evaluable/non-measurable by RECIST 1.1 criteria (13). **HT should be continued until there is clear evidence of disease progression or new lesions. Some patients with ER/PR+ MBC may experience prolonged periods of disease stability (years) while HT is continued and quality of life is preserved.** Our approach is to proceed with first disease assessment/restaging no sooner than 3 to 4 months into HT, especially if the patient has bone only metastasis. During this period of time we follow patients clinically and assess their symptoms (bone pain).

Tumor flare with HT has been reported in some patients with MBC with bone metastases during the first weeks of treatment with tamoxifen and toremifene (20). Tumor flare is a syndrome of diffuse musculoskeletal pain with increased size of tumor lesions rather than regression. It is often associated with hypercalcemia. Tumor flare does not imply failure of HT or represent tumor progression; rather, it suggests that the tumor will respond to HT. Symptoms should be treated while HT is continued. If hypercalcemia occurs, appropriate measures should be instituted (20).

SEQUENTIAL LINES OF HORMONAL THERAPY

It is important to remember that a patient with ER/PR+ MBC who responded well to first-line HT will likely respond to another line of HT, although the response rate and duration of response decrease.

When contemplating first or subsequent HTs in ER/PR+ MBC, our approach is to carefully assess patients' symptoms and the tumor's features such as degree of ER and/or PR expression, location of metastases (bone only vs. bone + limited visceral sites), disease burden (extent and number of metastases), and prior response to and length of benefit from HT. Asymptomatic patients, with low volume disease, even if visceral, but with high ER/PR expression and HER2– can be suitable candidates for further lines of HT.

> ➤ If there is no evidence of visceral crisis and there are available hormonal options, then we always consider another line of HT as the preferred systemic management.

Postmenopausal Women

Postmenopausal women with ER/PR+, HER2– MBC have a variety of options for treatment. Therapies include AIs (anastrozole, letrozole, exemestane), SERMs (tamoxifen, toremifene), fulvestrant, and combination therapies with the CDK 4/6 inhibitor palbociclib and the mTOR inhibitor everolimus.

Selective Estrogen Receptor Modulators (tamoxifen, toremifene)

Tamoxifen (20 mg daily) is a nonsteroidal SERM with potent antiestrogenic properties, which are related to its ability to compete with estrogen for binding sites in target tissues. Tamoxifen is an established treatment option for ER/PR+ MBC in postmenopausal women. Tamoxifen is extensively metabolized after oral administration with N-desmethyl tamoxifen as the major metabolite found in plasma. Tamoxifen is a substrate of cytochrome P-450 3A, 2C9 and 2D6, and an inhibitor of P-glycoprotein (21). It is important to take into consideration drug interactions when prescribing.

Toremifene (60 mg daily) is another ER receptor agonist/antagonist indicated for the treatment of MBC in postmenopausal women with ER+ or unknown tumors. Three prospective, randomized, controlled clinical studies (North American, Eastern European, and Nordic) were conducted to evaluate the efficacy of toremifene for the treatment of MBC in ER+ postmenopausal women. Two of the three studies showed similar results for all effectiveness end points, while the Nordic Study showed a longer time to progression (TTP) for tamoxifen (22). Based on these findings and the availability of newer hormonal agents and combinations, toremifene is rarely used in treatment of advanced ER/PR+ BC.

Aromatase Inhibitor (AI)

FIRST-LINE TREATMENT

AIs have compared favorably to tamoxifen with improvements in overall response rates (ORR), progression-free survival (PFS), and overall survival (OS). One of the largest phase III trials that included 916 women showed a significant benefit of first-line treatment with letrozole (2.5 mg daily) compared to tamoxifen in terms of PFS (9.4 vs. 6.0 months; HR 0.72; $P < .0001$) and RR (32% vs. 21%; $P = .0002$) with a non-significant increase in OS (23). An analysis of two phase III trials comparing anastrozole (1 mg daily) to tamoxifen showed a similar significant improvement in PFS

(10.7 vs. 6.4 months; $P = .022$) in the ER/PR+ subgroup (24). Exemestane (25 mg daily) has been compared to tamoxifen in a nonblinded phase III trial of 371 women showing a similar significant improvement in RR (46% vs. 31%; $P = .005$) and PFS (9.9 vs. 5.8 months; $P = .028$ by Wilcoxon test) but no improvement in OS (25).

> ➤ A 2006 meta-analysis of 23 MBC trials with 8,504 women comparing AIs (first, second, and third generation agents) with tamoxifen showed a significant benefit in OS with the third generation AIs (HR 0.87, $P \leq .001$) (26). The significant survival benefit was maintained in both first-line and second-line trials in this meta-analysis.

Comparisons of AIs to one another have largely not shown differences in efficacy. Several studies compared exemestane to anastrozole, showing equal efficacy and no differences in ORR, PFS, or OS (27–29). Letrozole has been compared to anastrozole as second-line therapy in a phase III/IV trial with no difference in TTP, clinical benefit, or OS, albeit a significant improvement in ORR favoring letrozole was observed (19.1% vs. 12.3%; $P = .013$) (30). Consequently, no convincing data is available showing a preference of one AI over the other in the first- or second-line setting.

Fulvestrant is an SERD. It binds to the ER in a competitive mode with affinity comparable to estradiol and downregulates the ER protein in BC cells. It is Food and Drug Administration (FDA) approved for treatment of ER/PR+, MBC in postmenopausal women after disease progression on antiestrogen therapy, and for ER/PR+ HER2- advanced or MBC in combination with palbociclib after progression on endocrine therapy. Based on the FIRST trial, results that are discussed later, fulvestrant can also be considered for first-line treatment.

Fulvestrant dose is 500 mg intramuscularly on day 1, 15, 29, and then every 28 days. For patients with hepatic impairment (Child–Pugh class B), a dose of 250 mg is utilized but the same schedule is recommended.

FULVESTRANT VERSUS TAMOXIFEN

In an early first-line phase III trial of 587 women with ER/PR+ MBC, 250 mg of fulvestrant was compared to tamoxifen. There was no difference in PFS (6.8 vs. 8.3 months) or ORR (31.6% vs. 33.9%), respectively (31). These negative results were attributed to the lower dose of fulvestrant as subsequent prospective trials have shown a benefit to a higher 500 mg dose.

FULVESTRANT DOSAGE MATTERS

> ➤ **The CONFIRM trial** compared a 500 mg to 250 mg dose of fulvestrant in the second-line, AI refractory setting. A significant improvement in PFS was demonstrated with the higher dose which is now considered standard dose for treatment of MBC (32).

FULVESTRANT AS FIRST-LINE THERAPY COMPARED TO AI

The FIRST trial compared fulvestrant to anastrozole as first-line therapy. It showed a significant increase in PFS favoring fulvestrant (23.4 vs. 13.1 months, HR 0.66; $P = .01$) (33) and clinical benefit rate (CBR) of 72.5% and 62%, respectively (34).

A more recent update to the FIRST trial in 2015 suggests an OS benefit. Recently, the **phase III FALCON trial** was presented at the 2016 ESMO meeting; 462 patients (fulvestrant, n = 230; anastrozole, n = 232) were randomized. The primary endpoint was met showing statistically significant improvement in PFS with fulvestrant versus anastrozole (HR 0.797 [95% CI 0.637, 0.999]; P = .0486; median PFS, 16.6 versus 13.8 months, respectively) (35,36).

COMBINATION HORMONAL THERAPY WITH FULVESTRANT

The combination of fulvestrant and anastrozole has been compared to anastrozole alone in two trials with disparate results. Fulvestrant was given at 250 mg monthly, considered a nonstandard dose now. The *FACT trial* included 514 women and did not show any difference in PFS (10.8 vs. 10.2 months; HR 0.99; P = .91) (37). The *SWOG 0226 trial*, however, suggested the combination therapy was better in terms of PFS (15 vs. 13.5 months; HR 0.80; P = .007) and OS (47.7 vs. 41.3 months; HR 0.81; P = .049) (38). The FACT trial had more patients who received adjuvant chemotherapy and adjuvant tamoxifen therapy whereas the SWOG 0226 trial had more de novo metastatic disease.

Second-Line Therapy With Fulvestrant at 250 mg has been compared favorably to AIs, with no difference in OS (39). Fulvestrant has also been compared in combination with exemestane in the second-line setting in the **SoFEA trial**. No difference in PFS was found when the combination of fulvestrant and exemestane was compared to fulvestrant or exemestane alone (4.4 vs. 4.8 vs. 3.4 months, respectively; P = .98) (40).

MECHANISTIC TARGET OF RAPAMYCIN (mTOR) INHIBITORS IN MBC

The mTOR pathway mediates cell growth and metabolism and can be activated by a range of signaling factors such as ERs. Dysregulation of this pathway can lead to the resistance to endocrine therapy, whereby further targeted inhibition has been shown to restore endocrine sensitivity for clinical benefit (41). Everolimus 10 mg daily is FDA approved for treatment of ER/PR+ HER2− advanced breast cancer in combination with exemestane after failure of treatment with letrozole or anastrozole. Some of the most common adverse reactions with an incidence of ≥30% include stomatitis, infections, rash, fatigue, and diarrhea.

EVEROLIMUS AND EXEMESTANE

BOLERO-2 trial was a phase III trial that randomized 724 women who had progressed on AI therapy to combination therapy using exemestane + everolimus or exemestane + placebo. The combination treatment resulted in a significantly longer PFS (7.8 vs. 3.2 months, respectively; HR 0.45; P < .0001) and led to its FDA approval for use in this setting (42,43).

EVEROLIMUS AND TAMOXIFEN

TAMRAD trial was a phase II trial that assessed everolimus with tamoxifen compared to tamoxifen alone following progression on an AI. This showed superiority of the combination with a longer PFS (8.6 vs. 4.5 months; HR 0.54; P = .002) (44).

Toxicities notable in both mTOR studies included a higher rate of stomatitis, rash, fatigue, diarrhea, and anorexia (42–44).

TEMSIROLIMUS AND LETROZOLE

HORIZON trial was a phase III study that compared temsirolimus (an mTOR inhibitor) + letrozole to letrozole alone in the first-line setting. There was no benefit seen with the combination compared to letrozole alone (45).

The lack of benefit seen in HORIZON supports the restricted benefit of mTOR inhibition to those with acquired AI resistance.

TARGETED CYCLIN-DEPENDENT KINASE 4/6 INHIBITORS

Cyclin D1 and CDK4/6 are downstream of ER signaling pathways and activation of these pathways leads to cellular proliferation. In vitro, palbociclib reduces cellular proliferation of ER+ breast cancer cell lines by blocking progression of the cell cycle from G1 into S phase. CDK 4/6 inhibitors have recently been shown to be effective in the management of ER/PR+, HER2– MBC based on several clinical trials.

PALOMA-1 was a phase II study that showed that the combination of letrozole and palbociclib nearly doubled the PFS from 10.2 to 20.2 months compared to letrozole alone (HR 0.49; P = .0004) in the first-line setting in patients with ER/PR+ MBC (46). Notable toxicities in the experimental group were neutropenia, pulmonary embolism, diarrhea, and fatigue.

This led to the accelerated FDA approval of palbociclib in February 2015 contingent upon the confirmatory phase III *PALOMA-2 trial*.

PALOMA-3 was a phase III trial that compared palbociclib + fulvestrant to fulvestrant alone as second-line therapy following disease progression on prior endocrine therapy. It showed a similar doubling of PFS by 5.4 months (9.2 vs. 3.8 months, respectively; HR 0.42; P < .001) in the combination arm (47). This led to the FDA approval of palbociclib + fulvestrant in the second-line setting. What is not known, however, is the effectiveness of second- or third-line HT after palbociclib combinations.

PALOMA-2 was a phase III confirmatory trial of palbociclib + letrozole (P+LET) versus letrozole (LET) alone as first-line treatment of ER/PR+ MBC. The data from this trial was presented recently (48): the PFS was significantly longer for the combination of P+LET versus LET (HR 0.58, 95% CIs [0.46, 0.72]; P < .000001) and median PFS of 24.8 versus 14.5 mos, respectively.

Palbociclib for ER+ HER2+ disease is not currently approved for use given the lack of published clinical data; however, active clinical trials are under way. Preclinical data support that the combination may be effective (46).

Progestins

Megestrol acetate (MA) and medroxyprogesterone acetate are progestins with anti-estrogenic properties that disrupt the ER cycle, possibly through inhibition of aromatase activity or action through the glucocorticoid receptor, androgen receptor, or progesterone receptor. Early randomized trials showed activity in ER/PR+ MBC with an approximate response rate of 25% and median duration of response of 15 months with activity seen following progression on tamoxifen (49,50).

CALGB 8741 was a phase III study that assessed dose escalation of MA in the treatment of ER/PR+ MBC. The response rates were 23%, 27%, and 27% for MA 160 or 800 or 1,600 mg/d, respectively, and no significant differences in the treatment arms were noted for TTP or for survival; survival medians were 28 months dose), 24 months (mid-dose), and 29 months (high dose) (49). Side effects e notable for increased thromboembolic events, weight gain, and fluid retention. These agents have been compared to AIs following progression on tamoxifen herapy in several studies with similar response rates and PFS but an improved side-effect profile favoring AIs (51–54).

A combined updated analysis of the two prior trials by Buzdar et al demonstrated a significant OS advantage favoring anastrozole versus MA (26.7 vs. 22.5 months; HR 0.78; $P < .025$) (55). Exemestane was compared to MA in a trial of 769 women demonstrating an improvement in PFS (4.7 vs. 3.8 months; $P = .037$; respectively) and OS (median not yet reached vs. 28.5 months; $P = .039$; respectively) (56).

Use of progestins in treatment of ER/PR+ MBC is sporadic given their toxicity profile and availability of more effective targeted agents and combinations.

Estrogen Therapy for ER/PR+ MBC

Although counterintuitive and seemingly paradoxical, estrogen has been used successfully in the treatment of ER/PR+ BC. The treatment efficacy of a synthetic estrogen, diethylstilbestrol (DES), in postmenopausal women with BC was noted in the 1940s, suggesting that low estrogen levels associated with the menopause may sensitize BC to DES. Some women treated with intermittent therapy had repeated regressions of disease upon reintroduction of DES. In the 1980s, tamoxifen was FDA approved and DES was eventually withdrawn from use in treatment of BC. Estradiol is still occasionally used in treatment of BC after the failure of newer endocrine therapies (56).

A randomized phase II trial in postmenopausal women with ER/PR+, AI-resistant MBC was done to compare clinical benefit of 30 mg estradiol daily (10 mg TID) with 6 mg daily (2 mg TID) and to determine if prior exposure to AI treatment sensitizes ER+ MBC to lower, better tolerated, and safer doses of estradiol. A total of 66 patients were treated and clinical benefit rates (CBRs) were 28% (30-mg arm) and 29% (6-mg arm) (57). The frequency of grade 3+ adverse events was higher in the 30-mg versus 6-mg arm ($P = .03$). Seven patients with estradiol-sensitive disease were retreated with an AI upon progression, two had partial responses and one stable disease suggesting resensitization to estrogen deprivation.

> ➤ Low-dose estrogen is rarely considered for treatment of ER/PR+ MBC. It is important to remember and to consider it only in settings when hormone resistance is established after multiple lines of antiestrogen therapies.

Premenopausal Women With ER/PR+ MBC

In the following we discuss several effective treatment options for premenopausal women with ER/PR+ MBC including ovarian suppression/ablation, SERMS, combination therapy of ovarian suppression and SERM or AI, or SERD and other targeted agents.

Ovarian Suppression/Ablation

Ovarian suppression/ablation can be completed with luteinizing-hormone-releasing hormone (LHRH)/gonadotropin-releasing hormone (GnRH) agonists, radiotherapy to the ovaries, or oophorectomy. Ovarian suppression/ablation alone is effective therapy for premenopausal women with ER/PR+ MBC, with response rates ranging from 14% to 70% (58,59). In an early study of 136 premenopausal women randomly assigned to either ovarian suppression with goserelin or ovarian ablation with oophorectomy, no difference was seen in OS, failure-free survival, or RR (60). Ovarian suppression with hormone therapy in the advanced setting has been found to have increased PFS (HR 0.70; $P = .0003$) and OS (HR 0.78; $P = .02$) in a meta-analysis of GnRH alone or in combination with tamoxifen (61). Ovarian suppression induces a higher risk of osteoporosis, dyslipidemia, hot flashes, vaginal dryness, and mood swings, which are important factors to counsel the premenopausal population (61). Choice of therapy is largely based on patient and physician preference given the varied side-effect and long-term risk profiles.

For premenopausal women, we recommend ovarian suppression combined with a hormonal treatment that is the same as would be given for postmenopausal women (AI, SERD [62], targeted agent combinations) or treatment with a SERM alone for premenopausal women with MBC.

Selective Estrogen Receptor Modulators

SERMs such as tamoxifen have been used for many years for the treatment of MBC, although with limited data for the premenopausal population.

TAMOXIFEN

In prospective randomized studies comparing tamoxifen to ovarian ablation (oophorectomy or ovarian irradiation) in premenopausal women with MBC, the ORR, TTF, and OS were similar (63,64). Elevated serum and plasma estrogens have been observed in premenopausal women receiving tamoxifen, but the data from the randomized studies do not suggest an adverse effect of this increase. A limited number of premenopausal patients with progression of disease (PD) on tamoxifen responded to subsequent ovarian ablation.

Tamoxifen has shown to be equivalent to ovarian suppression in several trials conducted in premenopausal women with response rates of approximately 45% (18). A 1997 meta-analysis that evaluated 220 women showed no statistically significant difference in risk of disease progression or death (65).

Combination therapy of tamoxifen and ovarian suppression has shown an increased PFS (8.7 vs. 5.4 months; HR 0.70; $P = .0003$) and OS (2.9 vs. 2.5 years; HR 0.78; $P = .02$) when compared to ovarian suppression alone in a meta-analysis of four randomized trials (61). No trials have compared single agent tamoxifen with ovarian suppression and tamoxifen in MBC.

> ➤ Based on this data, our approach is to always utilize ovarian suppression in addition to tamoxifen in premenopausal women with ER/PR+ MBC.

Aromatase Inhibitors

AIs prevent the peripheral conversion of androgens to estrogens and are effective in many settings (chemoprevention, neoadjuvant, adjuvant, metastatic) for postmenopausal women. Their use is contraindicated in premenopausal women without the use of ovarian suppression due to the negative feedback loop from the pituitary, leading to an increase in estrogen production by the ovaries.

Limited phase II trials in premenopausal women have shown encouraging clinical benefit with ovarian suppression and AIs (66–69). It is important to remember that in the postmenopausal setting, AIs have showed superiority to tamoxifen as frontline therapy for ER/PR+ MBC, which has further supported their use in the premenopausal space, although direct evidence for this is lacking (26). Additionally, no trials have been published comparing ovarian suppression + AI to ovarian suppression alone; however, as mentioned previously, ovarian suppression and tamoxifen compared to ovarian suppression alone showed benefit for the combination with improved RR, PFS, and OS.

Cyclin-Dependent Kinase Inhibitor

The recently approved CDK 4/6-inhibitor, palbociclib, has shown clinical benefit in the large **PALOMA-3** trial where palbociclib + fulvestrant was compared to fulvestrant alone as second-line therapy following progression of disease on prior endocrine therapy. This randomized, phase III trial showed a statistically significant prolongation of PFS by 5.4 mos (9.2 vs. 3.8 mos, respectively; HR 0.42; $P <$ .001) in the combination arm (47). This trial included postmenopausal and premenopausal women on ovarian suppression comprising 20% of the study population. In subgroup analysis, premenopausal women had similar clinical benefit to postmenopausal women (HRs 0.44 and 0.41, respectively; $P =$ .94) (47). This trial led to the recent expanded FDA approval for second-line therapy with fulvestrant and included pre/perimenopausal women in the indication.

PALOMA-1 was a phase II trial comparing letrozole alone to letrozole + palbociclib in postmenopausal women with ER/PR+ MBC as first-line therapy. PALOMA-1 showed benefit in terms of prolongation of PFS in the combination arm (46).

PALOMA-2 is a phase III study to confirm the phase II findings. Although premenopausal women on ovarian suppression were not included in either trial, we feel it is reasonable to consider ovarian suppression + letrozole + palbociclib in the first-line setting.

Selected Novel Agents in Clinical Trials for ER/PR+ MBC

PI3K INHIBITORS

Many exciting novel agents are in development for ER/PR+ MBC. Of the many novel agents, PI3K inhibitors such as buparlisib (BKM120) show promising results. The PI3K/AKT/mTOR pathway is implicated in many malignancies and in breast cancer PI3K mutations are common. The initial **BELLE-2 (NCT01610284)** results were presented at the 2015 San Antonio Breast Cancer Symposium. In this phase III randomized trial of fulvestrant versus fulvestrant + buparlisib, PFS was increased in the combination arm (6.9 vs. 5 months, HR .78; $P <$ .001) (70). In evaluating the circulating tumor DNA, patients with mutant PIK3CA had an even greater benefit with combination therapy compared to fulvestrant alone (7 vs. 3.2 months, HR 0.56; $P <$ .001). **BELLE-3 (NCT01633060)** is still recruiting and is evaluating buparlisib + fulvestrant after progression on an mTOR inhibitor. Additional PI3K inhibitors such as **idelalisib, pictilisib, and alpelisib** are being evaluated in clinical trials.

CDK INHIBITORS SELECTIVE FOR CDK4 AND CDK6

Abemaciclib has shown promising initial results gaining a FDA breakthrough designation. Abemaciclib shows initial single agent activity with an objective response rate of 33.3% and clinical benefit rate of 61.1% (71). A single-arm phase II trial of abemaciclib in previously treated patients (**MONARCH-1-NCT02102490**) and two phase III combination trials (**MONARCH-2-NCT02107703** with fulvestrant and **MONARCH-3-NCT02246621 with an AI**) are ongoing. The results of the MONA-LEESA 2 trial (NCT01958021) were recently presented at the ESMO2016 meeting. In this trial, postmenopausal women (N = 668) with ER/PR+, HER2– MBC with no prior systemic treatment for MBC were randomized (1:1) to receive ribociclib (600 mg/day, 3-weeks-on/1-week-off) + letrozole (2.5 mg/day, continuous) or placebo + letrozole. The study met its primary objective: at the interim analysis, PFS was significantly improved in the ribociclib arm, with a HR of 0.556 (95% CI: 0.429–0.720; P = .00000329). Median PFS was not reached in the ribociclib arm (95% CI: 19.3–not estimable) versus 14.7 months in the placebo arm (95% CI: 13.0–16.5). In patients with measurable disease at baseline, ORR was 53% versus 37% (ribociclib vs. placebo arm; P = .00028) and CBR was 80% versus 72% (P = .02) (72).

HISTONE DEACETYLASE (HDAC) INHIBITOR

Entinostat is a novel class I HDAC inhibitor, which has been shown to inhibit growth factor signaling pathways that mediate hormone resistance. The **ENCORE 301** trial compared entinostat + exemestane to exemestane + placebo in 130 heavily pretreated patients who were resistant to AIs. The PFS was 4.28 versus 2.27 months (HR 0.73; P = .055) with an exploratory end point showing benefit in median OS, 28.1 versus 19.8 months (HR 0.59; P = .036) (73). A phase III trial E2112 (**NCT02115282**) with entinostat + exemestane versus exemestane + placebo in ER/PR+, HER2–, pre and post menopausal women and men who failed an AI therapy in first line setting is ongoing.

> **MANAGEMENT PEARLS—MBC HORMONAL THERAPY**

1. The presence and degree of tissue ER/PR expression strongly predicts response to hormonal treatments, with responses seen in approximately 60% of women with both ER+ and PR+ tumors, versus 30% in women with either ER+ or PR+ status alone, versus less than 10% of women with receptor negative (ER–/PR–) disease. Patients with both ER+ and PR+ tumors have a more favorable prognosis with longer OS than their counterpart single hormone receptor positive tumors.
2. HT should be continued until there is clear evidence of disease progression. Some patients with ER/PR+ MBC may experience prolonged periods of disease stability (years) while HT is continued and quality of life is preserved.
3. We do not recommend combining HT agents with chemotherapy in ER/PR+ MBC.
4. It is important to remember that a patient with ER/PR+ MBC who responded well to first-line HT may respond to another line of HT, although the response rate and duration of response decrease.
5. Not all visceral disease requires upfront chemotherapy. If there is no evidence of visceral crisis and there are available hormonal options, we always consider another line of HT as the preferred systemic management.

CHEMOTHERAPY

Single Agent Versus Combination Chemotherapy

There are no prospective data that demonstrate conclusively that combination chemotherapy improves survival when compared to single agent cytotoxic chemotherapy for treatment of MBC. However, combination chemotherapy has been shown to increase overall response rates in MBC. Therefore, when a higher response rate is vital, such as in patients with visceral crisis, combination chemotherapy may be appropriate. Otherwise, single agent therapy is preferred to avoid cross-resistance to multiple agents and to limit toxicities.

In a prospective randomized study comparing first-line single agent epirubicin (E) to combination cyclophosphamide, epirubicin, and fluorouracil (ECF), no significant difference in survival or TTP was appreciated between the two treatments (74). Similar results were shown comparing sequential versus concomitant administration of an anthracycline and taxane as first-line treatment of MBC (75). **ECOG 1193** did show that combination of doxorubicin and paclitaxel (AT) was associated with a higher ORR and longer median TTP than sequential therapy as first-line therapy for MBC, but with greater toxicity and no difference in OS (76).

The European MBC task force performed a literature review of different monotherapy versus combination therapy comparison studies. None of these studies showed meaningful differences in PFS or OS (77).

Single Agent Chemotherapy

Anthracyclines are active agents in the treatment of MBC. Cumulative cardiac toxicity inherent to prolonged use becomes a concern in the metastatic setting and limits its use in treatment of advanced breast cancer due to the frequent utilization of these agents in the adjuvant setting. However, in the setting of de novo presentation of advanced breast cancer, anthracycline as single agent or in combination (AC, EC, or TAC) can be considered when the visceral burden of disease is high and indications for chemotherapy are present (see p. 175).

DOXORUBICIN

In a phase III study, doxorubicin alone was compared to combination therapy with vinorelbine, and the treatments were found to be similar with respect to TTP and OS (78). The dosing schedule for doxorubicin alone is **60 to 75 mg/m^2 every 3 weeks or 20 mg/m^2 weekly.**

Epirubicin is a structural analog of doxorubicin with similar efficacy, but with some data to suggest a lower rate of cardiac toxicity (79). The half-life of epirubicin is much shorter than doxorubicin but the peak plasma concentration is similar. A prospective comparison study of epirubicin (85 mg/m^2) versus doxorubicin (60 mg/m^2) every 21 days in patients with advanced BC who failed nonanthracycline combination chemotherapy showed that ORR = 25% in both arms; median duration of response was 11.9 mos for epirubicin and 7.1 mos for doxorubicin. The median doses to the development of laboratory cardiotoxicity were estimated to be 935 mg/m^2 (epirubicin) and 468 mg/m^2 (doxorubicin) and the median cumulative dose at which congestive heart failure (CHF) was observed was 1,134 mg/m^2 (epirubicin) versus 492 mg/m² (doxorubicin) (79). Epirubicin just like doxorubicin can be dosed at 20 to 25 mg/m² weekly.

Pegylated liposomal doxorubicin (PLD) was developed to further improve the safety profile of anthracyclines. PLD is doxorubicin confined within liposomes stabilized by grafting polyethylene glycol onto its surface. PLD has a longer half-life (55 hours) prolonging the circulation time (80). In a study comparing PLD to doxorubicin, median PFS and OS were comparable in the two arms (80,81). PLD was associated with a decreased risk of cardiomyopathy, even in high-risk patients, although with a higher incidence of dose-related palmar plantar erythrodysesthesia (PPE) (80,81). PLD is commonly given at a dose of **40 to 50 mg/m² every 3 to 4 weeks**.

TAXANES

Taxane-containing regimens improve OS, TTP, and tumor ORR in women with MBC and are routinely prescribed as first- and later-line therapy in the metastatic setting due to high ORR noted in multiple studies (82–84). In a Cochrane review, taxanes were found to be superior to anthracycline and other nonanthracycline regimens in terms of PFS and OS (85). The combined HR for OS and TTP favored the taxane-containing regimens (HR 0.93; P = .002; 0.92; P = .002) respectively. For studies of first-line chemotherapy, this effect persisted for OS (HR 0.93; P = .03) but not for TTP (HR 0.96; P = .22). Response rates were also better with taxane-containing chemotherapy (HR 1.20; P < .00001).

Paclitaxel was initially given as a 250 mg/m² 96-hour infusion and demonstrated a response rate of 56% as initial chemotherapy (82). Further studies utilized shorter infusions of paclitaxel (**175 mg/m² by 3-hour infusion every 21 days**) in patients previously treated with the FEC as an adjuvant or first-line therapy for MBC and was associated with ORR of 54% for adjuvant FEC and 60% for 5-flurouracil/epirubicin/cyclophosphamide (FEC) as first-line treatment (86). Other phase II studies of paclitaxel have shown comparable results (83,84). Paclitaxel given weekly (**dose range 80–108 mg/m²**) was associated with the ORR of 53%, with 10% complete response (CR) (87). Median response duration was 7.5 months (range, 2 to 11+). Responses were observed in 50% of patients who had received prior anthracycline therapy, including in half of patients with disease progression on anthracycline within 1 year (87).

Paclitaxel is most commonly given on a **weekly schedule at 80 mg/m²**, based on a 2010 meta-analysis that showed improved OS and improved tolerability over an every 3-week schedule (88).

Docetaxel differs from paclitaxel in its pharmacokinetic profile. The cellular uptake is higher with docetaxel compared to paclitaxel, and the efflux rate is about thrice slower for docetaxel. This contributes to the greater cytotoxicity of docetaxel than paclitaxel. Data suggests there is only partial cross-resistance between paclitaxel and docetaxel. A phase II study that evaluated the response to **docetaxel (75–100 mg/m² every 21 days)** in patients with paclitaxel-resistant MBC showed an ORR of 17.4% (89). Weekly docetaxel at 40 mg/m² demonstrated an ORR of 41% in the metastatic setting in a phase II study (90). However, it is more commonly given on an every 3-week schedule, based on a study in the adjuvant setting, which demonstrated an improvement in DFS with this schedule (88).

When comparing these two taxanes, toxicities do differ. Generally paclitaxel results in more neuropathy and myalgia, whereas docetaxel generally causes more febrile neutropenia, edema (which can be ameliorated with the use of dexamethasone), and gastrointestinal side effects (diarrhea).

Nab-paclitaxel (albumin-bound solvent-free paclitaxel) was designed to overcome the infusion reactions experienced in relation to the solvents used in paclitaxel. These solvent vehicles were also thought to impair drug delivery to the tumor and be responsible for the disproportionate systemic drug exposure (91). Nab-paclitaxel and paclitaxel have been compared in xenograft tumor models at equitoxic doses, and nab-paclitaxel was found to have greater antitumor activity (92). When compared to docetaxel, nab-paclitaxel resulted in significantly longer PFS in the first-line setting (93–96). Nab-paclitaxel may be dosed at **100 to 150 mg/m² on days 1, 8, and 15 of a 28-day cycle or 260 mg/m² every 3 weeks (94–96)**.

OTHER AGENTS

Capecitabine is an oral prodrug and is converted to its active form 5-fluorouracil by the enzyme pyrimidine nucleoside phosphorylase. This enzyme is expressed at high levels by various tumor, which results in precise delivery of active drug to the tumor tissue and reduces bowel exposure to the active drug. A patient with MBC who does not want intravenous (IV) chemotherapy may choose to start with the oral capecitabine. The FDA-approved capecitabine at **(1,250 mg/m² twice daily orally for 2 weeks on and 1 week off)** but this dose is often difficult to tolerate and patients often require dose reductions. Many oncologists start with alternative dosing schedules and use **1,000 mg/m² bid × 14 days, 7 days off schedule**. Studies have shown these dose reductions do not impair efficacy of the drug (97). In a phase II study of patients with paclitaxel-refractory disease, ORR was approximately 20%. The most common adverse events reported include hand–foot syndrome, diarrhea, nausea, and vomiting. The median TTP was 93 days, and median duration of response was 8.1 months (96). In a first-line study, ORR was 26.1% with a dose of 2,000 mg/m² (98). In another first-line phase II randomized study, ORR was 30% with capecitabine compared to 16% with Cytoxan, methotrexate, and 5-fluorouracil (CMF). Median TTP was longer with capecitabine versus CMF (4.1 vs. 3 months) respectively but survival was similar in the two treatment arms (99).

Gemcitabine is a nucleoside analog that has shown significant antitumor activity across a wide range of tumors with low systemic toxicity. It is generally administered at a dose of **1,000 mg/m² weekly for 2 weeks followed by a 1-week rest**. In the first-line setting, a response rate of 37% was noted (100), and in the second-line, 26% (101). When given as third- or fourth-line treatment in MBC, it has an ORR of 17% to 19% (102).

Eribulin mesylate is a nontaxane microtubule inhibitor; it is active in cell lines that have become resistant to taxanes. It is generally administered at **a dose of 1.4 mg/m² on day 1 and 8 of a 21-day cycle**. In a phase II study, eribulin demonstrated an objective RR of 11.5% (103). In a phase III open-label randomized study, eribulin was compared to various therapies in heavily pretreated MBC (EMBRACE trial). The control arm consisted of treatment of physician's choice (TPC). There was a significant increase in OS for the eribulin group compared to the TPC group (13.1 months vs. 10.6 months). More common grade 3 or 4 adverse events that occurred with eribulin were neutropenia, leukopenia, and peripheral neuropathy (104).

Vinorelbine is a semisynthetic vinca alkaloid that inhibits microtubule assembly and interferes with formation of the mitotic spindle and prevents cell division. It is generally administered at a dose of **25–30 mg/m² weekly on days 1 and 8 in a 3-week cycle**. As first-line treatment in advanced breast cancer, objective ORR was shown to be 35% (105,106,107,108). It has an objective ORR of 47% as second- or third-line treatment in MBC and no cross-resistance was documented with prior anthracycline or taxane treatment (105). The mechanism of action of docetaxel and vinorelbine has been found to be synergistic in preclinical models. In a phase II study of first-line therapy for patients who were taxane-naïve, the combination of docetaxel and vinorelbine resulted in an ORR of 59% (109).

Ixabepilone is an epothilone B analog, nontaxane microtubule-stabilizing compound, that has activity in taxane-resistant patients. This drug was evaluated in a phase II study of patients who were resistant to anthracyclines, taxanes, and capecitabine. ORR was 18.3% in this heavily pretreated population and a manageable toxicity profile was noted (110). A randomized phase III trial in patients with locally advanced MBC with prior anthracycline and taxane exposure with ixabepilone (40 mg/m² IV q 3 weeks) and capecitabine (2,000 mg/m²/d days 1–14) versus capecitabine (2,500 mg/m²/d days 1–14) was done. Ixabepilone + capecitabine prolonged PFS compared to capecitabine alone (median, 5.8 vs. 4.2 mos), with a 25% reduction in the estimated risk of disease progression (HR, 0.75; P = .0003). Objective response rate was also increased (35% vs. 14%; P < .0001) (111, 208). The usual dose of Ixabepilone is 40 mg/m² IV every 21 days.

Platinum agents including cisplatin and carboplatin are usually administered as part of combination regimens as there are limited single agent responses noted with these drugs. This class of drugs may be particularly useful in patients who have tumors in which DNA damage repair pathways are impaired, such as with BRCA mutations. Platinum agents (carboplatin or cisplatin) are typically combined with paclitaxel or gemcitabine in MBC, standard doses of these agents are used.

MAINTENANCE CHEMOTHERAPY

A systematic meta-analysis of 11 randomized chemotherapy clinical trials for MBC including 2,269 patients showed that longer first-line chemotherapy duration resulted in a marginal improvement in OS (HR, 0.91, 95% CIs [0.84, 0.99]; P = .046) and a substantial improvement in PFS (HR, 0.64, 95% CIs [0.55, 0.76]; P < .001) (112). There were no differences in effect on either OS or PFS between subgroups defined by time of random assignment, study design, number of chemotherapy cycles in the control arm, or concomitant endocrine therapy. The number of cycles of chemotherapy in the standard duration groups (control arms) ranged from 3 to 8 while the number of maintenance chemotherapy cycles ranged from 6 to continuing until disease progression or unacceptable toxicity. In terms of clinical benefit on OS, the 9% reduction in the hazard of death for longer duration of chemotherapy was felt to be marginally beneficial. In practice, this needs to be considered against toxicity.

> ➤ **MANAGEMENT PEARLS—CHEMOTHERAPY** (Table 6.1)

1. There are no prospective data that demonstrate conclusively that combination cytotoxic chemotherapy meaningfully improves survival when compared to single agent sequential chemotherapy for treatment of MBC. However, combination chemotherapy has been shown to increase ORR.
2. When a higher response rate is vital, such as in patients with visceral crisis, combination chemotherapy may be appropriate. Otherwise, single agent therapy is preferred to avoid cross-resistance to multiple agents and to limit toxicities.
3. Maintenance chemotherapy: A systematic meta-analysis of 11 randomized chemotherapy clinical trials in MBC including 2,269 patients showed that longer first-line chemotherapy duration resulted in a marginal improvement in OS (HR, 0.91, 95% CIs [0.84, 0.99]; $P = .046$) and a substantial improvement in PFS. This marginal benefit has to be weighed against increased toxicities of maintenance cytotoxic chemotherapy.

HER2+ MBC

HER2 positivity, seen in approximately 20% of breast cancers, is a prognostic and predictive marker in MBC (122). Historically, tumor tissue overexpression of HER2 was associated with increased risk of recurrence and worse overall prognosis. Since the introduction of HER2 targeted agents, the disease course in metastatic setting has been altered with improvement in median survival now reaching 56 months as seen in the CLEOPATRA trial (123).

Anti-HER2 therapy indications follow the previously described immunohistochemistry and in situ hybridization guidelines as set by the American Society of Clinical Oncology/College of American Pathologists (ASCO/CAP) and previously described in Chapter 5. HER2 therapy is typically administered in combination with hormone and chemotherapy as described in the following.

Triple-Positive ER/PR/HER2+ MBC

Nearly 50% of all HER2-positive breast cancers will also coexpress ER or PR receptors (124,125). Triple-positive MBC can be treated with HER2 directed therapy, chemotherapy, and/or hormonal therapy (HT). Here we also do not recommend concurrent chemotherapy with HT and recommend sequential approaches using guidelines discussed in this chapter.

Society guidelines differ in the treatment algorithm for hormone positive HER2+ given the lack of evidence in randomized controlled trials.

- **ASCO guidelines support recommendations** for the upfront treatment in triple-positive MBC with differing "strengths" based on available evidence (126).
  - **HER2 targeted therapy combined with chemotherapy is a "strong" recommendation.**
  - HER2 targeted therapy combined with endocrine therapy is a "moderate" recommendation.

(*text continues on page 195*)

Table 6.1 Chemotherapy Regimens for Metastatic Breast Cancer

Author	No. of subjects	Randomization	Primary end point(s)	Efficacy	Grade 3/4 toxicities	Line of therapy and prior exposure to A/T
Norris et al (78)	300	Doxo + VNB vs. Doxo alone	ORR	ORR 38% on combination arm vs. 30% on doxorubicin alone ($P = .2$)	Granulocytopenia—69% in combo arm, neurotoxicity 6% on Doxo + VNB vs. 1% on Doxo alone, venous toxicity (22% on combo arm vs. 2% on single agent)	First- or second-line therapy for MBC No prior A exposure, prior T permitted
Perez et al (113)	212	NA paclitaxel alone	ORR, TTP	ORR 21.5% median TTP 4.7 months	Hematologic toxicity 15%, neurotoxicity 9%	Two prior lines of therapy permitted for MBC including prior A and/or T
Harvey et al (114)	527	Docetaxel 60, 75, or 100 mg/m^2	ORR	ORR 22.1%, 23.3%, 36% in each arm, respectively Higher response rate with 100 mg/m^2 ($P = .037$)	Neutropenia (49.3%, 67.9%, 86.3% respectively)	First- or second-line therapy for MBC

(continued)

Table 6.1 Chemotherapy Regimens for Metastatic Breast Cancer (*continued*)

Author	No. of subjects	Randomization	Primary end point(s)	Efficacy	Grade 3/4 toxicities	Line of therapy and prior exposure to A/T
Gradishar (95)	302	Nab-paclitaxel 300 mg/m^2 q3w, 100 mg/m^2 weekly, 150 mg/m^2 weekly, docetaxel 100 mg/m^2 q3w	ORR, PFS	Longer PFS on nab-paclitaxel than docetaxel (12.9 vs. 7.5 months; P = .0065). Higher ORR on nab-paclitaxel (49% on 150 mg/m^2, 45% on 100 mg/m^2, 35% on docetaxel)	Neutropenia (39% on 300 mg/m^2, 20% on 100 mg/m^2, 35% on 150 mg/m^2, 19% on docetaxel), sensory neuropathy (17% on 300 mg/m^2 vs. 12% on docetaxel), fatigue on docetaxel	No prior chemotherapy in metastatic setting
O'Shaughnessy et al (115)	95	Cape vs. CMF	ORR, TTP	ORR—30% on Cape vs. 16% on CMF, median TTP 4.1 months on Cape vs. 3 months on CMF	Hand–foot syndrome on Cape 34%, patients on Cape experienced treatment interruption due to severe adverse events	No prior chemotherapy in advanced/metastatic setting
Modi et al (116)	22	NA Gemcitabine alone	RR	PR 17% (95% CI 4%–41%)	Neutropenia, fatigue, neuropathy	MBC treated with 2–4 prior chemotherapy regimens that included an A and T

(*continued*)

Table 6.1 Chemotherapy Regimens for Metastatic Breast Cancer (*continued*)

Author	No. of subjects	Randomization	Primary end point(s)	Efficacy	Grade 3/4 toxicities	Line of therapy and prior exposure to A/T
Cortes et al (104)	762	Eribulin vs. TPC	OS	OS (13.1 vs. 10.6 months)	Fatigue (54% on eribulin and 40% on TPC), neutropenia (24% on eribulin vs. 7% on TPC), peripheral neuropathy (8% on eribulin, 2% on TPC)	Between 2 and 5 previous chemotherapy regimens (two or more for advanced disease), including A and T
Zelek et al (105)	40	NA VNB alone	Objective response	ORR 25%. Median time to failure 6 months (range 4–12)	Neutropenia, neuropathy, ileus, anemia	Anthracyclines and taxanes
Mavroudis et al (117)	286	Doc + Epi (DE) vs. Doc + Cape (DC)	TTP, OS	ORR 51.5% with DE vs. 52.9% with DC. Median TTP 10.6 months vs. 11 months, respectively	Neutropenia 57% with DE vs. 46% on DC (P = .069), anemia 20% vs. 7%, respectively	Previously untreated/previous anthracycline-based (neo)-adjuvant chemotherapy was allowed if completed >1 year before enrollment

(*continued*)

Table 6.1 Chemotherapy Regimens for Metastatic Breast Cancer (*continued*)

Author	No. of subjects	Randomization	Primary end point(s)	Efficacy	Grade 3/4 toxicities	Line of therapy and prior exposure to A/T
Albain et al (118)	529	Gem + Pacli (GT) vs. Pacli alone	OS, TTP	Median OS 18.6 months on GT versus 15.8 months on Pacli	Neutropenia 47.9% on GT vs. 11.5% on Pacli only. Febrile neutropenia 4.6% vs. 1.2%, respectively	Anthracycline-based adjuvant therapy
Canellos et al (119)	184	CMF vs. L-PAM	RR	CMF 49 (53%) complete (14 patients) or partial (35 patients) response, 18 of the 91 patients (20%) treated with L-PAM responded	Extent of myelosuppression was greater in the CMF arm	No prior chemotherapy
O'Shaughnessy et al (120)	511	Capecitabine/ docetaxel vs. docetaxel alone	TTP, OS	TTP (HR = 0.652; P = .0001, 6.1 vs. 4.2 months), OS (HR = 0.775; P = .0126, 14.5 vs. 11.5 months)	Gastrointestinal side effects and hand–foot syndrome more with combination	Anthracycline
Sparano et al (121)	1,221	Ixabepilone/ Cape vs. Cape	OS	HR = 0.85; P = .0231	Peripheral neuropathy 24% vs. 1.2%	Anthracycline/ Taxane in adjuvant or metastatic setting

A/T, anthracycline/taxane; Cape, Capecitabine; CMF, cyclophosphamide, methotrexate, 5-fluorouracil; Doc, docetaxel; Doxo, doxorubicin; Epi, epirubicin; HR, hazard ratio; L-PAM, melphalan; MBC, metastatic breast cancer; NA, not applicable; ORR, overall response rate; OS, overall survival; Pacli, paclitaxel; PFS, progression-free survival; PR, progesterone receptor; RR, response rate; TPC, treatment of physician's choice; TTP, time to progression; VNB, vinorelbine.

- ○ Endocrine therapy alone is a "weak" recommendation in carefully selected patients.
- ○ Endocrine therapy with HER2 therapy when chemotherapy ends and/or when cancer progresses is a "weak" recommendation.
- **The National Comprehensive Cancer Network (NCCN) guidelines recommend hormonal therapy** as a frontline approach and do not recommend combination therapy with HER2 directed agents (127). The NCCN supports endocrine therapy alone until progression through three sequential agents or symptomatic visceral disease, whereupon combination HER2 directed agents with chemotherapy is suggested.

> ➤ For ER/PR+ HER2+ MBC, our approach favors using HER2 directed therapy combined with chemotherapy initially, given its clear benefit in OS with the addition of HT after the completion of chemotherapy. For those who will not tolerate chemotherapy or who have low volume non visceral disease, HER2 therapy plus HT can be considered.

Hormone Therapy and HER2 Therapy

TRASTUZUMAB/AI

The TAnDEM trial was the first randomized phase III study to combine hormonal agents with trastuzumab as treatment for ER/PR+ HER2+ MBC. The study demonstrated a PFS benefit of 2.4 months (4.8 vs. 2.4 months; HR 0.63; $P = .0016$) with trastuzumab in combination with anastrozole compared to anastrozole alone; however, OS was not significantly different between the two treatment arms (128).

The eLecTRA trial showed a nonsignificant 11-month PFS benefit (14.1 vs. 3.3 months; HR 0.67; $P = .23$) when trastuzumab was combined with letrozole compared to letrozole alone, Clinical benefit rate was 39% for letrozole compared to 65% letrozole and trastuzumab (odds ratio 2.99, 95% CI 1.01–8.84). However, there was no difference in OS (129). This trial was hampered by slow accrual and had to be closed prematurely; thus, it did not have appropriate power for OS determination.

Another trial that compared the combination of lapatinib and letrozole to letrozole alone showed an increased PFS (8.2 vs. 3.0 months; HR 0.71; $P = .019$) but did not report OS (130).

HER2 Blockade and Chemotherapy

Trastuzumab is a bioengineered humanized monoclonal antibody against the extracellular domain of the HER2 protein in preclinical models trastuzumab inhibited tumor growth when used alone but also had synergistic or additive effects when combined with several chemotherapy agents (cisplatin, carboplatin, docetaxel, doxorubicin, cyclophosphamide, methotrexate, and paclitaxel). This promising preclinical data led to a pivotal trial (1995–1997) in women with MBC with HER2, 2+ and 3+ tissue expression by IHC; women were randomized to chemotherapy alone (AC or paclitaxel) or chemotherapy + trastuzumab. Treatment with trastuzumab was associated with a significantly higher rate of overall response (50% vs. 32%, $P < .001$), longer duration of response (median, 9.1 vs. 6.1 months; $P < .001$), and a longer time to treatment failure (median, 6.9 vs. 4.5 months; $P < .001$). Treatment with trastuzumab was also associated with a lower risk of death at one year (22% vs. 33%; $P = .008$). Based on the results of this study trastuzumab was FDA approved in September 1998 as first-line therapy in combination with paclitaxel and as single agent for those who received ≥ 1 chemotherapy regimens for MBC. Dako's Hercep tissue test was approved simultaneously to identify patients with HER2+ MBC (131,132).

Dual HER2 Blockade With Chemotherapy

Pertuzumab blocks the dimerization of the HER family molecules that activate the downstream signaling cascade and signals the immune system to initiate antibody-mediated cytotoxicity. A new standard of care in HER2 MBC was defined in 2012 when pertuzumab obtained FDA approval in combination with trastuzumab and docetaxel as first-line treatment of MBC.

CLEOPATRA WITH DOCETAXEL (THP)

Phase III trial evaluated pertuzumab + docetaxel + trastuzumab versus the control of docetaxel + trastuzumab alone in 808 women with HER2+ MBC. Patients were treated with trastuzumab (8 mg/kg loading dose, then 6 mg/kg IV) and docetaxel (75 mg/m² IV) and randomized to pertuzumab (840 mg loading dose, then 420 mg) or placebo (123). Treatment was administered every 3 weeks until PD or intolerable side effects. If side effects developed, the docetaxel could be stopped and the trastuzumab + pertuzumab continued until progression of disease (PD). The addition of pertuzumab increased PFS from 12.4 to 18.7 months (HR 0.62, 95% CIs [0.51, 0.75]) and OS from 40.8 to 56 months (HR 0.68; $P < .001$) (123,133). The addition of pertuzumab was very well tolerated with a mild increase in diarrhea, rash, pruritus, and upper respiratory infections, and the rate of cardiac dysfunction was less than 2% in each arm (123,133).

> ➤ The combination of pertuzumab, trastuzumab, and docetaxel has become the new standard first-line treatment for HER2+ MBC.

PACLITAXEL, TRASTUZUMAB, AND PERTUZUMAB

A phase II single-arm study evaluated weekly paclitaxel 80 mg/m² with standard dose every 3 weeks and trastuzumab and pertuzumab as first-line therapy in patients with metastatic disease. The PFS was 24.2 months and well tolerated (134).

Kadcyla/TDM1/Ado-Trastuzumab Emtansine

Kadcyla/TDM1/Ado-trastuzumab emtansine is an antibody drug conjugate of a microtubule inhibitor DM-1 bound by a thioester linker to trastuzumab.

TH3RESA study was a phase III study of ado-trastuzumab emtansine versus TPC for HER2+ MBC as third-line therapy in patients already treated with trastuzumab and lapatinib. TH3RESA showed that ado-trastuzumab emtansine resulted in an improvement in PFS (median 6.2 vs. 3.3 months; $P < .0001$) (135). The treatment was better tolerated with a lower incidence of grade 3 or worse adverse events with only an increase in grade 3 thrombocytopenia as compared to physician choice chemotherapy (5% vs. 2%) (135).

EMILIA study was a phase III trial that compared ado-trastuzumab emtansine at 3.6 mg/kg IV with lapatinib 1,250 mg orally + capecitabine 1,000 mg/m^2 twice daily for days 1 to 14 for second-line therapy. The ado-trastuzumab emtansine arm had a 4-month improvement in PFS of 10 versus 6 months (HR 0.65, 95% CIs [0.55, 0.77]) (136). Ado-trastuzumab emtansine resulted in better quality of life with lower rates of diarrhea (2% vs. 21%) and hand–foot syndrome (0% vs. 16%) (136). Increased rates of thrombocytopenia (13% vs. 0.2%) and elevated liver function enzymes (7% vs. 2%) were observed with ado-trastuzumab emtansine (136).

MARIANNE trial: Ado-trastuzumab emtansine was evaluated as first-line therapy for MBC. The phase III MARIANNE trial failed to show superiority of the ado-trastuzumab emtansine compared to trastuzumab/taxane or ado-trastuzumab emtansine/pertuzumab combination. The PFS for the three arms ranged from 13.7 to 15.2 months with ORR from 60% to 68% (137).

> ➤ Based on the positive results of the EMILIA study for second-line therapy and the negative results of the MARIANNE trial for first-line therapy, Kadcyla/TDM1/ado-trastuzumab emtansine has become standard treatment for second-line HER2+ MBC.

Lapatinib

Lapatinib is a potent and reversible inhibitor of the adenosine triphosphate (ATP) binding site at the tyrosine kinase domain of HER2 and became FDA approved as a second-line therapy option for HER2+ MBC in 2007 based on the EGF100151 study.

EGF100151 study was a large phase III trial that randomized women with HER2+ MBC who had progressed after an anthracycline, taxane, and trastuzumab to a combination of capecitabine 2,000 mg/m^2 on days 1 to 14 of a 21-day cycle + lapatinib 1,250 mg daily or capecitabine alone at 2,500 mg/m^2 on days 1 to 14 of a 21-day cycle. An interim analysis strongly favored the combination arm with an HR of 0.49 in TTP ($P < .001$) (138). The median TTP was 8.4 versus 4.4 months with an ORR of 22% versus 14% with the combination versus capecitabine alone group ($P = .09$) (138). Given these results, the study was halted early. A final survival analysis failed to show statistically significant improvements in survival (64 vs. 75 weeks, HR 0.87; $P = .21$), although there was significant crossover to lapatinib (139). After adjusting for crossover, analysis showed a 20% lower risk for death for patients treated with lapatinib + capecitabine (HR, 0.80; $P = .043$) (139).

As mentioned in this section, capecitabine and lapatinib remain third-line therapy, as the *EMILIA* study showed that the ado-trastuzumab emtansine arm had a 4-month improved PFS of 10 versus 6 months (HR 0.65, 95% CIs [0.55, 0.77]) with a better toxicity profile (136).

CNS METASTASES

Capecitabine and lapatinib are small molecules that cross the blood brain barrier.

The *LANDSCAPE study* was a phase II study that showed a 65% partial response of brain metastases in patients receiving lapatinib + capecitabine prior to whole brain radiation as a systemic therapy and a median TTP of 5.5 months (140).

Currently studies are looking at other approaches to treatment of HER2+ CNS disease. **PATRICIA trial (NCT02536339)** is a phase II study looking at pertuzumab + high-dose trastuzumab after progression in the CNS post radiotherapy (141).

Another study **(NCT02048059)** is looking at GRN1005, a novel peptide–drug conjugate composed of paclitaxel covalently linked to a peptide, angiopep-2, that targets the low-density lipoprotein receptor-related protein 1 in treatment of CNS disease in breast cancer patients with recurrent CNS metastases and leptomeningeal disease (142).

> ➤ Based on currently available data, we recommend lapatinib + capecitabine as third-line therapy for HER2+ MBC, but will consider using lapatinib + capecitabine as an earlier treatment if CNS metastases are present.

CONTINUED HER2 BLOCKADE BEYOND PROGRESSION

Continued HER2 blockade beyond progression is common practice. Trastuzumab and nonanthracycline chemotherapies (eribulin, vinorelbine, gemcitabine, and taxanes) may be combined despite previous progression on trastuzumab with continued benefit. Trastuzumab beyond progression was evaluated prospectively in multiple studies as well.

HERMINE STUDY

A French observational study in subset analysis evaluated 177 patients who progressed while on first-line treatment with trastuzumab. 107 patients remained on trastuzumab beyond progression while in 70 patients trastuzumab was discontinued. The study found significant improvement in outcomes in the women who remained on trastuzumab (OS of 27.8 vs. 16.9 months; $P < .001$) and longer median OS time from the date of progression (21.3 vs. 4.6 months; $P < .001$) (143). Of note, the women not receiving trastuzumab at progression seemed to have worse prognostic factors, but an exploratory subgroup analysis controlling for such imbalances continued to identify trastuzumab beyond progression as providing significant clinical benefit (143).

GERMAN BREAST GROUP AND BREAST INTERNATIONAL GROUP

Trastuzumab beyond progression was evaluated prospectively by the German Breast Group and Breast International Group and compared capecitabine to capecitabine + trastuzumab. The analysis showed improvement in TTP of 8.2 versus 5.6 mos favoring the capecitabine + trastuzumab group with an unadjusted HR of 0.69 (95% CIs [0.48, 0.97]; two-sided log-rank $P = .0338$) (144). ORR (27.0% vs. 48.1%; odds ratio, 2.50; $P = .0115$) and OS rates (20.4 vs. 25.5 mos; $P = .257$) favored the capecitabine + trastuzumab group with no increase in toxicity (144).

> ➤ For patients who will tolerate further chemotherapy, at progression we recommend the combination of trastuzumab with nonanthracycline single agent chemotherapy. Vinorelbine, eribulin, paclitaxel, docetaxel, and gemcitabine have been combined with trastuzumab in refractory HER2+ disease.

French cohort study LHORA described the clinical features of patients with HER2+ MBC who were long-term responders to first-line trastuzumab without further disease progression (145). **This study illustrates that a subset of patients** with HER2+ MBC achieve excellent disease stability while on maintenance trastuzumab with acceptable toxicity profile. This was a multicenter, noninterventional study conducted in 57 centers in France. Eligible patients were women with HER2+ metastatic or locally advanced breast cancer, treated with first-line therapy, and progression-free for ≥3 years after starting trastuzumab. In total, 128 patients were included in this analysis; the median age was 61 years (34,35,37–61,63–71, 73–90,92–96,98–100), and 58% were ER/PR+. The median duration of first-line trastuzumab was 4.5 years (0.8–12.10); median PFS was 6.4 years (5.7; not reached); no trastuzumab deaths were seen (145).

DUAL BLOCKADE WITHOUT CHEMOTHERAPY

Many patients cannot tolerate chemotherapy. Dual HER2 blockade without chemotherapy has been tested in multiple scenarios.

TRASTUZUMAB AND LAPATINIB

EGF104900 is a phase III study that demonstrated that lapatinib + trastuzumab significantly improved PFS and CBR versus lapatinib monotherapy (146). Patients (N = 291) with HER2+ MBC whose disease progressed during prior trastuzumab-based therapies were randomly assigned to receive lapatinib monotherapy or lapatinib and trastuzumab. Lapatinib and trastuzumab dual anti-HER2 therapy without chemotherapy showed superiority to lapatinib monotherapy in PFS (11 vs. 8 weeks) (HR 0.74; P = .011) and offered significant OS benefit (14 vs. 9 mos) (HR 0.74; P = .026), despite significant crossover in the study. Absolute improvements in OS rates were 10% at 6 months and 15% at 12 months in the combination arm compared to the monotherapy arm. Multiple baseline factors including PS, nonvisceral disease, and limited metastatic sites were associated with improved OS. EGF104900 revealed a significant, 4.5-month median, OS advantage with the combination therapy and supports dual HER2 blockade in patients with heavily pretreated HER2+ MBC.

Trastuzumab and Pertuzumab Without Chemotherapy

A single-arm phase II trial was done to assess the efficacy and safety profile of the combination in patients with HER2+ MBC whose disease had progressed during prior trastuzumab-based therapy (147). The objective response rate was 24.2% and the CBR was 50% (7.6% CR, 16.7% PR, and 25.8% stable disease of ≥6 months). Median PFS was 5.5 months. Overall, the combination of pertuzumab and trastuzumab was well tolerated and active, and adverse events were mild to moderate; there were no withdrawals as a result of cardiac-related adverse events.

Other Targets With Anti-HER2 Therapy

Preclinical data show that mTOR inhibition sensitizes PTEN deficient tumors and therefore reverses trastuzumab resistance via the hyperactivated PIK/AKT/mTOR pathway. The BOLERO-1 study was done to clinically test this concept.

   BOLERO-1 (NCT00876395) was a phase III, randomized, double-blind, multicenter study of the combination of everolimus 10 mg daily and weekly trastuzumab and paclitaxel 3 out of 4 weeks as first-line treatment for patients with HER2+ MBC. In all patients, median PFS was not statistically different between the treatment arms, 14.95 months (95% CIs [14.55, 17.91]) with everolimus versus

14.49 months with placebo (HR 0.89; P = .1166) (148). In the HR negative subpopulation (n = 311), median PFS with everolimus was 20 months compared to 13 months with placebo (HR 0.66; P = .0049); however, the protocol-specified significance threshold (P = .0044) was not crossed.

The most common adverse events with everolimus were stomatitis (67% vs. 32%) and diarrhea (57% vs. 47%) (148).

➤ MANAGEMENT PEARLS—HER2+ MBC

1. The combination trastuzumab/pertuzumab/docetaxel is recommended as first-line therapy. Ado-trastuzumab emtansine is second-line therapy and lapatinib with capecitabine is the third-line treatment option for HER2+ disease.
2. After failure of the previous treatments, it is acceptable to offer treatments with other single agent chemotherapy and trastuzumab.
3. Dual HER2 blockade with lapatinib and trastuzumab or trastuzumab and pertuzumab without chemotherapy has been associated with clinically meaningful responses and survival benefit and can be considered when chemotherapy is not indicated or declined by the patient.
4. ER/PR+ HER2+ patients may have endocrine therapy combined with anti-HER2 therapy in the absence of chemotherapy.
5. Lapatinib and capecitabine are small molecules and cross the blood–brain barrier. In the presence of CNS metastasis, capecitabine and lapatinib may be considered earlier in the course of therapy.
6. A higher than standard dose of trastuzumab is being tested in a phase II PATRICIA trial (NCT02536339) in patients with HER2+ MBC with CNS involvement.

Antiresorptive Therapy for Bone Metastases

Metastatic disease to bones is very common for many cancer types, yet the incidence of bone disease is highest for patients diagnosed with breast cancer. Between 70% and 80% of women diagnosed with MBC will have bone involvement and it is the first site of metastatic disease in approximately 40% of women (149). Coupled with the fact that patients with bone only metastases tend to have longer survival and bone metastases may be associated with significant morbidity, bone metastases present a diverse challenge in the treatment of MBC. Favorable prognostic factors include low grade, ER-positivity, prolonged DFS, and lack of additional sites of disease (150).

Bone metastases disrupt the normal homeostasis between bone formation and resorption by promoting osteoclast maturation and activity and increased bone resorption; this may lead to the development of skeletal-related events (SREs) (151). SREs are defined as fractures, spinal cord compression, need for surgery and/or radiation to relieve symptomatic disease, and hypercalcemia of malignancy. The use of osteoclast inhibitors (OIs) in MBC patients with bony metastases is crucial to prevent SREs (149,152).

Studies have shown that despite the wide availability of OIs, a large proportion of patients do not receive these treatments (153,154). Studies indicate, on average, it takes about 7 months from diagnosis of bone metastases to development of the first bone complication if the patient is not treated with an OI (155). Bone pain is not always a reliable indicator to assess the risk of bone complications in patients untreated with an OI. In a retrospective analysis of patients not treated with an OI, the same percentage of patients without bone pain at baseline experienced one or more bone complications compared to patients with bone pain at baseline within 24 months (nearly 50% in each group) (152).

There are two types of OIs: bisphosphonates (pamidronate and zoledronic acid [ZA]) and rank ligand inhibitors (denosumab).

The choice of OI is generally based on patient preference (subcutaneous vs. IV therapy), frequency of administration, tolerance, and cost.

BISPHOSPHONATE

ZA demonstrated the greatest efficacy of the available bisphosphonates. ZA is dosed at 4 mg, infused over no less than 15 minutes, every 3 to 4 weeks. Infusion time is shorter when compared to pamidronate (2 hours). In placebo-controlled trials, ZA effectively decreased the risk of SREs in women with bone metastases from breast cancer (30% vs. 50%) (156). Recent results indicate that for patients who received IV monthly ZA for 1 year or longer, the efficacy of continuing ZA every 12 weeks was noninferior to every 4-week dosing (157). For patients with impaired renal function with a calculated serum creatinine clearance of less than 60 mg/min, dose reductions are required.

RANK LIGAND INHIBITOR

Denosumab is a monoclonal antibody against receptor activator of nuclear factor kappa B ligand (RANKL). For bone metastasis, the recommended dosage is 120 mg every 4 weeks. Advantages of denosumab include subcutaneous dosing, lack of need for renal dosing, and decreased acute-phase reactions (158). Acute-phase reactions (flu-like symptoms) occur almost three times more frequently with ZA than with denosumab (159).

Compared to ZA, denosumab has been shown to result in a greater reduction in risk of SREs. These results were demonstrated in a meta-analysis of three phase III trials comparing the two agents (160). Denosumab reduced SRE by 17% (HR 0.83; $P < .001$) with median time to first event of 27.6 versus 19.5 months (160). However, given the difference in cost and no difference in OS or PFS, many continue to use ZA.

Serious adverse events associated with all antiresorptive agents are hypocalcemia and osteonecrosis of the jaw (ONJ). The antiresorptive agents inhibit osteoclastic bone resorption and reduce skeletal calcium release into circulation. With calcium supplementation, the risk of hypocalcemia is reduced from 27% to 40% (161). Therefore, supplemental calcium is recommended for patients receiving these agents for bone metastasis.

The other rare but serious complication from antiresorptive therapy is ONJ. In trials comparing ZA and denosumab, less than 2% of patients developed this complication and the difference was not statistically different between the two classes (162). All patients should receive a dental examination and appropriate preventive dentistry before bone-modifying agent therapy and maintain optimal oral health. In addition, all patients should be counseled to follow up with a dental provider at regular intervals during therapy to ensure oral health is maintained. ONJ was documented as early as 4 months after starting therapy and up to 30 months after the first dose of drug; the median time of drug exposure prior to the development of ONJ was 14 months with both ZA and denosumab (162). It is essential to assess vitamin D levels before starting OIs and to prescribe appropriate supplementation (1,000 IU daily) (163,164).

Bony metastases significantly impact quality of life; therefore, MBC patients should be offered OI therapy at diagnosis with bone metastases. Patients should be carefully monitored for side effects of these therapies.

LOCAL–REGIONAL THERAPY FOR MBC

Surgical resection and radiation of the primary tumor in patients with stage IV breast cancer is controversial. Historically, systemic therapy is the mainstay of treatment and surgery has generally been reserved for palliation of symptomatic primary tumors. However, given that improvements in systemic therapy have translated into a large portion of patients being alive several years after treatment, there has been renewed interest in local–regional treatment for patients with MBC. While the success of surgical resection of the primary tumor and limited metastatic disease in other cancers, including colorectal carcinoma (165) and renal cell carcinoma (166), is well documented and results of retrospective studies in breast cancer demonstrate a survival advantage with surgery, there is significant selection bias inherent in these studies (167). Until additional results from randomized clinical trials are available, surgery and radiation therapy (RT) in patients with MBC should be considered in the context of a multidisciplinary treatment plan or for palliation in patients with progressive, symptomatic disease.

Retrospective Data

Multiple retrospective institutional and large database series have been published documenting a survival benefit for local therapy in patients with MBC (Table 6.2). The majority of the early series focused on the use of surgery; however, more recent series also included breast conserving surgery (BCS) and RT alone (173–175). A recently published meta-analysis of 15 case series found that local therapy was associated with improved survival (HR 0.69; $P < .001$), independent of age, tumor burden, type of surgery, margin status, site of metastases, HR status, and HER2 status (176). However, caution is warranted in widespread adoption of local treatment for patients with MBC based on several factors: (a) limitations of retrospective studies, including patient selection bias, (b) lack of distinction in most studies of when metastatic disease was identified (pre- or postlocal therapy), (c) identification of the optimal sequence of therapies, and (d) early preclinical animal models suggesting that local therapy can lead to an accelerated growth of metastatic disease (177,178).

A matched pair analysis examining the records of stage IV breast cancer patients from Massachusetts General Hospital and Brigham and Women's Hospital showed that case matching reduced or eliminated the apparent survival benefit associated with surgery (179).

Table 6.2 Retrospective Studies Examining the Association of Surgery and Survival in Stage IV Breast Cancer

Study	Number of patients	Dates of treatment	Surgery Y—yes N—no	Median overall survival (months)	P value
Fields et al (168)	409	1996–2005	Y—187 N—222	26.8 12.6	<.0001
Blanchard et al (169)	395	1973–1991	Y—242 N—153	27.1 16.8	<.0001
Bafford et al (170)	147	1998–2005	Y—61 N—86	42 28	.093
Ruiterkamp et al (171)	728	1993–2004	Y—288 N—440	31 14	<.0001
Lang et al (172)	208	1997–2002	Y—74 N—134	56.1 37.2	.002

Two large database analyses using data from the National Cancer Database (NCDB) and the SEER database demonstrated a survival benefit in patients with stage IV breast cancer who underwent surgical resection. The NCDB analysis evaluated survival in 16,023 breast cancer patients with stage IV disease. This study showed that surgical resection of the primary tumor with partial mastectomy (3,513 patients, median OS 26.9 months) or total mastectomy (5,649 patients, median OS 31.9 months) resulted in a survival advantage compared to patients who did not have surgery (6,861 patients, median OS 19.3 months), $P < .0001$ (180). The SEER database analysis examined outcomes in 9,734 patients with stage IV breast cancer. Patients who had surgery had a significant improvement in OS compared to patients who did not have surgery, after controlling for variables associated with survival (181).

Trials Evaluating Surgical Removal of the Primary Tumor

At the 2013 San Antonio Breast Cancer Conference, the results from two randomized clinical trials examining the role of surgical removal of the primary tumor in patients with stage IV breast cancer were presented. The primary end point for both trials was OS; on initial reporting, both showed no survival advantage for patients undergoing surgical resection.

The first trial, which was conducted at the **Tata Memorial Centre in Mumbai, India (ClinicalTrials.gov ID NCT00193778)**, enrolled 350 patients with de novo MBC. Patients received induction chemotherapy and were then randomized to local–regional therapy or no local–regional therapy for the primary tumor. With a median follow-up of 23 months, there was no reported difference in median OS between the groups, 19.2 months in the local and systemic treatment group versus 20.5 months in the systemic treatment group (HR = 1.04; 95% CIs [0.81, 1.34]) (182). In addition, no significant differences in survival were seen between groups in the planned subset analyses including menopausal status, visceral versus bone metastases, >3 versus 1 to 3 metastases, and hormone receptor or HER2 status. The authors acknowledge several limitations, including the lower than expected survival for both groups, and minimal use of adjuvant HT (7% of eligible patients) and HER2 directed therapy (2% of eligible patients) (182).

The second trial (ClinicalTrials.gov ID NCT0055986), presented at interim analysis, was conducted by the Turkish Federation of Breast Diseases Societies and randomized 278 patients to either surgery first followed by systemic therapy or systemic therapy alone (183,184). With a mean follow-up of 21 months, no significant difference in survival was reported (35% in the surgery group vs. 31% in the systemic group, $P = .24$). However, on subset analysis an improvement in OS was shown for patients in the local therapy group with a solitary bone metastasis.

Prospective trials are ongoing in the **United States/Canada (ECOG 2108/ RTOG 1173)**, Japan (185), Thailand, and Australia. We await the results of the recently closed ECOG/RTOG trial, in which women without progressive disease 16 to 32 weeks after initial systemic chemotherapy were enrolled and randomly assigned to local–regional therapy versus continuation of systemic therapy. The primary end point is OS with secondary outcomes including PFS and quality of life (QoL). While the Japanese study will also test the benefit of local therapy after systemic treatment, the trials in Thailand and Australia will mirror the Turkish study and perform local therapy prior to initiation of systemic therapy.

Until further reporting from prospective clinical trials, our decision to offer local–regional surgery and RT in the MBC setting is made on an individualized basis after discussion in multidisciplinary conference. Factors used in our decision process include age, PS, systemic disease burden, and response to initial systemic therapy. The goal of local–regional therapy in these women is to reduce the risk of local–regional recurrence, as well as to potentially provide a survival benefit.

For those thought most likely to benefit from local–regional therapy, the guidelines for choosing between BCS and mastectomy are similar to those for early-stage disease. Whole breast RT is offered following BCS and the decision to treat the regional lymphatics following BCS mirrors that for nonmetastatic disease. For patients with MBC treated with mastectomy, local–regional radiation is offered if there are positive margins, LN-positive disease, and/or initial T4 disease. We prefer to offer shorter courses of radiation for patients with metastatic disease. Therefore, for patients in which we recommend whole breast RT only, we strongly prefer use of a hypofractionated regimen (40–42.5 Gy in 15–16 fractions) (186) with consideration of a boost for patients with positive margins and young patients. When treating the breast and regional nodes, we prefer comprehensive breast and nodal RT with standard fractionation (40 in 15 fractions). For patients who are not surgical candidates, we treat gross disease to a radiobiologic equivalent dose of 70 Gy.

OLIGOMETASTATIC DISEASE IN MBC

Oligometastatic disease refers to the presence of metastatic disease at a limited number of sites, either at initial presentation (synchronous) or after definitive therapy (metachronous). Advances in detection of metastatic lesions using high resolution CT and MRI, along with the routine use of PET, have allowed for more definitive identification of metastatic disease and patients with oligometastatic disease. Local therapy with surgical metastasectomy or RT to oligometastatic sites can potentially increase the progression-free interval by removal or ablation of residual disease and neoplastic clones resistant to systemic therapies (187). Advances in delivery of radiation have allowed for more aggressive treatments (ie, higher doses of radiation) with rapid dose drop-off, resulting in reduced dose to nearby normal tissues and lower risk of toxicities.

Single fraction high-dose ablative radiation treatment, termed stereotactic radiosurgery (SRS), was pioneered for small intracranial lesions. This concept has been advanced to the treatment of extracranial lesions with stereotactic body radiotherapy (SBRT) with typical regimens containing one to five fractions. SRS and SBRT to oligometastatic sites allow for short course treatments and can be performed prior to or interdigitated with systemic therapy, which remains the cornerstone of treatment. High-dose ablative RT is also hypothesized to have additional immune-mediated effects, which may become more pronounced with the increasing use of immunomodulatory agents (188).

In patients with oligometastatic disease, improved outcomes are generally seen in patients with good response to systemic treatments, fewer and smaller metastases, lack of intracranial disease, and metachronous lesions with long disease-free intervals (189). Specific to breast cancer, improved outcomes are seen in female patients with ER-positive disease, bone only metastases, and single metastases (190). The University of Rochester investigators published a retrospective pooled analysis of women with oligometastatic disease and reported a 4-year actuarial OS of 59%, PFS of 38%, and local control of 89% (190). To directly test whether ablative therapy to oligometastases in breast cancer improves survival, the NRG has an open phase IIR/III protocol (NRG-BR002) for the use of SBRT in breast cancer with ≤2 metachronous metastatic sites. If PFS is improved with local therapy, the trial will expand patient numbers and test whether local therapy improves OS. A current phase I trial (NRG-BR001) is assessing the safety of SBRT for up to four metastatic lesions.

Similar to the data on stereotactic radiotherapy, there are case series of surgical metastasectomy. Surgery is generally reserved for patients who respond to systemic therapy, who have control of other sites of metastatic disease, and in whom an R0 resection can be achieved.

Hepatic resection for breast cancer metastases has been examined in multiple single-institution studies with 5-year survival rates ranging from 18% to 61% (191). The largest series reported in the literature evaluated patients treated at the Paul Brousse Hospital in France from 1984 to 2004 (192). A total of 85 patients with MBC underwent hepatic resection. The majority of patients received systemic therapy prior to surgery. At a median follow-up of 38 months, the median survival after surgery was 32 months and the 5-year survival was 37%. Factors associated with poor survival on multivariable analysis were lack of response to preoperative systemic therapy, R2 resection, and lack of repeat surgery for recurrent hepatic disease.

Other emerging liver-directed therapies are being used in patients with unresectable MBC with liver metastases. The two primary therapies we use include transarterial chemoembolization (TACE) and selective internal radiation (SIRT). These were initially used in primary liver malignancies and metastatic colorectal cancer, but are being more widely used in breast cancer. In 208 patients with MBC with unresectable hepatic metastases treated with TACE, response was demonstrated in 63.5% of patients with median survival of 18.5 months (193). Coldwell et al investigated the use of Yttrium-90-based SIRT in patients with chemorefractory MBC with unresectable liver metastases in 44 patients. CT response was demonstrated in 47% and PET response in 95% of patients with improved survival in responders (194).

PULMONARY METASTASIS RESECTION

Studies examining resection of pulmonary metastases in patients with stage IV breast cancer report 5-year survival rates ranging from 27% to 54% and median survival of 35 to 97 months (191). Data from the International Registry of Lung Metastases on 467 women with MBC who underwent surgical resection of lung metastases showed a median survival of 37 months and 5-year, 10-year, and 15-year survival rates of 38%, 22%, and 20% in patients who underwent complete resection (195). Factors associated with increased survival in these patients included a long disease-free interval and RO resection.

In clinical practice, identification of patients who are likely to benefit from surgical or ablative therapies remains challenging. We currently evaluate these cases individually and, if possible, prefer enrollment in a clinical trial examining this treatment paradigm. Our preference is to discuss patients in a multidisciplinary setting and offer clinical trials to eligible patients. Decisions are based on patient and disease characteristics, which have retrospectively been shown to impact patient outcomes with aggressive therapy.

CENTRAL NERVOUS SYSTEM DISEASE AND CORD COMPRESSION

CNS Disease

The occurrence of brain metastases in women with breast cancer has risen in recent years and may occur in up to 10% to 15% of all women diagnosed (196). The increase is likely due to improvements in cancer treatments and supportive care measures along with increased resolution and use of MRI. Risk factors for the development of brain metastases in breast cancer include younger age, increased nodal disease burden, higher grade tumors, larger primary tumor size, HER2 positivity, and ER-negativity. Triple-negative patients appear to be at particularly high risk.

Recently, a breast cancer-specific graded prognostic assessment (GPA) was generated to aid in prognosis for patients with brain metastases. Improved outcomes were seen in patients with high Karnofsky performance status (KPS), younger age, HER2 positivity, and ER/PR-positivity. Based on these factors, median survival can range from 3.4 months to 25.3 months (Table 6.3) (197).

Because of the heterogeneity in which patients present with brain metastases, treatment decisions are based on a number of factors including presence of neurological symptoms, concern for herniation, number and size of metastases, extent of extracranial disease, PS, and patient preference. Traditional treatment approaches include surgery and adjuvant radiation or radiation alone, which can include a combination of whole brain radiotherapy (WBRT) and SRS. There is growing controversy regarding the use of WBRT for patients with limited intracranial disease, particularly a solitary lesion.

Table 6.3 Diagnosis-Specific Graded Prognostic Assessment

Factor	Points				
	0	0.5	1.0	1.5	2.0
KPS	≤50	60	70–80	90–100	–
Subtype	Basal (triple negative)	–	Luminal A	HER2+	Luminal B
Age	≥60	<60			

GPA score	Median overall survival (months)
0–1.0	3.4
1.5–2.0	7.7
2.5–3.0	15.1
3.5–4.0	25.3

GPA, graded prognostic assessment; KPS, Karnofsky performance status.

Surgery for Brain Metastasis

Surgical resection of brain metastases is useful in many scenarios, including relief of mass effect, to improve local control, to confirm diagnosis, and as salvage treatment in previously treated patients. Of patients with brain metastases, approximately 30% are surgical candidates (minimal number of brain metastases in favorable locations with good PS) (198). In an effort to improve upon outcomes of WBRT alone, Patchell et al randomized 48 patients with solitary brain metastases to WBRT plus biopsy alone versus WBRT plus surgical resection. Of the initial 56 patients evaluated, 6 (11%) were found to have nonmetastatic lesions (primary brain tumors or abscess/inflammation). Patients who underwent surgical resection had improved local control (80% vs. 48%), functional independence (9 vs. 2 months), and median OS (9 vs. 3 months) compared to WBRT alone (199). In an attempt to decrease the role for WBRT, a subsequent study randomized patients with a solitary metastasis to resection with or without WBRT. The addition of WBRT decreased the risk of local failure (10% vs. 46%), any brain recurrence (18% vs. 70%), and neurological death (14% vs. 44%) but there was no OS benefit (200).

Radiation for Brain Metastasis

SRS

For brain metastases treated with SRS alone, local control is approximately 70% to 80% and in-brain progression is approximately 60% to 70%. Local control for patients treated with WBRT and SRS is improved to 90+% and in-brain progression decreases to 30% to 40% (201). A retrospective analysis of 132 consecutive breast cancer patients treated with SRS for brain metastases at Massachusetts General Hospital demonstrated that CNS progression was associated on multivariate analysis with omission of WBRT and triple-negative and luminal B subtypes. Factors significantly associated with OS on multivariate analysis were KPS, progressive extracranial disease, and triple-negative subtype, but not the addition of WBRT (202). Memorial Sloan Kettering retrospectively reviewed breast cancer patients with one to three brain metastases treated with SRS alone and reported median OS of 17.6 months with a local failure rate of 10% and in-brain failure rate of 45% at 1 year. On multivariate analysis, OS was impacted by triple-negative receptor status, active extracranial disease, and KPS (203). While these reports are biased due to their retrospective nature, they do suggest that SRS alone must be used with particular caution in patients with triple-negative subtype and active extracranial disease. Also, patients treated with SRS alone for breast cancer brain metastases require close surveillance.

WBRT ALONE

WBRT has been used extensively in the treatment of brain metastases for over 50 years. Initial studies in the 1960s and 1970s documented improvement in survival compared to no treatment. Modern reports on the use of WBRT show local control rates of 50% to 70% and distant brain failure of 20% (80% brain control at 1 year) (204). Modern fractionation schedules of radiation include 30 Gy in 10 fractions and 37.5 Gy in 15 fractions. Because larger fraction sizes can be associated with worse long-term cognitive toxicities, it is our preference to perform 37.5 Gy in 15 fractions, when patients have good PS and control of systemic disease.

> ## ➤ MANAGEMENT PEARLS FOR BRAIN METASTASES

Our institutional practice is to tailor treatments based on patient and disease characteristics.

1. For patients with large lesions that are symptomatic or associated with significant edema or mass effect, we recommend initial surgical resection followed by adjuvant WBRT.
2. Patients with limited systemic disease burden, 1 to 4 brain metastases, and good PS are candidates for WBRT and/or SRS. Typically, we administer 37.5 Gy in 15 fractions WBRT and utilize the SRS dose scheme per RTOG 9508 except for tumors <2 cm, where we use 20 Gy (196).
3. If patients are not candidates for frame-based radiosurgery, our institutional preference is to perform LINAC-based frameless fractionated stereotactic radiotherapy with three fractions to a total dose of 27 Gy (maximal diameter 2 cm), 24 Gy (2–3 cm), and 21 Gy (3–4 cm).
4. For patients with diffuse intracranial disease and/or a poor PS, our initial treatment of choice is WBRT, often 30 Gy in 10 fractions, although 20 Gy in 5 fractions is a good option for particularly poor performers.
5. In those patients with a modest PS who improve after WBRT, we will often consolidate larger lesions with SRS in an effort to prevent local recurrence.

Spinal Cord Compression

Another common problem from metastatic disease that compromises neurological function is vertebral body bony metastases that result in spinal cord compression. Spinal cord compression is an emergent condition best treated with multimodality treatments. Patchell et al randomized patients to radiation versus surgical decompression and subsequent radiation. Patients who received surgery had improved functional outcomes with 84% versus 57% able to walk and 122 versus 13 days of treatment response (206).

> ➤ We strongly recommend surgical decompression prior to radiation for spinal cord compression in operable patients. We typically use 30 Gy in 10 fractions to treat the cord compression with the RT portal including one vertebral body above and below the site of disease.

Bone Metastases

RT is an integral component of the treatment of bone metastases and is typically indicated for relief of pain. Use of radiation for pain associated with bone metastases results in up to a 70% to 80% RR and resolution of pain in around half of patients. The benefit typically starts 1 to 2 weeks after treatment and maximal effect is achieved 6 to 8 weeks after treatment. A prospective trial in the United States randomized 898 patients to 30 Gy in 10 fractions or 8 Gy in 1 fraction. The overall response was 66% and comparable between arms. There was more acute toxicity in the 30 Gy arm (17% vs. 10%); however, patients treated to 30 Gy required retreatment less frequently (9% vs. 18%) (207).

More recently, several prospective trials have assessed whether shorter courses of RT are equivalent to two to three treatments. For patients with MBC, shorter schedules allow for quicker reinitiation of systemic therapy and decreased transportation to the hospital. In total, 1,157 patients in the Netherlands with painful bone metastases were randomized to receive either 24 Gy in six fractions or 8 Gy in a single fraction. There was no statistically significant difference in analgesia consumption, subjective pain response, toxicities, or quality of life.

> ➤ **MANAGEMENT PEARLS FOR BONE METASTASES**
>
> 1. In our clinical practice, we generally recommend and perform short courses of palliative treatment for bone metastases (one fraction).
> 2. However, we favor more prolonged courses (2 weeks) in areas of retreatment or for patients with long life expectancy with the goal of decreasing retreatment.
> 3. Spine SBRT is typically reserved for breast cancer patients who have failed conventional RT.

REFERENCES

1. Siegel RL, Miller KD, Jemal A. Cancer statistics, 2015. *Can J Clin.* 2015;65(1):5–29.

2. Cardoso F, Harbeck N, Fallowfield L, et al. Locally recurrent or metastatic breast cancer: ESMO clinical practice guidelines for diagnosis, treatment and follow-up. *Ann Oncol.* 2012;23(suppl 7):vii11–vii19.

3. Howlader N, Noone AM, Krapcho M, et al. *SEER Stat fact sheets: female breast cancer, 1975-2013.* Bethesda, MD: National cancer institute. http://seer.cancer.gov/csr/1975_2013

4. Greenberg PA, Hortobagyi GN, Smith TL, et al. Long-term follow-up of patients with complete remission following combination chemotherapy for metastatic breast cancer. *J Clin Oncol.* 1996;14(8):2197–2205.

5. Dawood S, Broglio K, Ensor J, et al. Survival differences among women with de novo stage IV and relapsed breast cancer. *Ann Oncol.* 2010;21(11):2169–2174.

6. Andre F, Slimane K, Bachelot T, et al. Breast cancer with synchronous metastases: trends in survival during a 14-year period. *J Clin Oncol.* 2004;22(16):3302–3308.

7. Dawood S, Broglio K, Esteva FJ, et al. Defining prognosis for women with breast cancer and CNS metastases by HER2 status. *Ann Oncol.* 2008;19(7):1242–1248.

8. Simmons C, Miller N, Geddie W, et al. Does confirmatory tumor biopsy alter the management of breast cancer patients with distant metastases? *Ann Oncol.* 2009;20(9):1499–1504.

9. Schnipper LE, Smith TJ, Raghavan D, et al. American Society of Clinical Oncology identifies five key opportunities to improve care and reduce costs: the top five list for oncology. *J Clin Oncol.* 2012;30(14):1715–1724.

10. Cristofanilli M, Budd GT, Ellis MJ, et al. Circulating tumor cells, disease progression, and survival in metastatic breast cancer. *N Engl J Med.* 2004;351(8):781–791.

11. Hortobagyi GN, Smith TL, Legha SS, et al. Multivariate analysis of prognostic factors in metastatic breast cancer. *J Clin Oncol.* 1983;1(12):776–786.

12. Legha SS, Buzdar AU, Smith TL, et al. Response to hormonal therapy as a prognostic factor for metastatic breast cancer treated with combination chemotherapy. *Cancer.* 1980;46(3):438–445.

13. Eisenhauer E, Therasse P, Bogaerts J, et al. New response evaluation criteria in solid tumours: revised RECIST guideline (version 1.1). *Eur J Cancer.* 2009;45(2):228–247.

14. Wilcken N, Hornbuckle J, Ghersi D. Chemotherapy alone versus endocrine therapy alone for metastatic breast cancer. *Cochrane Database Syst Rev.* 2003;(2):CD002747.

15. Fossati R, Confalonieri C, Torri V, et al. Cytotoxic and hormonal treatment for metastatic breast cancer: a systematic review of published randomized trials involving 31,510 women. *J Clin Oncol.* 1998;16(10):3439–3460.

16. Stockler M, Wilcken N, Ghersi D, Simes RJ. Systematic reviews of chemotherapy and endocrine therapy in metastatic breast cancer. *Cancer Treat Rev.* 2000;26(3):151–168.

17. Clark GM, Osborne CK, McGuire WL. Correlations between estrogen receptor, progesterone receptor, and patient characteristics in human breast cancer. *J Clin Oncol.* 1984;2(10):1102–1109.

18. Osborne CK, Yochmowitz MG, Knight WA, McGuire WL. The value of estrogen and progesterone receptors in the treatment of breast cancer. *Cancer.* 1980;46(S12):2884–2888.

19. Stuart-Harris R, Shadbolt B, Palmqvist C, Ross HC. The prognostic significance of single hormone receptor positive metastatic breast cancer: an analysis of three randomised phase III trials of aromatase inhibitors. *Breast.* 2009;18(6):351–355.

20. Arumugam GP, Sundravel S, Shanthi P, Sachdanandam P. Tamoxifen flare hypercalcemia: an additional support for gallium nitrate usage. *J Bone Miner Metab.* 2006;24(3):243–247.

21. AstraZeneca Pharmaceuticals LP. *Nolvadex* (Tamoxifen Citrate). Wilmington, DE: Delaware. 2004. http://www.accessdata.fda.gov/drugsatfda_docs/label/2005/17970s053lbl.pdf

22. Pyrhönen S, Ellmen J, Vuorinen J, et al. Meta-analysis of trials comparing toremifene with tamoxifen and factors predicting outcome of antiestrogen therapy in postmenopausal women with breast cancer. *Breast Cancer Res Treat.* 1999;56(2):131–141.

23. Mouridsen H, Gershanovich M, Sun Y, et al. Phase III study of letrozole versus tamoxifen as first-line therapy of advanced breast cancer in postmenopausal women: analysis of survival and update of efficacy from the International Letrozole Breast Cancer Group. *J Clin Oncol.* 2003;21(11):2101–2109.

24. Bonneterre J, Buzdar A, Nabholtz JM, et al. Anastrozole is superior to tamoxifen as first-line therapy in hormone receptor positive advanced breast carcinoma. *Cancer.* 2001;92(9):2247–2258.

25. Paridaens RJ, Dirix LY, Beex LV, et al. Phase III study comparing exemestane with tamoxifen as first-line hormonal treatment of metastatic breast cancer in postmenopausal women: the European Organisation for Research and Treatment of Cancer Breast Cancer Cooperative Group. *J Clin Oncol.* 2008;26(30):4883–4890.

26. Mauri D, Pavlidis N, Polyzos NP, Ioannidis JPA. Survival with aromatase inhibitors and inactivators versus standard hormonal therapy in advanced breast cancer: meta-analysis. *J Natl Cancer Inst.* 2006;98(18):1285–1291.

27. Campos SM, Guastalla JP, Subar M, et al. A comparative study of exemestane versus anastrozole in patients with postmenopausal breast cancer with visceral metastases. *Clin Breast Cancer.* 2009;9(1):39–44.

28. Llombart-Cussac A, Ruiz A, Anton A, et al. Exemestane versus anastrozole as front-line endocrine therapy in postmenopausal patients with hormone receptor-positive, advanced breast cancer: final results from the Spanish Breast Cancer Group 2001-03 phase 2 randomized trial. *Cancer.* 2012;118(1):241–247.

29. Iwata H, Masuda N, Ohno S, et al. A randomized, double-blind, controlled study of exemestane versus anastrozole for the first-line treatment of postmenopausal Japanese women with hormone-receptor-positive advanced breast cancer. *Breast Cancer Res Treat.* 2013;139(2):441–451.

30. Rose C, Vtoraya O, Pluzanska A, et al. An open randomised trial of second-line endocrine therapy in advanced breast cancer: comparison of the aromatase inhibitors letrozole and anastrozole. *Eur J Cancer.* 2003;39(16):2318–2327.

31. Howell A, Robertson JFR, Abram P, et al. Comparison of fulvestrant versus tamoxifen for the treatment of advanced breast cancer in postmenopausal women previously untreated with endocrine therapy: a multinational, double-blind, randomized trial. *J Clin Oncol.* 2004;22(9):1605–1613.

32. Leo AD, Jerusalem G, Petruzelka L, et al. Final overall survival: fulvestrant 500 mg vs. 250 mg in the randomized confirm trial. *J Natl Cancer Inst.* 2014;106(1):1–7.

33. Robertson JFR, Llombart-Cussac A, Rolski J, et al. Activity of fulvestrant 500 mg versus anastrozole 1 mg as first-line treatment for advanced breast cancer: results from the FIRST study. *J Clin Oncol.* 2009;27(27):4530–4535.

34. Robertson JFR, Lindemann JPO, Llombart-Cussac A, et al. Fulvestrant 500 mg versus anastrozole 1 mg for the first-line treatment of advanced breast cancer: follow-up analysis from the randomized 'FIRST' study. *Breast Cancer Res Treat.* 2012;136(2):503–511.

35. Ellis MJ, Llombart-Cussac A, Feltl D, et al. Fulvestrant 500 mg versus anastrozole 1 mg for the first-line treatment of advanced breast cancer: overall survival analysis from the phase II first study. *J Clin Oncol.* 2015;33(32):3781–3786.

36. Ellis MJ, Bondarenko I, Trishkina E, et al. FALCON: A phase III randomised trial of fulvestrant 500 mg vs. anastrozole for hormone receptor-positive advanced breast cancer. Breast Cancer/Anticancer Agents & Biologic Therapy. October 8, 2016. http://www.esmo.org/Conferences/ESMO-2016-Congress/Press-Media/Targeting-Estrogen-Receptor-Improves-Progression-free-Survival-in-Advanced-Breast-Cancer

37. Bergh J, Jonsson PE, Lidbrink EK, et al. FACT: an open-label randomized phase III study of fulvestrant and anastrozole in combination compared with anastrozole alone as first-line therapy for patients with receptor-positive postmenopausal breast cancer. *J Clin Oncol.* 2012;30(16):1919–1925.

38. Mehta RS, Barlow WE, Albain KS, et al. Combination anastrozole and fulvestrant in metastatic breast cancer. *N Engl J Med.* 2012;367:435–444.

39. Chia S, Gradishar W, Mauriac L, et al. Double-blind, randomized placebo controlled trial of fulvestrant compared with exemestane after prior nonsteroidal aromatase inhibitor therapy in postmenopausal women with hormone receptor-positive, advanced breast cancer: results from EFECT. *J Clin Oncol.* 2008;26(10):1664–1670.

40. Johnston SRD, Kilburn LS, Ellis P, et al. Fulvestrant plus anastrozole or placebo versus exemestane alone after progression on non-steroidal aromatase inhibitors in postmenopausal patients with hormone-receptor-positive locally advanced or metastatic breast cancer (SoFEA): a composite, multicentre, phase 3 randomised trial. *Lancet Oncol.* 2013;14(10):989–998.

41. Johnston SRD. Enhancing endocrine therapy for hormone receptor-positive advanced breast cancer: co-targeting signaling pathways. *J Natl Cancer Inst.* 2015;107(10):1–10.

42. Baselga J, Campone MF, Piccart M, et al. Everolimus in postmenopausal hormone-receptor-positive advanced breast cancer. *N Engl J Med.* 2012;366(6):520–529.

43. Piccart M, Hortobagyi GN, Campone M, et al. Everolimus plus exemestane for hormone-receptor-positive, human epidermal growth factor receptor-2-negative advanced breast cancer: overall survival results from BOLERO-2. *Ann Oncol.* 2014;25(12):2357–2362.

44. Bachelot T, Bourgier C, Cropet C, et al. Randomized phase II trial of everolimus in combination with tamoxifen in patients with hormone receptor-positive, human epidermal growth factor receptor 2-negative metastatic breast cancer with prior exposure to aromatase inhibitors: a GINECO study. *J Clin Oncol.* 2012;30(22):2718–2724.

45. Wolff AC, Lazar AA, Bondarenko I, et al. Randomized phase III placebo-controlled trial of letrozole plus oral temsirolimus as first-line endocrine therapy in postmenopausal women with locally advanced or metastatic breast cancer. *J Clin Oncol.* 2013;31(2):195–202.

46. Finn RS, Crown JP, Lang I, et al. The cyclin-dependent kinase 4/6 inhibitor palbociclib in combination with letrozole versus letrozole alone as first-line treatment of oestrogen receptor-positive, HER2-negative, advanced breast cancer (PALOMA-1/TRIO-18): a randomised phase 2 study. *Lancet Oncol.* 2015;16(1):25–35.

47. Turner NC, Ro J, Andre F, et al. Palbociclib in hormone-receptor-positive advanced breast cancer. *N Engl J Med.* 2015:1–11.

48. Finn RS, Martin M, Rugo HS, et al. PALOMA-2: primary results from a phase III trial of palbociclib (P) with letrozole (L) compared with letrozole alone in postmenopausal women with ER+/HER2– advanced breast cancer (ABC). [abstract 507, Meeting: 2016 ASCO Annual Meeting]. *J Clin Oncol.* 2016;34.

49. Abrams J, Aisner J, Cirrincione C, et al. Dose-response trial of megestrol acetate in advanced breast cancer: cancer and leukemia group B phase III study 8741. *J Clin Oncol.* 1999;17(1):64–73.

50. Willemse PH, van der Ploeg E, Sleijfer DT, et al. A randomized comparison of megestrol acetate (MA) and medroxyprogesterone acetate (MPA) in patients with advanced breast cancer. *Eur J Cancer*. 1990;26(3):337–343.

51. Buzdar AU, Jones SE, Vogel CL, et al. A phase III trial comparing anastrozole (1 and 10 milligrams), a potent and selective aromatase inhibitor, with megestrol acetate in postmenopausal women with advanced breast carcinoma. Arimidex study group. *Cancer*. 1997;79(4):730–739.

52. Buzdar AU, Jonat WF, Howell A, et al. Anastrozole versus megestrol acetate in the treatment of postmenopausal women with advanced breast carcinoma: results of a survival update based on a combined analysis of data from two mature phase III trials. Arimidex study group. *Cancer*. 1998;83(6):1142–1152.

53. Jonat W, Howell AF, Blomqvist CF, et al. A randomised trial comparing two doses of the new selective aromatase inhibitor anastrozole (arimidex) with megestrol acetate in postmenopausal patients with advanced breast cancer. *Eur J Cancer*. 1996;32(3):404–412.

54. Dombernowsky P, Smith I, Falkson G, et al. Letrozole, a new oral aromatase inhibitor for advanced breast cancer: double-blind randomized trial showing a dose effect and improved efficacy and tolerability compared with megestrol acetate. *J Clin Oncol*. 1998;16(2):453–461.

55. Buzdar A, Douma J, Davidson N, et al. Phase III, multicenter, double-blind, randomized study of letrozole, an aromatase inhibitor, for advanced breast cancer versus megestrol acetate. *J Clin Oncol*. 2001;19(14):3357–3366.

56. Kaufmann M, Bajetta E, Dirix LY, et al. Exemestane is superior to megestrol acetate after tamoxifen failure in postmenopausal women with advanced breast cancer: results of a phase III randomized double-blind trial. The exemestane study group. *J Clin Oncol*. 2000;18(7):1399–1411.

57. Ellis MJ, Gao F, Dehdashti F, et al. Lower-dose vs. high-dose oral estradiol therapy of hormone receptor–positive, aromatase inhibitor–resistant advanced breast cancer: a phase 2 randomized study. *JAMA*. 2009;302(7):774–780.

58. Prowell TM, Davidson NE. What is the role of ovarian ablation in the management of primary and metastatic breast cancer today? *Oncologist*. 2004;9(5):507–517.

59. Robertson J, Blamey R. The use of gonadotrophin-releasing hormone (GnRH) agonists in early and advanced breast cancer in pre-and perimenopausal women. *Eur J Cancer*. 2003;39(7):861–869.

60. Taylor CW, Green S, Dalton WS, et al. Multicenter randomized clinical trial of goserelin versus surgical ovariectomy in premenopausal patients with receptor-positive metastatic breast cancer: an intergroup study. *J Clin Oncol*. 1998;16(3):994–999.

61. Klijn JG, Blamey RW, Boccardo F, et al. Combined tamoxifen and luteinizing hormone-releasing hormone (LHRH) agonist versus LHRH agonist alone in premenopausal advanced breast cancer: a meta-analysis of four randomized trials. *J Clin Oncol*. 2001;19(2):343–353.

62. Bartsch R, Bago-Horvath Z, Berghoff A, et al. Ovarian function suppression and fulvestrant as endocrine therapy in premenopausal women with metastatic breast cancer. *Eur J Cancer*. 2012;48(13):1932–1938.

63. Sawka CA, Pritchard KI, Shelley W, et al. A randomized crossover trial of tamoxifen versus ovarian ablation for metastatic breast cancer in premenopausal women: a report of the National Cancer Institute of Canada Clinical Trials Group (NCIC CTG) trial MA. 1. *Breast Cancer Res Treat*. 1997;44(3):211–215.

64. Buchanan RB, Blamey RW, Durrant KR, et al. A randomized comparison of tamoxifen with surgical oophorectomy in premenopausal patients with advanced breast cancer. *J Clin Oncol.* 1986;4(9):1326–1330.

65. Crump M, Sawka CA, DeBoer G, et al. An individual patient-based meta-analysis of tamoxifen versus ovarian ablation as first line endocrine therapy for premenopausal women with metastatic breast cancer. *Breast Cancer Res Treat.* 1997;44(3):201–210.

66. Cheung KL, Agrawal A, Folkerd EJ, et al. Suppression of ovarian function in combination with an aromatase inhibitor as treatment for advanced breast cancer in pre-menopausal women. *Eur J Cancer.* 2010;46(16):2936–2942.

67. Park IH, Ro J, Lee KS, et al. Phase II parallel group study showing comparable efficacy between premenopausal metastatic breast cancer patients treated with letrozole plus goserelin and postmenopausal patients treated with letrozole alone as first-line hormone therapy. *J Clin Oncol.* 2010;28(16):2705–2711.

68. Carlson RW, Theriault R, Schurman CM, et al. Phase II trial of anastrozole plus goserelin in the treatment of hormone receptor-positive, metastatic carcinoma of the breast in pre-menopausal women. *J Clin Oncol.* 2010;28(25):3917–3921.

69. Wang J, Xu B, Yuan P, et al. Phase II trial of goserelin and exemestane combination therapy in premenopausal women with locally advanced or metastatic breast cancer. *Medicine.* 2015;94(26):1–6.

70. PIK3CA status in circulating tumor DNA predicts efficacy of buparlisib plus fulvestrant in postmenopausal women with endocrine-resistant HR+/HER2- advanced breast cancer: first results from the randomized, phase III BELLE-2 trial (SABCS Oral Presentation #S6-01; December 11, 3:15 PM CST).

71. Tolaney S, Rosen L, Beeram M, et al. Clinical activity of abemaciclib, an oral cell cycle inhibitor, in metastatic breast cancer. San Antonio Breast Cancer Symposium. 2014(P5-19-13).

72. Hortobagyi GN, Stemmer SM, Burris HA, et al. First-line ribociclib + letrozole for post-menopausal women with hormone receptor-positive (HR+), HER2-negative (HER2−), advanced breast cancer (ABC). Breast Cancer/Anticancer Agents & Biologic Therapy. October 8, 2016. http://www.esmo.org/Conferences/ESMO-2016-Congress/Press-Media/Ribociclib-Improves-Progression-free-Survival-in-Advanced-Breast-Cancer

73. Yardley Da, Ismail-Khan R, Melichar B, et al. Randomized phase II, double-blind, placebo-controlled study of exemestane with or without entinostat in postmenopausal women with locally recurrent or metastatic estrogen receptor-positive breast cancer progressing on treatment with a nonsteroidal aromata. *J Clin Oncol.* 2013;31(17):2128–2135.

74. Joensuu H, Holli K, Heikkinen M, et al. Combination chemotherapy versus single-agent therapy as first- and second-line treatment in metastatic breast cancer: a prospective randomized trial. *J Clin Oncol.* 1998;16(12):3720–3730.

75. Alba E, Martín M, Ramos M, et al. Multicenter randomized trial comparing sequential with concomitant administration of doxorubicin and docetaxel as first-line treatment of metastatic breast cancer: a Spanish Breast Cancer Research Group (GEICAM-9903) phase III study. *J Clin Oncol.* 2004;22(13):2587–2593.

76. Sledge GW, Neuberg D, Bernardo P, et al. Phase III trial of doxorubicin, paclitaxel, and the combination of doxorubicin and paclitaxel as front-line chemotherapy for metastatic breast cancer: an intergroup trial (E1193). *J Clin Oncol.* 2003;21(4):588–592.

77. Cardoso F, Bedard PL, Winer EP, et al. International guidelines for management of metastatic breast cancer: combination vs sequential single-agent chemotherapy. *J Natl Cancer Inst.* 2009;101(17):1174–1181.

78. Norris B, Pritchard KI, James K, et al. Phase III comparative study of vinorelbine combined with doxorubicin versus doxorubicin alone in disseminated metastatic/recurrent breast cancer: National Cancer Institute of Canada clinical trials group study MA8. *J Clin Oncol.* 2000;18(12):2385–2394.

79. Jain KK, Casper ES, Geller NL, et al. A prospective randomized comparison of epirubicin and doxorubicin in patients with advanced breast cancer. *J Clin Oncol.* 1985;3(6):818–826.

80. O'Brien ME, Wigler N, Inbar M, et al. Reduced cardiotoxicity and comparable efficacy in a phase III trial of pegylated liposomal doxorubicin HCl (CAELYX/Doxil) versus conventional doxorubicin for first-line treatment of metastatic breast cancer. *Ann Oncol.* 2004;15(3):440–449.

81. Symon Z, Peyser A, Tzemach D, et al. Selective delivery of doxorubicin to patients with breast carcinoma metastases by stealth liposomes. *Cancer.* 1999;86(1):72–78.

82. Holmes FA, Walters RS, Theriault RL, et al. Phase II trial of taxol, an active drug in the treatment of metastatic breast cancer. *J Natl Cancer Inst.* 1991;83(24):1797–1805.

83. Ravdin PM, Burris HA, 3rd, Cook G, et al. Phase II trial of docetaxel in advanced anthracycline-resistant or anthracenedione-resistant breast cancer. *J Clin Oncol.* 1995;13(12):2879–2885.

84. Wilson WH, Berg SL, Bryant G, et al. Paclitaxel in doxorubicin-refractory or mitoxantrone-refractory breast cancer: a phase I/II trial of 96-hour infusion. *J Clin Oncol.* 1994;12(8):1621–1629.

85. Ghersi D, Willson ML, Chan MM, et al. Taxane-containing regimens for metastatic breast cancer. *Cochrane Database Syst Rev.* 2015;(6):CD003366.

86. Pugliese P, Brugnatelli S, Giordano M, et al. Paclitaxel in anthracycline-treated breast cancer patients. *Oncol Rep.* 1998;5(4):915–918.

87. Seidman AD, Hudis CA, Albanell J, et al. Dose-dense therapy with weekly 1-hour paclitaxel infusions in the treatment of metastatic breast cancer. *J Clin Oncol.* 1998;16(10):3353–3361.

88. Sparano JA, Wang M, Martino S, et al. Weekly paclitaxel in the adjuvant treatment of breast cancer. *N Engl J Med.* 2008;358(16):1663–1671.

89. Eisenhauer EA, Vermorken JB. The taxoids. Comparative clinical pharmacology and therapeutic potential. *Drugs.* 1998;55(1):5–30.

90. Valero V, Jones SE, Von Hoff DD, et al. A phase II study of docetaxel in patients with paclitaxel-resistant metastatic breast cancer. *J Clin Oncol.* 1998;16(10):3362–3368.

91. Desai N, Trieu V, Yao Z, et al. Increased antitumor activity, intratumor paclitaxel concentrations, and endothelial cell transport of cremophor-free, albumin-bound paclitaxel, ABI-007, compared with cremophor-based paclitaxel. *Clin Cancer Res.* 2006;12(4): 1317–1324.

92. Burstein HJ, Manola J, Younger J, et al. Docetaxel administered on a weekly basis for metastatic breast cancer. *J Clin Oncol.* 2000;18(6):1212–1219.

93. Gradishar WJ, Tjulandin S, Davidson N, et al. Phase III trial of nanoparticle albumin-bound paclitaxel compared with polyethylated castor oil-based paclitaxel in women with breast cancer. *J Clin Oncol.* 2005;23(31):7794–7803.

94. Nyman DW, Campbell KJ, Hersh E, et al. Phase I and pharmacokinetics trial of ABI-007, a novel nanoparticle formulation of paclitaxel in patients with advanced nonhematologic malignancies. *J Clin Oncol.* 2005;23(31):7785–7793.

95. Gradishar WJ, Krasnojon D, Cheporov S, et al. Significantly longer progression-free survival with nab-paclitaxel compared with docetaxel as first-line therapy for metastatic breast cancer. *J Clin Oncol.* 2009;27(22):3611–3619.

96. Rugo HS, Barry WT, Moreno-Aspitia A, et al. Randomized phase III trial of paclitaxel once per week compared with nanoparticle albumin-bound nab-paclitaxel once per week or ixabepilone with bevacizumab as first-line chemotherapy for locally recurrent or metastatic breast cancer: CALGB 40502/NCCTG N063H (Alliance). *J Clin Oncol.* 2015;33(21):2361–2369.

97. Kaufmann M, Maass N, Costa SD, et al. First-line therapy with moderate dose capecitabine in metastatic breast cancer is safe and active: results of the MONICA trial. *Eur J Cancer.* 2010;46(18):3184–3191.

98. Bajetta E, Procopio G, Celio L, et al. Safety and efficacy of two different doses of capecitabine in the treatment of advanced breast cancer in older women. *J Clin Oncol.* 2005;23(10):2155–2161.

99. Mackean M, Planting A, Twelves C, et al. Phase I and pharmacologic study of intermittent twice-daily oral therapy with capecitabine in patients with advanced and/or metastatic cancer. *J Clin Oncol.* 1998;16(9):2977–2985.

100. Blackstein M, Vogel CL, Ambinder R, et al. Gemcitabine as first-line therapy in patients with metastatic breast cancer: a phase II trial. *Oncology.* 2002;62(1):2–8.

101. Kim MK, Kim SB, Ahn JH, et al. Gemcitabine single or combination chemotherapy in post anthracycline and taxane salvage treatment of metastatic breast cancer: retrospective analysis of 124 patients. *Cancer Res Treat.* 2006;38(4):206–213.

102. Rha SY, Moon YH, Jeung HC, et al. Gemcitabine monotherapy as salvage chemotherapy in heavily pretreated metastatic breast cancer. *Breast Cancer Res Treat.* 2005;90(3):215–221.

103. Vahdat LT, Pruitt B, Fabian CJ, et al. Phase II study of eribulin mesylate, a halichondrin B analog, in patients with metastatic breast cancer previously treated with an anthracycline and a taxane. *J Clin Oncol.* 2009;27(18):2954–2961.

104. Cortes J, O'Shaughnessy J, Loesch D, et al. Eribulin monotherapy versus treatment of physician's choice in patients with metastatic breast cancer (EMBRACE): a phase 3 open-label randomised study. *Lancet.* 2011;377(9769):914–923.

105. Zelek L, Barthier S, Riofrio M, et al. Weekly vinorelbine is an effective palliative regimen after failure with anthracyclines and taxanes in metastatic breast carcinoma. *Cancer.* 2001;92(9):2267–2272.

106. Terenziani M, Demicheli R, Brambilla C, et al. Vinorelbine: an active, non cross-resistant drug in advanced breast cancer. Results from a phase II study. *Breast Cancer Res Treat.* 1996;39(3):285–291.

107. Martin M, Ruiz A, Muñoz M, et al. Gemcitabine plus vinorelbine versus vinorelbine monotherapy in patients with metastatic breast cancer previously treated with anthracyclines and taxanes: final results of the phase III Spanish Breast Cancer Research Group (GEICAM) trial. *Lancet Oncol.* 2007;8(3):219–225.

108. Weber BL, Vogel C, Jones S, et al. Intravenous vinorelbine as first-line and second-line therapy in advanced breast cancer. *J Clin Oncol.* 1995;13(11):2722–2730.

109. Gralow JR, Barlow WE, Lew D, et al. A phase II study of docetaxel and vinorelbine plus filgrastim for HER-2 negative, stage IV breast cancer: SWOG S0102. *Breast Cancer Res Treat.* 2014;143(2):351–358.

110. Perez EA, Lerzo G, Pivot X, et al. Efficacy and safety of ixabepilone (BMS-247550) in a phase II study of patients with advanced breast cancer resistant to an anthracycline, a taxane, and capecitabine. *J Clin Oncol.* 2007;25(23):3407–3014.

111. Thomas ES, Gomez HL, Li RK, et al. Ixabepilone plus capecitabine for metastatic breast cancer progressing after anthracycline and taxane treatment. *J Clin Oncol.* 2007;25(33):5210–5217.

112. Gennari, A, Stockler M, Puntoni M, et al. Duration of chemotherapy for metastatic breast cancer: a systematic review and meta-analysis of randomized clinical trials. *J Clin Oncol.* 2011;29(16):2144–2149.

113. Perez EA, Vogel CL, Irwin DH, et al. Multicenter phase II trial of weekly paclitaxel in women with metastatic breast cancer. *J Clin Oncol.* 2001;19(22):4216–4223.

114. Harvey V, Mouridsen H, Semiglazov V, et al. Phase III trial comparing three doses of docetaxel for second-line treatment of advanced breast cancer. *J Clin Oncol.* 2006;24(31):4963–4970.

115. O'Shaughnessy JA, Blum J, Moiseyenko V, et al. Randomized, open-label, phase II trial of oral capecitabine (Xeloda) vs. a reference arm of intravenous CMF (cyclophosphamide, methotrexate and 5-fluorouracil) as first-line therapy for advanced/metastatic breast cancer. *Ann Oncol.* 2001;12(9):1247–1254.

116. Modi S, Currie VE, Seidman AD, et al. A phase II trial of gemcitabine in patients with metastatic breast cancer previously treated with an anthracycline and taxane. *Clin Breast Cancer.* 2005;6(1):55–60.

117. Mavroudis D, Papakotoulas P, Ardavanis A, et al. Randomized phase III trial comparing docetaxel plus epirubicin versus docetaxel plus capecitabine as first-line treatment in women with advanced breast cancer. *Ann Oncol.* 2010;21(1):48–54.

118. Albain KS, Nag SM, Calderillo-Ruiz G, et al. Gemcitabine plus paclitaxel versus paclitaxel monotherapy in patients with metastatic breast cancer and prior anthracycline treatment. *J Clin Oncol.* 2008;26(24):3950–3957.

119. Canellos GP, Pocock SJ, Taylor SG 3rd, et al. Combination chemotherapy for metastatic breast carcinoma. Prospective comparison of multiple drug therapy with L-phenylalanine mustard. *Cancer.* 1976;38(5):1882–1886.

120. O'Shaughnessy J, Miles D, Vukelja S, et al. Superior survival with capecitabine plus docetaxel combination therapy in anthracycline-pretreated patients with advanced breast cancer: phase III trial results. *J Clin Oncol.* 2002;20(12):2812–2823.

121. Sparano JA, Vrdoljak E, Rixe O, et al. Randomized phase III trial of ixabepilone plus capecitabine versus capecitabine in patients with metastatic breast cancer previously treated with an anthracycline and a taxane. *J Clin Oncol.* 2010;28(20):3256–3263.

122. Harris L, Fritsche H, Mennel R, et al. American Society of Clinical Oncology 2007 update of recommendations for the use of tumor markers in breast cancer. *J Clin Oncol.* 2007;25(33):5287–5312.

123. Swain SM, Baselga J, Kim S, et al. Pertuzumab, trastuzumab, and docetaxel in HER2-positive metastatic breast cancer. *N Engl J Med.* 2015;372(8):724–734.

124. Konecny G, Pauletti G, Pegram M, et al. Quantitative association between HER-2/neu and steroid hormone receptors in hormone receptor-positive primary breast cancer. *J Natl Cancer Inst.* 2003;95(2):142–153.

125. Dowsett M, Dunbier AK. Emerging biomarkers and new understanding of traditional markers in personalized therapy for breast cancer. *Clin Cancer Res.* 2008;14(24):8019–8026.

126. Giordano, SH, Temin S, Kirshner JJ, et al. Systemic therapy for patients with advanced human epidermal growth factor receptor 2–positive breast cancer: American Society of Clinical Oncology clinical practice guideline. *J Clin Oncol.* 2014;32(19):2078–2099.

127. National Comprehensive Cancer Network. Breast cancer (version 1). http://www.nccn.org/professionals/physician_gls/pdf/breast.pdf. Published 2016.

128. Kaufman B, Mackey JR, Clemens MR, et al. Trastuzumab plus anastrozole versus anastrozole alone for the treatment of postmenopausal women with human epidermal growth factor receptor 2-positive, hormone receptor-positive metastatic breast cancer: results from the randomized phase III TAnDEM study. *J Clin Oncol.* 2009;27(33):5529–5537.

129. Huober J, Fasching PA, Barsoum M, et al. Higher efficacy of letrozole in combination with trastuzumab compared to letrozole monotherapy as first-line treatment in patients with HER2-positive, hormone-receptor-positive metastatic breast cancer—results of the eLEcTRA trial. *Breast.* 2012;21(1):27–33.

130. Johnston S, Pippen J, Pivot X, et al. Lapatinib combined with letrozole versus letrozole and placebo as first-line therapy for postmenopausal hormone receptor—positive metastatic breast cancer. *J Clin Oncol.* 2009;27(33):5538–5546.

131. Trastuzumab. [package insert]. https://www.gene.com/download/pdf/herceptin_prescribing.pdf

132. Slamon DJ, Leyland-Jones B, Shak S, et al. Use of chemotherapy plus a monoclonal antibody against HER2 for metastatic breast cancer that overexpresses HER2. *N Engl J Med.* 2001;344(11):783–792.

133. Swain SM, Kim S, Cortés J, et al. Pertuzumab, trastuzumab, and docetaxel for HER2-positive metastatic breast cancer (CLEOPATRA study): overall survival results from a randomised, double-blind, placebo-controlled, phase 3 study. *Lancet Oncol.* 2013;14(6):461–471.

134. Dang C, Iyengar N, Datko F, et al. Phase II study of paclitaxel given once per week along with trastuzumab and pertuzumab in patients with human epidermal growth factor receptor 2–positive metastatic breast cancer. *J Clin Oncol.* 2014;33(5):442–447.

135. Krop IE, Kim S, González-Martín A, et al. Trastuzumab emtansine versus treatment of physician's choice for pretreated HER2-positive advanced breast cancer (TH3RESA): a randomised, open-label, phase 3 trial. *Lancet Oncol.* 2014;15(7):689–699.

136. Verma S, Miles D, Gianni L, et al. Trastuzumab emtansine for HER2-positive advanced breast cancer. *N Engl J Med.* 2012;367(19):1783–1791.

137. Ellis PA, Barrios CH, Eiermann W, et al. *Phase III, randomized study of trastuzumab emtansine (T-DM1){/-} pertuzumab (P) vs trastuzumab taxane (HT) for first-line treatment of HER2-positive MBC: primary results from the MARIANNE study.* ASCO Annual Meeting Proceedings. 2015.

138. Geyer CE, Forster J, Lindquist D, et al. Lapatinib plus capecitabine for HER2-positive advanced breast cancer. *N Engl J Med.* 2006;355(26):2733–2743.

139. Cameron D, Casey M, Oliva C, et al. Lapatinib plus capecitabine in women with HER-2-positive advanced breast cancer: final survival analysis of a phase III randomized trial. *Oncologist.* 2010;15(9):924–934.

140. Bachelot T, Romieu G, Campone M, et al. Lapatinib plus capecitabine in patients with previously untreated brain metastases from HER2-positive metastatic breast cancer (LANDSCAPE): a single-group phase 2 study. *Lancet Oncol.* 2013;14(1):64–71.

141. Pertuzumab with high-dose trastuzumab in human epidermal growth factor receptor 2 (HER2)-positive metastatic breast cancer (MBC) with central nervous system (CNS) progression post-radiotherapy, ClinicalTrials.gov Identifier:NCT02536339

142. ANG1005 in breast cancer patients with recurrent brain metastases, ClinicalTrials.gov Identifier:NCT02048059

143. Extra JM, Antoine EC, Vincent-Salomon A, et al. Efficacy of trastuzumab in routine clinical practice and after progression for metastatic breast cancer patients: the observational Hermine study. *Oncologist.* 2010;15(8):799–809.

144. von Minckwitz G, du Bois A, Schmidt M, et al. Trastuzumab beyond progression in human epidermal growth factor receptor 2-positive advanced breast cancer: a German breast group 26/breast international group 03-05 study. *J Clin Oncol.* 2009;27(12):1999–2006.

145. Spano JP, Beuzeboc P, Coeffic D, et al. Long term HER2+ metastatic breast cancer survivors treated by trastuzumab: results from the French cohort study LHORA. *Breast.* 2015;24(4):376–383. doi:10.1016/j.breast.2015.02.035

146. Blackwell KL, Burstein HJ, Storniolo AM, et al. Overall survival benefit with lapatinib in combination with trastuzumab for patients with human epidermal growth factor receptor 2–positive metastatic breast cancer: final results from the EGF104900 study. *J Clin Oncol.* 2012;30(21):2585–2592.

147. Baselga J, Gelmon KA, Verma S, et al. Phase II trial of pertuzumab and trastuzumab in patients with human epidermal growth factor receptor 2–positive metastatic breast cancer that progressed during prior trastuzumab therapy. *J Clin Oncol.* 2010;28:1138–1144.

148. Hurvitz SA, Andre F, Jiang Z, et al. Combination of everolimus with trastuzumab plus paclitaxel as first-line treatment for patients with HER2-positive advanced breast cancer (BOLERO-1): a phase 3, randomised, double-blind, multicentre trial. *Lancet Oncol.* 2015;16(7):816–829.

149. Coleman RE. Clinical features of metastatic bone disease and risk of skeletal morbidity. *Clin Cancer Res.* 2006;12(20, pt 2):6243s–6249s.

150. Coleman RE, Smith P, Rubens RD. Clinical course and prognostic factors following bone recurrence from breast cancer. *Br J Cancer.* 1998;77(2):336–340.

151. Domchek SM, Younger J, Finkelstein DM, Seiden MV. Predictors of skeletal complications in patients with metastatic breast carcinoma. *Cancer.* 2000;89(2):363.

152. Saad F, Eastham J. Zoledronic acid improves clinical outcomes when administered before onset of bone pain in patients with prostate cancer. *Urology.* 2010;76(5):1175–1181.

153. Oster G, Lamerato L, Glass AG, et al. Use of intravenous bisphosphonates in patients with breast, lung, or prostate cancer and metastases to bone: a 15-year study in two large US health systems. *Support Care Cancer.* 2014;22(5):1363–1373.

154. Mortimer JE, Schulman K, Kohles JD. Patterns of bisphosphonate use in the United States in the treatment of metastatic bone disease. *Clin Breast Cancer.* 2007;7(9):682–689.

155. Rosen LS, Gordon D, Tchekmedyian NS, et al. Long-term efficacy and safety of zoledronic acid in the treatment of skeletal metastases in patients with nonsmall cell lung carcinoma and other solid tumors: a randomized, phase III, double-blind, placebo-controlled trial. *Cancer.* 2004;100(12):2613–2621.

156. Kohno N, Aogi K, Minami H, et al. Zoledronic acid significantly reduces skeletal complications compared with placebo in Japanese women with bone metastases from breast cancer: a randomized, placebo-controlled trial. *J Clin Oncol.* 2005;23(15):3314.

157. Hortobagyi GN, Lipton A, Chew HK, et al. Efficacy and safety of continued zoledronic acid every 4 weeks versus every 12 weeks in women with bone metastases from breast cancer: results of the OPTIMIZE-2 trial. *J Clin Oncol.* 2014;32:5s.

158. XGEVA® (denosumab) prescribing information. http://pi.amgen.com/united_states/prolia/prolia_pi.pdf

159. Stopeck AT, Lipton A, Body JJ, et al. Denosumab compared with zoledronic acid for the treatment of bone metastases in patients with advanced breast cancer: a randomized, double-blind study. *J Clin Oncol.* 2010;28(35):5132–5139.

160. Lipton A, Fizazi K, Stopeck AT, et al. Superiority of denosumab to zoledronic acid for prevention of skeletal-related events: a combined analysis of 3 pivotal, randomised, phase 3 trials. *Eur J Cancer*. 2012;48(16):3082–3092.

161. Body JJ, Bone HG, de Boer RH, et al. Hypocalcaemia in patients with metastatic bone disease treated with denosumab. *Eur J Cancer*. 2015;51(13):1812–1821.

162. Saad F, Brown JE, Van Poznak C, et al. Incidence, risk factors, and outcomes of osteonecrosis of the jaw: integrated analysis from three blinded active-controlled phase III trials in cancer patients with bone metastases. *Ann Oncol*. 2012;23(5):1341.

163. Wang-Gillam A, Miles DA, Hutchins LF. Evaluation of vitamin D deficiency in breast cancer patients on bisphosphonates. *Oncologist*. 2008;13(7):821–827.

164. Van Poznak CH, Temin S, Yee GC, et al. American Society of Clinical Oncology executive summary of the clinical practice guideline update on the role of bone-modifying agents in metastatic breast cancer. *J Clin Oncol*. 2011;29(9):1221–1227.

165. Ruo L, Gougoutas C, Paty PB. Elective bowel resection for incurable stage IV colorectal cancer: prognostic variables for asymptomatic patients. *J Am Coll Surg*. 2003;196(5):722–728.

166. Flanigan RC, Salmon SE, Blumenstein BA, et al. Nephrectomy followed by interferon alfa-2b compared with interferon alfa-2b alone for metastatic renal-cell cancer. *N Engl J Med*. 2001;345(23):1655–1659.

167. Hartmann S, Reimer T, Gerber B, Stachs A. Primary metastatic breast cancer: the impact of locoregional therapy. *Breast Care (Basel)*. 2014;9(1):23–28.

168. Fields RC, Jeffe DB, Trinkaus K, et al. Surgical resection of the primary tumor is associated with increased long-term survival in patients with stage IV breast cancer after controlling for site of metastasis. *Ann Surg Oncol*. 2007;14(12):3345–3351.

169. Blanchard DK, Shetty PB, Hilsenbeck SG, Elledge RM. Association of surgery with improved survival in stage IV breast cancer patients. *Ann Surg*. 2008;247(5):732–738.

170. Bafford AC, Burstein HJ, Barkley CR, et al. Breast surgery in stage IV breast cancer: impact of staging and patient selection on overall survival. *Breast Cancer Res Treat*. 2009;115(1):7–12.

171. Ruiterkamp J, Ernst MF, van de Poll-Franse LV, et al. Surgical resection of the primary tumour is associated with improved survival in patients with distant metastatic breast cancer at diagnosis. *Eur J Surg Oncol*. 2009;35(11):1146–1151.

172. Lang JE, Tereffe W, Mitchell MP, et al. Primary tumor extirpation in breast cancer patients who present with stage IV disease is associated with improved survival. *Ann Surg Oncol*. 2013;20(6):1893–1899.

173. Le Scodan R, Stevens D, Brain E, et al. Breast cancer with synchronous metastases: survival impact of exclusive locoregional radiotherapy. *J Clin Oncol*. 2009;27(9):1375–1381.

174. Bourgier C, Khodari W, Vataire AL, et al. Breast radiotherapy as part of loco-regional treatments in stage IV breast cancer patients with oligometastatic disease. *Radiother Oncol*. 2010;96(2):199–203.

175. Leung AM, Vu HN, Nguyen KA, et al. Effects of surgical excision on survival of patients with stage IV breast cancer. *J Surg Res*. 2010;161(1):83–88.

176. Petrelli F, Barni S. Surgery of primary tumors in stage IV breast cancer: an updated meta-analysis of published studies with meta-regression. *Med Oncol*. 2012;29(5):3282–3290.

177. Fisher B, Gunduz N, Saffer EA. Influence of the interval between primary tumor removal and chemotherapy on kinetics and growth of metastases. *Cancer Res*. 1983;43(4):1488–1492.

178. Fisher B, Gunduz N, Coyle J, et al. Presence of a growth-stimulating factor in serum following primary tumor removal in mice. *Cancer Res.* 1989;49(8):1996–2001.

179. Cady B, Nathan NR, Michaelson JS, et al. Matched pair analyses of stage IV breast cancer with or without resection of primary breast site. *Ann Surg Oncol.* 2008;15(12):3384–3395.

180. Khan SA, Stewart AK, Morrow M. Does aggressive local therapy improve survival in metastatic breast cancer? *Surgery.* 2002;132:620–626.

181. Gnerlich J, Jeffe DB, Deshpande AD, et al. Surgical removal of the primary tumor increases overall survival in patients with metastatic breast cancer: analysis of the 1988–2003 SEER data. *Ann Surg Oncol.* 2007;14:2187–2194.

182. Badwe R, Hawaldar R, Nair N, et al. Locoregional treatment versus no treatment of the primary tumour in metastatic breast cancer: an open-label randomised controlled trial. *Lancet Oncol.* 2015;16(13):1380–1388.

183. Soran A, Ozbas S, Kelsey SF, Gulluoglu BM. Randomized trial comparing locoregional resection of primary tumor with no surgery in stage IV breast cancer at the presentation (Protocol MF07-01): a study of Turkish Federation of the National Societies for Breast Diseases. *Breast J.* 2009;15(4):399–403.

184. Soran A, Ozmen V, Ozbas S, et al. Abstract S2-03: early follow up of a randomized trial evaluating resection of the primary breast tumor in women presenting with de novo stage IV breast cancer; Turkish study (protocol MF07-01). *Cancer Research.* 2013;73(suppl 24):S2-03.

185. Shien T, Nakamura K, Shibata T, et al. A randomized controlled trial comparing primary tumour resection plus systemic therapy with systemic therapy alone in metastatic breast cancer (PRIM-BC): Japan clinical oncology group study JCOG1017. *Jap J Clin Oncol.* 2012;42(10):970–973.

186. Whelan TJ, Pignol JP, Levine MN, et al. Long-term results of hypofractionated radiation therapy for breast cancer. *N Engl J Med.* 2010;362(6):513–520.

187. Macdermed DM, Weichselbaum RR, Salama JK. A rationale for the targeted treatment of oligometastases with radiotherapy. *J Surg Oncol.* 2008;98(3):202–206.

188. Tree AC, Khoo VS, Eeles RA, et al. Stereotactic body radiotherapy for oligometastases. *Lancet Oncol.* 2013;14(1):e28–e37.

189. de Vin T, Engels B, Gevaert T, et al. Stereotactic radiotherapy for oligometastatic cancer: a prognostic model for survival. *Ann Oncol.* 2014;25(2):467–471.

190. Milano MT, Zhang H, Metcalfe SK, et al. Oligometastatic breast cancer treated with curative-intent stereotactic body radiation therapy. *Breast Cancer Res Treat.* 2009;115(3): 601–608.

191. Pockaj BA, Wasif N, Dueck AC, et al. Metastasectomy and surgical resection of the primary tumor in patients with stage IV breast cancer: time for a second look? *Ann Surg Oncol.* 2010;17(9):2419–2426.

192. Adam R, Aloia T, Krissat J, et al. Is liver resection justified for patients with hepatic metastases from breast cancer? *Ann Surg.* 2006;244:897–907.

193. Vogl TJ, Naguib NN, Nour-Eldin NE, et al. Transarterial chemoembolization (TACE) with mitomycin C and gemcitabine for liver metastases in breast cancer. *Eur Radiol.* 2010;20(1):173–180.

194. Coldwell DM, Kennedy AS, Nutting CW. Use of yttrium-90 microspheres in the treatment of unresectable hepatic metastases from breast cancer. *Int J Radiat Oncol Biol Phys.* 2007;69:800–804.

195. Friedel G, Pastorino U, Ginsberg RJ, et al. Results of lung metastasectomy from breast cancer: prognostic criteria on the basis of 467 cases of the International Registry of Lung Metastases. *Eur J Cardiothorac Surg.* 2002;22:335–344.

196. Lin NU, Bellon JR, Winer EP. CNS metastases in breast cancer. *J Clin Oncol.* 2004;22(17):3608–3617.

197. Sperduto PW, Kased N, Roberge D, et al. The effect of tumor subtype on the time from primary diagnosis to development of brain metastases and survival in patients with breast cancer. *J Neurooncol.* 2013;112(3):467–472.

198. Kalkanis SN, Kondziolka D, Gaspar LE, et al. The role of surgical resection in the management of newly diagnosed brain metastases: a systematic review and evidence-based clinical practice guideline. *J Neurooncol.* 2010;96(1):33–43.

199. Patchell RA, Tibbs PA, Walsh JW, et al. A randomized trial of surgery in the treatment of single metastases to the brain. *N Engl J Med.* 1990;322(8):494–500.

200. Patchell RA, Tibbs PA, Regine WF, et al. Postoperative radiotherapy in the treatment of single metastases to the brain: a randomized trial. *JAMA.* 1998;280(17):1485–1489.

201. Linskey ME, Andrews DW, Asher AL, et al. The role of stereotactic radiosurgery in the management of patients with newly diagnosed brain metastases: a systematic review and evidence-based clinical practice guideline. *J Neurooncol.* 2010;96(1):45–68.

202. Dyer MA, Kelly PJ, Chen YH, et al. Importance of extracranial disease status and tumor subtype for patients undergoing radiosurgery for breast cancer brain metastases. *Int J Radiat Oncol Biol Phys.* 2012;83(4):e479–e486.

203. Yang TJ, Oh JH, Folkert MR. Outcomes and prognostic factors in women with 1 to 3 breast cancer brain metastases treated with definitive stereotactic radiosurgery. *Int J Radiat Oncol Biol Phys.* 2014;90(3):518–525.

204. Gaspar LE, Mehta MP, Patchell RA, et al. The role of whole brain radiation therapy in the management of newly diagnosed brain metastases: a systematic review and evidence-based clinical practice guideline. *J Neurooncol.* 2010;96(1):17–32.

205. Andrews DW, Scott CB, Sperduto PW, et al. Whole brain radiation therapy with or without stereotactic radiosurgery boost for patients with one to three brain metastases: phase III results of the RTOG 9508 randomised trial. *Lancet.* 2004;363(9422):1665–1672.

206. Patchell RA, Tibbs PA, Regine WF, et al. Direct decompressive surgical resection in the treatment of spinal cord compression caused by metastatic cancer: a randomised trial. *Lancet.* 2005;366(9486):643–648.

207. Hartsell WF, Scott CB, Bruner DW, et al. Randomized trial of short- versus long-course radiotherapy for palliation of painful bone metastases. *J Natl Cancer Inst.* 2005;97(11):798–804.

208. Roche H, Conte P, Perez EA, et al. Ixabepilone plus capecitabine in metastatic breast cancer patients with reduced performance status previously treated with anthracyclines and taxanes: a pooled analysis by performance status of efficacy and safety data from 2 phase III studies. *Breast Cancer Res Treat.* 2011125(3):755–765.

Ewa Mrozek, Susan B. Kesmodel, and Katherine H. R. Tkaczuk

INTRODUCTION

The incidence of pregnancy-associated breast cancer (PABCa) has been increasing during the last few decades because of the rising breast cancer incidence and the delay in childbearing to the fourth decade of life (1). PABCa is defined as breast cancer diagnosed during pregnancy or within 1 year of delivery; however, the primary difficulty in managing these patients occurs when they are diagnosed during pregnancy. Pregnant and lactating women should undergo a breast examination as part of the routine prenatal examination. All palpable breast masses should be evaluated by imaging studies, and biopsy of suspicious masses should be performed without delay. Management of breast cancer during pregnancy requires a careful balance between using standard therapies to effectively treat the mother while minimizing the potential toxicities to the fetus. PABCa should be treated according to guidelines for young nonpregnant patients in highly qualified and experienced centers (2,3). A multidisciplinary collaboration between the surgical oncologist, medical oncologist, radiologist, obstetrician specializing in high-risk pregnancies, and perinatologist is required due to concerns for congenital malformations, effects of treatment on fetal growth, preterm delivery, and long-term side effects from cancer treatments in children.

EPIDEMIOLOGY

Breast cancer, the most common cancer in pregnant women, occurs in approximately 1 in 3,000 pregnant women (4). It is estimated that 10% of breast cancers in women ≤40 years of age are pregnancy-related, and approximately 1 in 5 breast cancers diagnosed in women aged 25 to 29 years is associated with a pregnancy (5).

No specific risk factors for breast cancer in pregnancy are known. Genetic and environmental risk factors are similar to those for age-adjusted breast cancer in the general population.

PABCa presents in more advanced stages with larger primary tumors and more frequent lymph node involvement when compared to nonpregnant women (6). However, the largest cohort study of 313 patients showed that after controlling for stage, prognostic factors, and adjuvant treatment, the disease-free survival and overall survival were similar for patients with breast cancer diagnosed during pregnancy compared to nonpregnant patients with breast cancer (7). In contrast, a large meta-analysis of 30 studies showed that the diagnosis of breast cancer in the postpartum period was associated with significantly poorer outcomes compared to diagnosis during pregnancy (8).

PABCa has more unfavorable histological features: high tumor grade, lower rate of hormone receptor expression, and higher rate of HER2 expression (9).

FETAL RISKS DURING PREGNANCY

A maternal fetal medicine consultation and follow-up is necessary to document fetal growth and development, as well as fetal age. Consultation should also include the review of antecedent maternal risks such as hypertension, diabetes, and complications during prior pregnancies. Estimation of the date of delivery is necessary to plan for systemic chemotherapy and breast surgery.

Fetal exposure to chemotherapy in the first trimester, especially during the gestational age of 2 to 8 weeks when organogenesis occurs, is associated with an increased risk of spontaneous miscarriage, fetal death, and major birth defects (10). First-trimester exposure to cytotoxic drugs has been associated with a 10% to 20% risk of major malformations (11). After organogenesis, several organs including the eyes, genitals, hematopoietic system, and the central nervous system remain vulnerable to chemotherapy (12).

The use of chemotherapy in the second and third trimesters of pregnancy does not increase the risk of fetal malformations, but is associated with intrauterine growth retardation (IUGR), prematurity, lower birthweight, and higher rate of stillbirth (13). The international registry data, which included 197 pregnant women with breast cancer who received chemotherapy during the second and third trimesters of pregnancy, showed that chemotherapy in utero lowered birthweight, with a slight increase in the incidence of premature deliveries and obstetric and neonatal adverse events compared to women who were not treated with chemotherapy while pregnant (14).

A significantly higher incidence of IUGR observed with chemotherapy given during pregnancy indicates a potentially toxic influence on placental development via incomplete trophoblast invasion into the uterus, resulting in a decreased transfer of nutrients to the fetus (15). Data on transplacental transfer rates of cytotoxic drugs are very limited in humans. Animal models indicate that the placenta acts as a barrier for the transfer of most chemotherapeutic drugs, reducing fetal exposure (16). Ionizing radiation greatly interferes with cell proliferation. Fetal exposure and damage can occur during diagnostic imaging studies and therapeutic radiotherapy. Timing of the exposure to radiation relative to the gestational age of the fetus is more important than the actual dose of radiation delivered (17). Radiation exposure >0.1 Gy during the first trimester may lead to congenital malformations, mental retardation, and increased relative risk of carcinogenesis (18). These risks are the reasons that pregnancy is an absolute contraindication to the use of therapeutic radiation.

The data on long-term outcomes of children exposed to chemotherapy in utero are limited, and there are currently no specific guidelines for monitoring such children (19). A recently published multicenter case–control study showed that prenatal exposure to maternal cancer and treatment with chemotherapy did not impair the cognitive, cardiac, or general development of children in early childhood (20).

Medical termination of pregnancy may be discussed when a diagnosis of PABCa is made early in the pregnancy. Generally, however, we do not recommend termination of pregnancy, as in most cases it is acceptable to delay surgery and chemotherapy until the patient is in her second trimester of pregnancy. In some cases neoadjuvant chemotherapy can be given to patients in the second or third trimester while surgery and radiation are performed after delivery. We typically recommend delaying chemotherapy until ≥20 weeks of pregnancy. The patient and her partner should be informed about the different treatment options and the physician should explain that termination of pregnancy has not been shown to improve the overall outcome of the cancer (21).

CHEMOTHERAPY

Since many pregnant patients present with biologically aggressive and/or large, locally advanced tumors, chemotherapy, given either before or after breast surgery, is often required. Unless the woman is diagnosed with breast cancer in the late third trimester of pregnancy, postponing chemotherapy treatment until after delivery is not recommended. Data in pregnant young women indicate that delaying or postponing chemotherapy might increase the risk of relapse (22).

The physiological alterations associated with pregnancy, such as changes in plasma volume, serum albumin, increased hepatic and renal clearance, and third spacing of drugs in the amniotic sac fluid, result in lower maximal concentrations of chemotherapy and a lower area under the concentration–time curve (23). The increased activity of major enzymes involved in the metabolism of taxanes and anthracyclines (including cytochrome p450 isoforms, such as CYP3A4 and CYP2C8) observed during the late trimesters of pregnancy, can further decrease the drug exposure (24). Despite those concerns, the same dose of chemotherapy is recommended for pregnant women compared to nonpregnant women. The dosing should be based on actual bodyweight and body surface area (25).

There are no randomized controlled trials evaluating the safety of the various chemotherapy regimens in breast cancer. There is only one single-institution prospective study published on pregnant patients with breast cancer, who were treated with 5-fluorouracil, doxorubicin, and cyclophosphamide (FAC) (26). The study enrolled 81 patients and showed that pregnant women with breast cancer can be treated safely with FAC during the second and third trimesters without concerns for serious complications or short-term health concerns for their offspring.

Anthracyclines, cyclophosphamide, and taxanes, the standard adjuvant or neoadjuvant combination that is recommended for nonpregnant patients, is also recommended for treatment of PABCa after the first trimester (26–29). Taxanes are substrates for the P glycoprotein (Pgp/MDR1/ABCB1), which is highly expressed on the maternal compartment of the placenta (30). The Pgp protects the fetus against xenobiotics and might therefore reduce the transplacental transfer of taxanes. There are limited data on the use of taxanes during pregnancy; however, a published review of literature that included 23 publications describing 40 women—27 with breast cancer, 10 with ovarian cancer, and 3 with non–small-cell lung cancer—and 42 neonates showed that taxanes do not appear to increase the risk of fetal or maternal complications when administered in the second and third trimesters of pregnancy (27). Paclitaxel was administered in 21 cases, docetaxel in 16 cases, and both drugs in 3 cases; except for 2 cases, taxanes were administered concomitantly or sequentially with other cytotoxic agents such as anthracyclines, cyclophosphamide, and platinum derivatives.

The use of anthracycline- or taxane-free regimens is not considered to be standard in nonpregnant women and therefore is not recommended in pregnant women. Since a recently published study found that fluorouracil does not add any benefit to an anthracycline–taxane-based regimen, it is no longer indicated for breast cancer therapy (31). In view of the third-space effect of methotrexate, the combination of this drug with cyclophosphamide and fluorouracil should not be used in pregnant women (32). Currently, there are limited reports of use of dose dense regimens for PABCa (33).

Targeted therapy. Trastuzumab use is not recommended during pregnancy. HER2 is strongly expressed in the fetal renal epithelium (34). A recent review identified 18 reports in the literature of trastuzumab use during pregnancy (35). The most frequent adverse effect, occurring in 33% of reported cases, was oligohydramnios and anhydramnios. Most of the pregnancies ended prematurely and four of the newborns died from complications of prematurity (mainly respiratory failure). However, the use of trastuzumab may be discussed in special, high-risk situations. In the neoadjuvant setting, treatment with pertuzumab in addition to trastuzumab and chemotherapy increases the pathological complete response rate in patients with HER2-positive breast cancer, but currently there are no data on use of pertuzumab during pregnancy and we would not recommend this approach in pregnant women. New breast cancer drugs, such as tyrosine kinase inhibitors, should not be used in pregnant patients because they have not been tested in this group. For HER2-positive pregnant patients receiving neoadjuvant therapy we typically recommend initiating standard chemotherapy before delivery and delaying the anti-HER2 therapy until after delivery, at which point a full course of trastuzumab +/− pertuzumab every 3 weeks for 17 cycles can be completed.

Supportive treatment for chemotherapy can be given to pregnant women according to general recommendations. The typical side effects and risks of chemotherapy in pregnant women are similar to those risks in nonpregnant women. There is consensus on the safe use of antiemetics like metoclopramide, the 5-HT-3 antagonist ondansetron, and corticosteroids during pregnancy (36,37). No data are available on the use of neurokinin 1 (NK-1) antagonists. Regarding corticosteroids, the use of methylprednisolone or hydrocortisone is preferred over dexa/betamethasone. Hydrocortisone and methylprednisolone are extensively metabolized in the placenta, so relatively small amounts of these drugs cross into the fetal compartment (38).

Granulocyte colony stimulating factor (G-CSF) is frequently used in nonpregnant patients to manage chemotherapy-induced neutropenia. The effectiveness and safety profile of G-CSF are not clearly established in pregnancy. Although data on the use of G-CSF in pregnant women are limited, we found no conclusive evidence that G-CSF use increases the rates of fetal death or congenital malformations, but feel that G-CSF should only be recommended when chemotherapy is recommended with curative intent after consideration of the overall risks and benefits. In an observational study in women with cyclic, idiopathic, or autoimmune neutropenia, the use of G-CSF during pregnancy was associated with no significant increase in adverse events, considering all pregnancies or individual mothers and adverse events in the neonates were similar between pregnancies with or without G-CSF therapy (39). Filgrastim carries the Food and Drug Administration (FDA) pregnancy category C and is not recommended unless the benefit outweighs the risk to the developing fetus. This generally means that animal studies have showed some evidence of maternal toxicity, embryolethality, and fetotoxicity; there are no controlled data in human pregnancy. Women who become pregnant during treatment with filgrastim should enroll in Amgen's Pregnancy Surveillance Program—1-800-77-AMGEN (1-800-772-6436). Nonetheless, the administration of G-CSF in pregnancy should only be considered when the benefits of managing maternal neutropenia outweigh the unknown fetal risks.

Chemotherapy should be avoided after 35 weeks of gestation due to the risk of spontaneous delivery before the recovery of bone marrow. In addition, delivery postponement after chemotherapy will facilitate fetal drug clearance via the placenta. This is most important in preterm babies who have immature liver and kidneys and thus limited capacity to metabolize and excrete the drugs.

HORMONAL THERAPY

Tamoxifen is the standard hormonal agent used for the treatment of premenopausal women with endocrine-responsive breast cancer, but it is a teratogenic agent. Studies using adjuvant hormonal therapy for breast cancer in pregnant women are very limited. Animal models have shown that tamoxifen can cause genitourinary developmental defects (40). Other birth defects associated with use of tamoxifen include Goldenhar syndrome (oculoauriculovertebral dysplasia), ambiguous genitalia, and Pierre Robin sequence, the triad of small mandible, cleft palate, and glossoptosis (41,42). A review of Astra Zeneca files identified 50 cases that were exposed to tamoxifen during pregnancy, with 10 congenital defects identified (43). Therefore, hormonal therapy should be started after delivery and after completion of chemotherapy. Delaying hormonal treatment will not reduce the efficacy of tamoxifen.

SURGERY IN PREGNANCY

Surgery can be performed during all trimesters of pregnancy (43). However, in the first trimester there is an increased risk of pregnancy loss and concern for potential exposure of the fetus to teratogens. The risk of miscarriage and preterm labor is lowest in the second trimester and increases during the third trimester.

When performing surgery in pregnant women, it is important to maintain venous return to the heart, which may be compromised due to pressure from the uterus. Patients who are at 20 weeks or greater gestation should be positioned in a left lateral tilt position to reduce compression on the inferior vena cava.

Surgical options that are available to pregnant women are the same as those that are available to nonpregnant patients and depend on the size of the tumor and extent of lymph node involvement. If breast conserving surgery is performed during pregnancy then adjuvant radiation therapy needs to be delayed until after delivery.

For early-stage breast cancer patients having surgery during pregnancy, sentinel lymph node biopsy typically with radiotracer alone may be considered (44). The radiation exposure to the fetus is low with this procedure. However, the options of sentinel lymph node biopsy and axillary lymph node dissection and the risks of each procedure should be clearly discussed with the patient. We currently discuss the option of sentinel lymph node biopsy using low-dose (10 MBq) lymphoscintig-raphy using (99m)Tc human serum albumin nanocolloids, radiotracer alone with pregnant patients who have clinically negative lymph nodes (45).

For patients with locally advanced tumors, we consider neoadjuvant systemic therapy, when appropriate, prior to surgery.

It is always important for the surgeon to speak with anesthesia and maternal fetal medicine so that a plan for anesthesia and fetal monitoring (when necessary) can be discussed and arranged prior to surgery.

➤ MANAGEMENT PEARLS

Anticancer treatment approaches should be individualized and adapted to the clinical presentation (breast cancer stage at presentation) and the trimes-ter of the pregnancy. Patients should be treated as closely as possible to the standard of care for nonpregnant patients and for the particular stage at diag-nosis. We always recommend a multidisciplinary approach to management from the initial diagnosis of breast cancer in a pregnant patient. Our specific approaches are discussed and reviewed as follows.

1. Surgery can be performed during all trimesters of pregnancy; however, it is preferred to wait until the second trimester when possible. Anesthe-sia risks during pregnancy should be considered and discussed with the patient's high-risk OB/GYN.
2. Surgical options in pregnant patients are the same as those for nonpreg-nant patients.
3. Standard anthracycline- and taxane-based chemotherapies can be used during the second and third trimesters. Dosing is similar to that for nonpregnant women. However, the use of growth factors (Neupogen or Neulasta) is less well defined, although studies have shown acceptable maternal and fetal safety in noncancer settings.
4. Monoclonal antibody therapy such as trastuzumab and pertuzumab and tyrosine kinase inhibitors have to be postponed until after delivery. For HER2-positive pregnant patients receiving neoadjuvant therapy we typically recommend initiating standard chemotherapy before delivery and delaying the anti-HER2 therapy until after delivery, at which point a full course of trastuzumab +/− pertuzumab every 3 weeks for 17 cycles can be completed.
5. Radiation therapy and hormonal treatments should be postponed until after delivery.
6. Delivery should not be induced before 37 weeks of pregnancy.

REFERENCES

1. Balasch J, Gratacós E. Delayed childbearing: effects on fertility and the outcome of preg-nancy. *Curr Opin Obstet Gynecol.* 2012;24(3):187–193.
2. Loibl S, Schmidt A, Gentilini O, et al. Breast cancer diagnosed during pregnancy: adapt-ing recent advances in breast cancer care for pregnant patients. *JAMA Oncol.* 2015;1(8):1145–1153.

3. Gradishar WJ, Anderson BO, Balassanian R, et al. Breast cancer version 2.2015. *J Natl Compr Canc Netw.* 2015;13(4):448–475.

4. Anders CK, Johnson R, Litton J, et al. Breast cancer before age 40 years. *Semin Oncol.* 2009;36(3):237–249.

5. Lee YY, Roberts CL, Dobbins T, et al. Incidence and outcomes of pregnancy-associated cancer in Australia, 1994-2008: a population-based linkage study. *BJOG.* 2012;119(13):1572–1582.

6. Stensheim H, Møller B, van Dijk T, Fosså SD. Cause-specific survival for women diagnosed with cancer during pregnancy or lactation: a registry-based cohort study. *J Clin Oncol.* 2009;27(1):45–51.

7. Amant F, von Minckwitz G, Han SN, et al. Prognosis of women with primary breast cancer diagnosed during pregnancy: results from an international collaborative study. *J Clin Oncol.* 2013;31(20):2532–2539.

8. Azim HA, Jr, Santoro L, Russell-Edu W, et al. Prognosis of pregnancy-associated breast cancer: a meta-analysis of 30 studies. *Cancer Treat Rev.* 2012;38(7):834–842.

9. Middleton LP, Amin M, Gwyn K, et al. Breast carcinoma in pregnant women: assessment of clinicopathologic and immunohistochemical features. *Cancer.* 2003;98(5):1055–1060.

10. Williams SF, Schilsky RL. Antineoplastic drugs administered during pregnancy. *Semin Oncol.* 2000;27(6):618–622.

11. Weisz B, Meirow D, Schiff E, Lishner M. Impact and treatment of cancer during pregnancy. *Expert Rev Anticancer Ther.* 2004;4(5):889–902.

12. Cardonick E, Iacobucci A. Use of chemotherapy during human pregnancy. *Lancet Oncol.* 2004;5(5):283–291.

13. Van Calsteren K, Heyns L, De Smet F, et al. Cancer during pregnancy: an analysis of 215 patients emphasizing the obstetrical and the neonatal outcomes. *J Clin Oncol.* 2010;28(4): 683–689.

14. Loibl S, Han SN, von Minckwitz G, et al. Treatment of breast cancer during pregnancy: an observational study. *Lancet Oncol.* 2012;13(9):887–896.

15. Cardonick E, Dougherty R, Grana G, et al. Breast cancer during pregnancy: maternal and fetal outcomes. *Cancer J.* 2010;16(1):76–82.

16. Van Calsteren K, Verbesselt R, Van Bree R, et al. Substantial variation in transplacental transfer of chemotherapeutic agents in a mouse model. *Reprod Sci.* 2011;18(1):57–63.

17. Kal HB, Struikmans H. Radiotherapy during pregnancy: fact and fiction. *Lancet Oncol.* 2005;6(5):328–333.

18. Needleman S, Powell M. Radiation hazards in pregnancy and methods of prevention. *Best Pract Res Clin Obstet Gynaecol.* 2016;33:108–116.

19. Hahn KM, Johnson PH, Gordon N, et al. Treatment of pregnant breast cancer patients and outcomes of children exposed to chemotherapy in utero. *Cancer.* 2006;107:1219–1226.

20. Amant F, Vandenbroucke T, Verheecke M, et al. Pediatric outcome after maternal cancer diagnosed during pregnancy. *N Engl J Med.* 2015;373(19):1824–1834.

21. Amant F, Loibl S, Neven P, Van Calsteren K. Breast cancer in pregnancy. *Lancet.* 2012;379(9815):570–579.

22. Beadle BM, Woodward WA, Middleton LP, et al. The impact of pregnancy on breast cancer outcomes in women ≤35 years. *Cancer.* 2009;115(6):1174–1184.

23. van Hasselt JG, van Calsteren K, Heyns L, et al. Optimizing anticancer drug treatment in pregnant cancer patients: pharmacokinetic analysis of gestation-induced changes for doxorubicin, epirubicin, docetaxel and paclitaxel. *Ann Oncol.* 2014;25(10):2059–2065.

24. Isoherranen N, Thummel KE. Drug metabolism and transport during pregnancy: how does drug disposition change during pregnancy and what are the mechanisms that cause such changes? *Drug Metab Dispos.* 2013;41:256–262.

25. Van Calsteren K, Verbesselt R, Ottevanger N, et al. Pharmacokinetics of chemotherapeutic agents in pregnancy: a preclinical and clinical study. *Acta Obstet Gynecol Scand.* 2010;89(10):1338–1345.

26. Murthy RK, Theriault RL, Barnett CM, et al. Outcomes of children exposed in utero to chemotherapy for breast cancer. *Breast Cancer Res.* 2014;16:500.

27. Mir O, Berveiller P, Goffinet F, et al. Taxanes for breast cancer during pregnancy: a systematic review. *Ann Oncol.* 2010;21(2):425–426.

28. Germann N, Goffinet F, Goldwasser F. Anthracyclines during pregnancy: embryo-fetal outcome in 160 patients. *Ann Oncol.* 2004;15(1):146–150.

29. Ring AE, Smith IE, Jones A, et al. Chemotherapy for breast cancer during pregnancy: an 18-year experience from five London teaching hospitals. *J Clin Oncol.* 2005;23:4192–4197.

30. Mir O, Berveiller P, Ropert S, et al. Emerging therapeutic options for breast cancer chemotherapy during pregnancy. *Ann Oncol.* 2008;19:607–613.

31. Del Mastro L, De Placido S, Bruzzi P, et al. Fluorouracil and dose-dense chemotherapy in adjuvant treatment of patients with early-stage breast cancer: an open-label, 2 × 2 factorial, randomised phase 3 trial. *Lancet.* 2015;385(9980):1863–1872.

32. Amant F, Deckers S, Van Calsteren K, et al. Breast cancer in pregnancy: recommendations of an international consensus meeting. *Eur J Cancer.* 2010;46(18):3158–3168.

33. Cardonick E, Gilmandyar D, Somer RA. Maternal and neonatal outcomes of dose-dense chemotherapy for breast cancer in pregnancy. *Obstet Gynecol.* 2012;120(6):1267–1272.

34. Press MF, Cordon CC, Slamon DJ. Expression of the HER-2/neu proto-oncogene in normal human adult and fetal tissues. *Oncogene.* 1990;5(7):953–962.

35. Zagouri F, Sergentanis TN, Chrysikos D, et al. Trastuzumab administration during pregnancy: a systematic review and meta-analysis. *Breast Cancer Res Treat.* 2013;137(2):349–357.

36. Matok I, Gorodischer R, Koren G, et al. The safety of metoclopramide use in the first trimester of pregnancy. *N Engl J Med.* 2009;360:2528–2535.

37. Pasternak B, Svanström H, Hviid A. Ondansetron in pregnancy and risk of adverse fetal outcomes. *N Engl J Med.* 2013;368(9):814–823.

38. Crowther CA, Doyle LW, Haslam RR, et al. Outcomes at 2 years of age after repeat doses of antenatal corticosteroids. *N Engl J Med.* 2007;357(12):1179–1189.

39. Boxer LA, Bolyard AA, Kelley ML, et al. Use of granulocyte colony-stimulating factor during pregnancy in women with chronic neutropenia. *Obstet Gynecol.* 2015;125(1):197–203.

40. Iguchi T, Hirokawa M, Takasugi M. Occurrence of genital tract abnormalities and bladder hernia in female mice exposed neonatally to tamoxifen. *Toxicology.* 1986;42:1:1–11.

41. Tewari K, Bonebrake RG, Asrat T, Shanberg AM. Ambiguous genitalia in infant exposed to tamoxifen in utero. *Lancet.* 1997;350(9072):183.

42. Isaacs RJ, Hunter W, Clark K. Tamoxifen as systemic treatment of advanced breast cancer during pregnancy—case report and literature review. *Gynecol Oncol.* 2001;80(3):405–408.

43. Barthelmes L, Gateley CA. Tamoxifen and pregnancy. *Breast.* 2004;13(6):446–451.

44. Cardonick, E. Pregnancy associated breast cancer: optimal treatment options. *Int J Womens Health.* 2014;6:935–943.

45. Gentili O, Cremonesi M, Toesca A, et al. Sentinel lymph node biopsy in pregnant patients with breast cancer. *Eur J Nucl Med Mol Imaging.* 2010;37(1):78–83.

Rachel Bluebond-Langner, Erin M. Rada, and Sheri Slezak

INTRODUCTION
Goals of Reconstruction
Breast reconstruction is usually not a single operation but rather a process that is an integral part of holistic care of the breast cancer patient. While women are initially concerned with their cancer diagnosis, most will go on to live long, normal lives. Over these years, many women find that breast reconstruction improves their ability to participate in desired activities, recover from cancer diagnosis, and ultimately achieve "wholeness." Nationally, approximately 50% of patients choose to undergo breast reconstruction (1). Regardless, all patients should be educated by a plastic surgeon about their reconstructive options at the time of their diagnosis and counseled appropriately. Studies find that information given before surgery by both the oncologic surgeon and a plastic surgeon about reconstruction can mitigate some of the imagined fears of recurrence, pain, and out of pocket costs (2). Patients' education impacts their quality of life, not only before surgery, but also long after finishing treatment.

Types of Reconstruction
In general, there are three types of breast reconstruction: autologous (utilizing the patient's own tissue), implant-based (ultimately utilizing a breast implant), and oncoplastic reduction (preserving and reshaping breast tissue remaining after a partial mastectomy). Decision making regarding reconstruction requires a discussion between the patient and surgeon to determine a patient's candidacy for various options based upon her body habitus, breast cancer treatment plan, medical and surgical comorbidities, and patient preferences. This makes the ultimate type of reconstruction a highly individualized decision for each patient. Differences between the implant and the autologous tissue breast reconstruction are shown in Table 8.1.

No Reconstruction/External Prosthesis
Approximately half of patients who undergo mastectomy choose no reconstruction (1). Many of these patients make this decision because they wanted to avoid further surgery; however, access to a plastic surgeon and preoperative counseling may also affect this decision. Patients who choose not to undergo reconstructive surgery may choose to wear an external prosthesis in their bra or other padded undergarments. There are, however, drawbacks to prostheses. Some women find them hot, heavy, and they may be displaced with movement or sports activities.

Table 8.1 Differences Between Expander/Implant and Autologous Tissue Reconstruction

Type of reconstruction	Expander/implant	Autologous tissue reconstruction
Surgery	2 or 3 operations	Usually 2 operations
General anesthesia	Yes	Yes
Hospitalization	First stage: 1–2 days Second stage: outpatient	Usually 3–5 days
Recovery period	2–3 weeks	4–8 weeks
Need for multiple office visits	Yes (for expansion)	Yes
Scars	Mastectomy scar only	Mastectomy scar and donor site scar
Shape and consistency	No natural sag, may be firm	More natural shape, soft
Potential problems	Breast hardening with shape change, skin ripples, infection, rupture	Abdominal weakness or bulge (TRAM), partial breast hardening, total flap loss
Skin sensation	Altered in surgical areas	Altered in surgical areas

TRAM, transverse rectus abdominis myocutaneous.

IMPLANT-BASED RECONSTRUCTION

Implant-based reconstruction refers to reconstruction ultimately utilizing a breast implant. At the time of mastectomy, either a permanent implant may be placed (sometimes referred to as "direct to implant") or, more commonly, a tissue expander is placed. The tissue expander acts as a temporary placeholder and is serially expanded with saline over several weeks to months in the outpatient setting. It is ultimately replaced with a permanent implant in a second-stage outpatient operation.

Choosing Implant-Based Reconstruction

According to statistics reported by the American Society of Plastic Surgeons (ASPS), 106,338 women underwent breast reconstruction in 2015 (www.plasticsurgery.org/news/plastic-surgery-statistics). Seventy-three percent of these women opted to have tissue expansion and subsequent placement of an implant. In a survey of female board certified plastic surgeons in the United States, 66% reported that they would personally choose implant-based reconstruction if they underwent mastectomy (3). Of the female plastic surgeons who primarily perform implant-based surgery, 87% would choose expander-based reconstruction for themselves. Of the female surgeons who perform autologous reconstruction for the majority of their patients, about half would choose expanders for their own surgery.

Implants and Devices Used for Reconstruction
TISSUE EXPANDERS

Tissue expanders consist of a silicone outer membrane and an internal cavity that expands with the injection of filler. They come in a wide variety of sizes, shapes, and designs. Some surgeons use a one-shape-fits-all approach (since this is a temporary device) whereas others utilize a base diameter measurement or a target volume. Other choices include round, profiled, or dual chamber. Tissue expander ports are either integrated or remote.

If the mastectomy flaps allow, it is preferable to fill the expander to about half of the mastectomy breast weight so that the patient is not flat postoperatively. The amount of fill in the operating room can be varied given the thickness of the flaps, the quality of the muscle coverage, and the size of the breast. If the mastectomy flaps are thin or of questionable blood supply, then the expander can be left empty to place less stress on the flaps. A 50% fill in the operating room is typically enough for the patient to see some shape but not enough to give the patient severe pain or to compromise the flaps and incision.

Postoperatively, tissue expanders are then filled in the office by the physician or by an appropriate physician extender. The valve is found with a magnet and 60 to 180 mL of fluid is placed per session based upon patient tolerance. If too much is placed at once, patients can have considerable pain from stretching of the muscle. Muscle relaxants may be useful in these cases. Fills are continued every week or two until the desired size is obtained, or until the breast is a bit larger than the contralateral side. Often, chemotherapy or radiation therapy may be needed in the postoperative period. Expansion can be continued during chemotherapy, but the shape of the breast should not be altered during radiation therapy because the dosimetric plan would be compromised. Depending on the radiation techniques utilized at a given institution, a tissue expander may be deflated so that superficial electron beam radiation can effectively target the internal mammary nodes. There is no time limit in which expansion must be completed; expanders have been left in place for extended periods without difficulty. Alternative methods of expansion with air or carbon dioxide activated by the patient are currently being explored.

When expansion is complete, secondary surgery is scheduled to remove the expander and perform the definitive reconstruction with a permanent implant, autologous tissue, or autologous tissue and an implant.

BREAST IMPLANTS

In the United States, breast implants are either saline- or silicone-filled. They are either profiled (form stable) or round, with a moderate to high projection, and have either textured or smooth surfaces. Current silicone implants are made with cohesive gel filler that has more crosslinking between silicone molecules than the silicone filler of previous generations. If cut in half, all currently available silicone implants remain intact like gelatin rather than leaking out. The vast majority of mastectomy (Figure 8.1) patients prefer silicone implants to saline because these

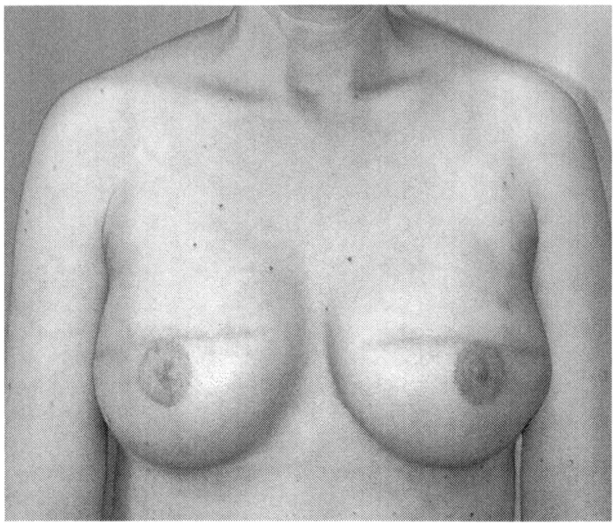

Figure 8.1 Bilateral mastectomy with implant reconstruction; nipples are tattooed.

implants are softer, feel more like normal tissue, move with the patient, and are more comfortable. Sizes range from 100 to 800 mL. Generally, the amount of saline placed in the expander is recorded and this is approximately the size of the implant chosen.

Acellular Dermal Matrix Sling for Inferior Implant Coverage

The implant or the expander is most commonly placed below the pectoralis major muscle. Traditionally, it was covered by the pectoralis muscle, serratus, and rectus fascia. More commonly now, a prosthetic or bioprosthetic sling is used to bridge the gap between the lower edge of the pectoralis muscle and the inframammary fold. While acellular dermal matrix (ADM) is the most common sling material, there are alternatives including bovine, porcine, and poly vicryl substitutes.

The sling gives complete coverage of the implant, prevents displacement of the implant above the muscle or laterally into the axilla, pulls the pectoralis muscle down to prevent window shading up, defines the inframammary fold, and allows greater intraoperative fill volume. There is also data that ADMs decrease the incidence of capsular contracture. Ibrahim et al demonstrated improved breast contour and cosmetic appearance with an ADM sling, allowing the implant to sit lower with a more natural shape, better lower pole projection, and inframammary fold definition (4). Increased risk of complication with slings is still debated. Lee did a meta-analysis of 23 studies representing 6,199 cases (5). He found that the use of ADM significantly elevated the risks of infection, seroma, and mastectomy flap necrosis, but did not affect the risks of implant loss, unplanned reoperation, and total complications. Critics of acellular matrixes also cite its significant cost.

Advantages of Implant-Based-Reconstruction

1. There are no additional scars. Implant-based reconstruction uses the mastectomy defect only, and does not have any donor site morbidity or scars elsewhere in the body.
2. There is a faster overall recovery period. The operation is only 30 to 60 minutes longer than the mastectomy and the postoperative length of stay is the same—typically one day.

Disadvantages of Implant-Based Reconstruction

1. If tissue expanders are utilized, the patient must go through a period of expansion in the outpatient setting over several weeks to months depending upon the desired size followed by a *second operation* to replace the tissue expanders with permanent breast implants.
2. Expanders are typically placed below the pectoralis major muscle, which may cause more postoperative pain with expansion compared to some alternatives.
3. Breast implants tend to sit higher on the chest and do not descend as naturally over time. In patients with unilateral mastectomy, this may cause significant asymmetry requiring contralateral procedures.
4. Patients must be counseled that implants are not meant to be lifelong devices. Given the young age of many breast cancer patients, most will require implant exchange at least once over the course of their lifetime. Implants last about 15 years, but the range is variable.
5. The largest implant currently available on the market is 800 mL though many implant companies plan to expand their lines to include larger sizes. For women with large breasts prior to mastectomy, 800 mL may not be adequate.

Complications of Implant-Based Surgery

INFECTION

Infection of an implant poses a serious threat to the success of expander/implant-based reconstruction. Incidence is 3.4% to 34.4% (6–8). Risk factors for infection include breast size larger than "C," previous irradiation, and repeat tissue expander placements (9). Organisms are most commonly staphylococcus species but may also include gram-negative rods and anaerobes. Cultures taken from the drains may help when choosing a course of antibiotics for patients with implant/expander-related infections. Treatment was historically implant removal followed by several months delay prior to a repeat reconstruction attempt. More recently, studies have shown successful treatment of up to 64.4% of patients with less severe infections using a combination of operative treatment and/or antibiotics (10,11). Patients successfully treated were stable with a normal white count and localized infection.

CAPSULAR CONTRACTURE

Capsular contracture has been a challenging complication since breast implants were introduced in 1960. Scarring around the implant causes a firm, high-riding breast that may be uncomfortably tight. *Grade* of capsular contracture is measured clinically according to the Baker Scale (Table 8.2) (12).

Table 8.2 Baker Capsular Contracture Scale After Prosthetic Breast Reconstruction

IA	Absolutely natural, cannot tell breast was reconstructed
IB	Soft, but the implant is detectable by physical examination or inspection because of mastectomy
II	Mildly firm reconstructed breast with an implant that may be visible and detectable by physical examination
III	Moderately firm reconstructed breast. The implant is readily detectable, but the result may still be acceptable
IV	Severe capsular contracture with unacceptable aesthetic outcome and/or significant patient symptoms requiring surgical intervention

The rate of capsular contracture has improved with newer model implants. In recent studies, grade III/IV contracture ranges from 8.3% to 16.3% (6,8). Rates of contracture are higher in irradiated breasts.

The cause of capsular contracture is not well understood but various theories have been postulated including silicone bleed, subclinical infection, bacterial biofilm formation, foreign body reaction, allergy, and patient factors. In Del Pozo's study of explanted breast prostheses, those with capsular contracture had a positive culture rate of 33% whereas those removed for other reasons had a 5% positive culture rate (13). Schreml et al found a 66.7% colonization rate for Baker III and IV capsules whereas no colonization was detected for Baker I and II capsules (14). Physicians have tried various strategies to avoid this complication including submuscular implant placement, textured implant shells, saline instead of silicone filler, ADM coverage, leukotriene antagonist administration, vitamin E therapy, ultrasound therapy, massage, and capsulectomy, all with various degrees of success.

MASTECTOMY FLAP ISCHEMIA

Flap ischemia can lead to necrosis, dehiscence, and loss of an expander. Implant-based surgery will only succeed if there is an adequate skin envelope to surround it. Extremely thin flaps are prone to necrosis and unlikely to succeed. Patients have different levels of adipose tissue, and some flaps are thinner in areas of the tumor. Methods of intraoperative perfusion assessment are becoming increasingly popular to assess perfusion to the mastectomy flaps. Newer technology provides an accurate and real-time intraoperative assessment of skin flap viability. If flow is inadequate, the plastic surgeon can excise the questionable area, place less fluid in the expander, delay the reconstruction, or plan to bring in new tissue with the use of autologous flaps.

FLUID COLLECTION

Hematoma and seroma are both complications that can occur after a large dead space is created during mastectomy. Rates of hematoma are lower than seroma, 1.3% and 4.9%, respectively (6,8).

Prevention of seromas is attempted with the use of closed suction drains at the time of mastectomy and expander placement. They are typically removed when drainage is less than 30 mL daily for three consecutive days. Persistent and high drainage may be a sign of a subclinical infection or a lymphatic leak. Other ways to prevent seromas that are less commonly performed include progressive tension sutures between the inferior pectoralis muscle or ADM and the skin flap, the use of new expanders with integral drain ports, and use of tissue glues.

While seromas may be aspirated, there is no conclusive data to guide the decision to aspirate secondary seromas or to let them resolve passively. The increased pressure of the seroma can make the process self-limiting, but this fluid is also a good medium for infection.

IMPLANT RUPTURE

Implant rupture may eventually occur in all patients. There is no evidence that a ruptured implant causes any health issues. It may present as a deflation (saline) or a change in firmness or contour (silicone). Many silicone ruptures are silent, so silicone implant ruptures must be evaluated with MRI. The Food and Drug Administration (FDA) recommends that any ruptured implant be replaced or removed because it is not in the state that the manufacturer tested it.

The expander can deflate from a mechanical fault at a seam, or it can be accidentally injured at the time of surgery or during injections in the office. If close to the goal volume, one may simply proceed to implant exchange. If not, the expander must be replaced. Some expanders have flipped and the valve becomes inaccessible. Fixation of the tabs can make this less likely.

VISIBLE RIPPLING OR WRINKLING OF THE IMPLANT

Implant rippling has been reported in 3% to 10% of patients in several studies (8). Many mastectomy flaps are very thin, making the folds in the implant visible. There are several strategies to correct this. Silicone implants show fewer ripples than saline implants. Form stable implants have the least visible rippling. The surgeon can attempt to disguise ripples by placing ADM beneath the mastectomy flap to increase the thickness or tighten the muscle and capsule. Fat injections into the flaps can also disguise ripples. A latissimus dorsi flap can be rotated under the skin to provide more coverage. It is generally only ripples in the cleavage area that are bothersome to the patient.

Surveillance

Expanders and implants are typically placed below the pectoralis major muscle, deep to the breast, so cancer surveillance is performed via palpation. No further mammograms are needed. FDA recommendations for implant surveillance (in all cosmetic and reconstructive surgery patients) are baseline MRI 3 years postoperatively followed by every 2 years thereafter. With rupture rates under 8% at 10 years, some feel that this is overly aggressive and expensive. High-resolution ultrasounds may also provide adequate surveillance.

Direct-to-Implant Reconstruction

When women have small to moderate sized breasts with minimal to moderate ptosis and wish to remain the same size or smaller after reconstruction, it is possible to avoid the expansion process and go immediately to permanent implants. The maximum size of the implant that can be placed at the time of mastectomy depends on the mastectomy flap thickness, the available muscle, the patient's desired size, and the use of local dermal flaps or ADM. A meta-analysis of 13 studies comparing direct-to-implant breast reconstructions with standard two-stage reconstructions revealed that wound infection, seroma, and capsular contracture risk were similar (15). Direct-to-implant reconstruction, however, had a higher risk for skin flap necrosis (OR, 1.43) and reoperation (OR, 1.25). It is imperative to choose the appropriate candidate for this procedure, but it is attractive in that it offers a one operation mastectomy and reconstruction. Tissue expanders should also be on hand in the operating room in case the flaps are thin or the perfusion to the flaps is questionable.

AUTOLOGOUS RECONSTRUCTION

Autologous reconstruction refers to procedures that utilize the patient's own tissue to recreate the absent breast. Historically, autologous reconstruction referred to only pedicled flaps including transverse rectus abdominis myocutaneous (TRAM) flaps and latissimus dorsi flaps. With advances in microsurgical techniques, free tissue transfer has become a mainstay of breast reconstruction.

Choosing Autologous Reconstruction

As with implant-based reconstruction, women choose to undergo autologous reconstruction for various reasons. While there is an additional donor site with a separate incision, many women like removal of excess skin and fat (ie, abdomen). While implants are safe, some women still develop unknown systemic complications from silicone. Other women do not like the idea of a foreign body and want their own tissue.

Donor Sites

The selection of donor site is based on the patient's body habitus as well as desire. The abdomen and back are the two most common donor sites for autologous tissue. A flap from the abdomen can be harvested with skin, fat, and muscle (TRAM flap) or with only skin and fat, sparing the muscle (deep inferior epigastric perforator [DIEP] or superficial inferior epigastric artery [SIEA] flaps). The latissimus dorsi muscle (Figure 8.2) can be harvested with skin and fat that sits in the bra line and rotated around to the chest. Generally, an implant is needed behind the flap for adequate size and projection. The buttock tissue (superior or inferior gluteal artery perforator [SGAP/IGAP] flap) and inner thigh tissue (transverse upper gracilis [TUG] flap) are less common donor sites and usually reserved for women who are very thin but want their own tissue and do not want to use their back or in whom autologous tissue is needed but other donor sites are not available.

Advantages

1. Some patients need a large skin paddle to replace resected skin.
2. In unilateral breast reconstruction cases it is often easier to match a large and ptotic breast with the patient's own fat.
3. Autologous tissue will produce more natural ptosis over time.

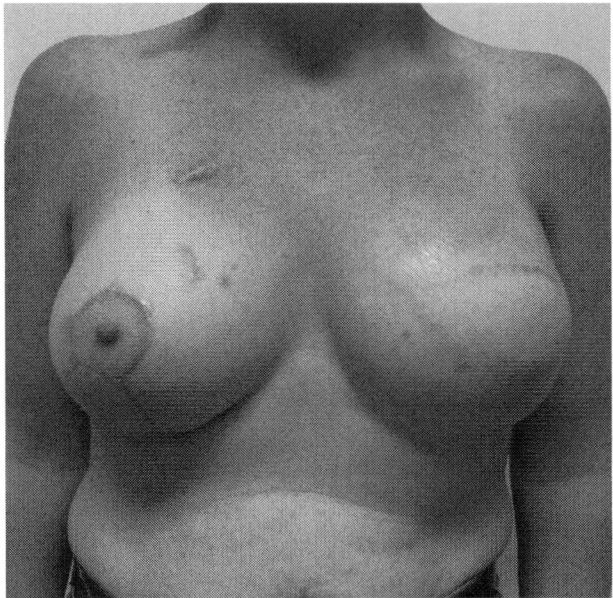

Figure 8.2 Left mastectomy with radiation; left latissimus dorsi and implant reconstruction; right mastopexy and augmentation.

4. One can avoid some of the prosthesis-related complications such as implant rupture, capsular contracture, and infection. If autologous tissue becomes infected it can be treated with antibiotics and occasionally wash out but the whole reconstruction is usually not lost.
5. While there is a donor site scar, many women like the idea of skin and fat being removed from another area of the body, particularly the abdomen.
6. Autologous tissue does not need to be replaced in 10 to 20 years.

Disadvantages

1. Longer operative time: Autologous tissue reconstruction has a longer operative time compared to implant reconstruction. Of the donor sites, the latissimus dorsi is the shortest, but a bilateral microsurgical reconstruction can be 10 to 12 hours or more. Longer operative times increase the risk of perioperative complications overall. Some patients, due to their comorbidities, may not be good candidates for microvascular reconstructions.
2. Flap failure: Microsurgical free tissue transfer has a failure rate of 1% to 10%. If the flap fails, an alternate form of reconstruction will need to be selected. Depending on the patient's needs, this may be immediate placement of an implant, a latissimus dorsi with implant, or another free flap. This may require a second operation once the patient has healed. This can be very disappointing for both the patient and the surgeon.

3. Donor site morbidity: With all autologous reconstruction there will be some donor site morbidity although it may be minimal. The potential for donor site complications such as wound infection, abdominal weakness, bulge, or hernia (TRAM or DIEP) needs to be discussed with the patient preoperatively. While some people will counsel patients that a TRAM or a DIEP is just like a tummy tuck, the incision may be higher than in a cosmetic abdominoplasty and the abdominal musculature may be weakened, leading to a bulge or hernia in up to 10% of cases (16).
4. Longer recovery: While implant reconstruction is an outpatient procedure, autologous tissue reconstruction requires a one-night (latissimus dorsi) or three- to five-night (DIEP, TRAM, and SGAP) inpatient stay. The postoperative recovery is 3 weeks (latissimus dorsi) to 6 weeks (TRAM, DIEP, and SGAP).

AUTOLOGOUS/IMPLANT COMBINED RECONSTRUCTION

In addition to the implant-based and autologous breast reconstruction modalities described here, some patients will require both. This combination reconstruction is used when autologous tissue is required to provide adequate healthy soft tissue but the volume and projection of the breast with the flap alone are inadequate. The most common scenario is the use of a latissimus dorsi rotational flap with an implant.

Difference Between TRAM and DIEP

A TRAM flap takes some or all of the rectus abdominis muscle. Patients may have hernias, bulges, or weakness in sports or heavy lifting activities. A DIEP flap (Figure 8.3) spares the muscle although it is divided to get to the vessels. More muscle function is preserved.

ONCOPLASTIC BREAST RECONSTRUCTION TECHNIQUES

One of the greatest advances of the past 10 years has been the incorporation of plastic surgery techniques in breast conservation with excellent cosmesis. Although most lumpectomy patients need only primary closure, there are some difficult resections that will leave large deficits and gross asymmetry or leave defects in cosmetically sensitive locations, such as the areola or upper inner quadrant. Breast conserving therapy can be offered to more people with superior cosmetic results when oncoplastic reconstruction is considered.

In oncoplasty, there are two basic different approaches:

1. *Volume-removal procedures,* which combine resection with breast reduction and reshaping techniques, and
2. *Volume-replacement* techniques, using fat grafting, local flaps (glandular, fasciocutaneous, or latissimus dorsi), or implants to fill in the lumpectomy cavity.

These procedures are generally needed if more than 20% of the breast will be excised, or if the patient is a D or larger cup size and desires reduction. These risks are small and can be reduced by waiting a full 6 to 8 weeks for radiation, and leaving the affected breast a bit larger than the contralateral side so that radiation shrinkage will be negated (Table 8.3).

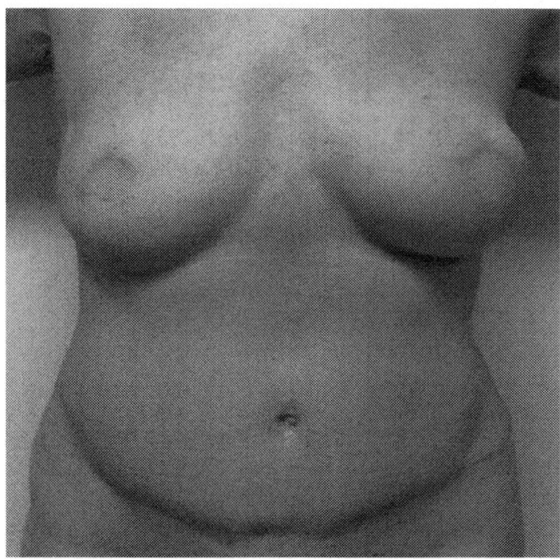

Figure 8.3 Bilateral deep inferior epigastric perforator (DIEP) flap reconstruction.

Fat necrosis or changes in mammogram are possible after rearrangement of breast tissue. Some authors report increased need for biopsy but others find no difference. Piper et al found no significant difference in abnormal mammographic findings prompting biopsy between oncoplastic reduction patients and lumpectomy alone patients at 6 months, 2 years, and 5 years postoperatively ($P > .05$). Biopsy rates over the 5-year period did not differ significantly between the two cohorts (18% lumpectomy, 24% oncoplastic cohort, $P = .46$) (19).

Table 8.3 Advantages/Disadvantages of Volume-Reduction Techniques	
Advantages	**Disadvantages**
Breast is saved and blood supply is intact before radiation, so healing is better (17,18)	A slightly longer operative time (3 hours)
Radiation is easier with fewer skin complications; less severe radiation dermatitis due to less redundant skin folds	The need for two surgical specialists in the operating room (breast and plastic surgeons) simultaneously
Allows better local control, with wider margins, and there is less repeat surgery for positive margins. The opposite breast is sampled	The possibility of wound complications delaying chemotherapy or radiation
Relief of neck, back, and shoulder pain and inframammary rashes	

In a large meta-analysis by Losken et al, oncoplastic reductions were compared to patients undergoing lumpectomy alone. Oncoplastic reductions had a larger specimen (4 times), a lower positive margin rate (12% vs. 21%), fewer reexcisions (4% vs. 14%), and higher patient satisfaction (90% positive vs. 83%) (20). In patients with ptosis who want to maintain as much volume as possible, a mastopexy will tighten the skin and lessen the volume defect by shaping the remaining tissue. A contralateral small reduction can be done to match the lumpectomy weight plus 10% to 20%.

Volume-Replacement Techniques

If a patient is small-breasted or does not wish to be smaller, then it is best to use a volume-replacement technique such as fat grafting, local breast glandular flap, a latissimus dorsi myocutaneous flap, a lateral thoracodorsal flap, or local abdominal advancement flaps. The larger lower abdominal free flaps are generally not needed and should be saved if total mastectomy is needed for positive margins or recurrence.

If the defect is central and requires the resection of the nipple–areolar complex (NAC), local flaps are useful to replace this area and avoid a depression. A new nipple can be reconstructed and areolar tattoos can be used after healing. Among oncoplastic approaches, a less utilized technique is the use of an implant. Although this can easily correct a local volume deficit, the cosmetic effects after radiation can be variable, and many patients will get a capsular contracture that causes firmness and distortion.

Silverstein et al recently described "extreme oncoplasty," which he defines as "breast conservation using oncoplastic techniques in a patient who, in most physicians' opinions, requires a mastectomy" (21). He studied patients with large (>5 cm) multifocal or multicentric tumors, positive nodes, and patients who will require radiation therapy, even if treated with mastectomy. He compared 66 such extreme patients with 245 consecutive patients with unifocal or multifocal tumors less than 5 cm. Complete resection rates were 96% standard versus 83% extreme and median tumor size was 21 mm versus 62 mm. Margins equal or greater than 1 mm were achieved in 88.6% versus 54%. Seventeen (6.9%) standard patients underwent reexcision versus 9% of extreme patients to achieve wider margins. One patient (0.4%) was converted to mastectomy versus four (6%) extreme patients. With 24 months of median follow-up, three patients (1.2%) in the standard group experienced local recurrence versus one patient (1.5%) in the extreme group. It is expected that the local recurrence will be somewhat higher in the extreme group but that there will be little or no impact on survival. Women who wish to save their breasts may try oncoplastic techniques and go on to mastectomy only if local control is not obtained. Similarly many patients treated with neoadjuvant therapy may be able to undergo breast conserving surgery with good margin control. Longer term studies are needed of local recurrence and survival.

Timing of Reconstruction

Treatment of breast cancer patients requires a multidisciplinary team approach. Breast reconstruction is one aspect of that care and must be planned in conjunction with the patient's overall oncologic treatment and goals. Breast cancer reconstruction may occur immediately (at the time of mastectomy) or in a delayed fashion.

IMMEDIATE RECONSTRUCTION

The definitive reconstruction with an implant, a latissimus dorsi with implant, or an autologous flap is performed at the time of mastectomy. Immediate reconstruction can be very appealing as it reduces the number of operations. The disadvantages of immediate breast reconstruction include longer operative time; fresh mastectomy flaps, which may have unapparent ischemia and subsequent necrosis; uncertainty about the need for postoperative radiation; and the need to heal quickly if chemotherapy is recommended. Complications are reported to be higher in immediate reconstruction as compared to delayed reconstruction, but this may be partially explained by the fact that immediate reconstruction will include the complications of both surgeries: the mastectomy and the reconstruction. This is generally done in patients in whom radiation is not needed (ie, prophylactic mastectomy, small area of ductal carcinoma in situ [DCIS]).

DELAYED IMMEDIATE RECONSTRUCTION

It is most common for tissue expanders to be placed at the time of mastectomy, await the final pathology, determine the need for chemotherapy and radiation, and then proceed with the definitive reconstructive plan. The disadvantage is that reconstruction occurs in two stages and that the tissue expander may be removed.

DELAYED RECONSTRUCTION

Some women do not have reconstruction at the time of mastectomy for a variety of reasons: stage of the cancer, medical comorbidities, or patient choice. Reconstruction can be performed months or years after mastectomy if the patient's medical circumstances or desire changes. Disadvantages include more operations and the resection of more skin in an unreconstructed breast. When reconstruction is performed later, additional skin is needed via expansion or autologous tissue.

Radiation Therapy and Breast Reconstruction

There have been great changes in radiation techniques over the last 20 years, and there are often no residual changes in a radiated patient's skin as compared to the other breast. Radiation oncologists target the breast parenchyma with tangential beams, and spare the skin, giving better long-term results. However, for the majority of patients, radiation makes breast reconstruction more difficult and increases the risk of complications for both implant-based reconstruction and microsurgical reconstruction. The skin envelope of the radiated breast will be tighter and the breast will never sag in the same way. Implant-based reconstruction in the setting of radiation has a higher incidence of infection, capsular contracture, and even implant extrusion. Radiation is not an absolute contraindication to tissue expander placement or implant-based reconstruction; however, the patient needs to be counseled about the potential increased risk for complication. Radiation can also make autologous reconstruction more challenging and increase the risk of flap failure as the vessels to which the flap is being anastomosed may have been damaged by the radiation. If the patient's skin has severe radiation changes such as telangiectasia, hyperpigmentation, parenchymal asymmetry, and/or skin thickening, then it is doubtful that this skin will successfully expand or be able to support an implant long term. In these cases, autologous tissue should be used: either a free flap or a latissimus dorsi with an implant.

However, radiation is not a contraindication for tissue expansion or implant-based reconstruction. The current evidence is divided with regard to radiation and the development of complications during breast reconstruction. In the Michigan Breast Reconstruction Outcome Study, radiotherapy, both before and after surgery, was associated with at least one complication; however, this trend did not reach statistical significance (6). McCarthy et al performed a retrospective comparative study of 1,170 expander/implant patients over 2 years and determined that pre-operative and postoperative chest wall irradiations were not significant predictors of complications (7). However, other studies differ in their findings. Contant et al studied 103 women with BRCA gene mutations undergoing prophylactic mastectomy with immediate expander/implant reconstruction. Radiation was found to be a significant risk factor, both for complications and for implant removal (22). It seems that some radiated patients do well and others do not. They must, however, be warned that some capsular contracture is seen in approximately 40% of these reconstructions. If the contracture is Baker grade II, it may be acceptable, but if it is Baker grade III or IV, patients will usually pursue capsulectomy to address the tightness.

Some patients wait to have reconstruction because of fear of recurrence in the first several years. Many patients (and some doctors) worry that reconstruction will hide a recurrence, but studies have not shown this (23). Since reconstruction does not affect surveillance or survival, immediate reconstruction or delayed immediate reconstruction (tissue expanders) saves the patient additional surgery, anesthesia, and recovery time by starting the reconstruction at the same time as the mastectomy. The patient does not have to endure a period of deformity and can move forward. In a study by Morrow et al, of the women who elected to undergo implant-based reconstruction, 82% underwent immediate reconstruction whereas only 18% selected a delayed reconstruction (1). Studies show less mourning and a faster return to daily activities if women have some form of reconstruction started at the time of the mastectomy. The Michigan Breast Reconstruction Outcome Study reviewed psychosocial outcomes at 1 and 2 years. That study found that both immediate and delayed reconstruction with implant and TRAM methods provided substantial psychosocial benefits to patients as measured by the Short Form-36 and the Functional Assessment of Cancer Therapy-Breast (24).

Secondary Reconstruction Procedures

NIPPLE RECONSTRUCTION

This is usually the last step in breast reconstruction. It can be done under local analgesia alone. The nipple projection is created from local tissue flaps. ADM or cartilage can be added for additional projection if desired. The areola is then tattooed (Figure 8.4). Recently many women have been electing not to have nipple reconstruction and elect for three-dimensional tattoos only. When done by a professional tattoo artist the results are outstanding.

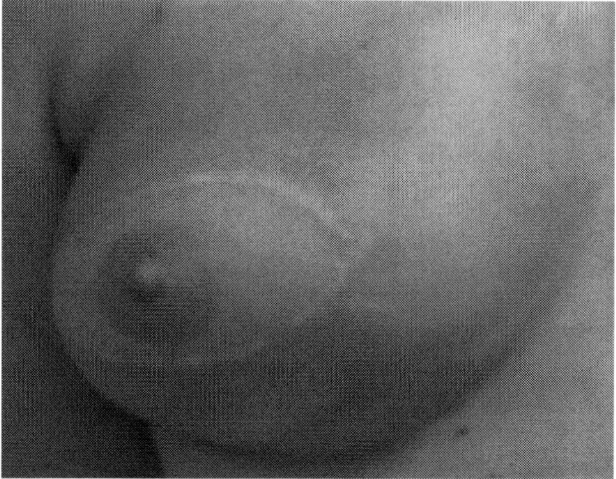

Figure 8.4 Nipple reconstruction with tattoo (latissimus dorsi w/implant).

In the past 5 years, there has been more interest in saving the NAC in mastectomy. There are considerable cosmetic advantages to NAC preservation. Metcalfe et al studied 157 women and found that on the BREAST-Q, women with NAC-sparing mastectomy had significantly higher levels of satisfaction with their breasts (P = .01), satisfaction with outcome (P = .02), and sexual well-being (P < .001) compared to skin-sparing mastectomy (SSM) (25). Advocates argue that only 1% or 2% of breast tissue in the nipple is retained and that this tissue is in a known location and can be followed by clinical examination.

Present criteria for preservation include tumors greater than 2 cm from the areola, no skin involvement, and no nipple discharge or disease. Relative contraindications to this procedure are ptotic breasts, large breast size, smoking, diabetes, and prior radiation therapy—each of these factors makes the flaps longer with more risk of ischemia. This can lead to skin and nipple necrosis, which is reported to be about 5% to 10% (26). Skin incisions for nipple-sparing mastectomy (NSM) may be periareolar, lateral, or inframammary. Inframammary incisions are the best concealed but require an incision length of 8 to 10 cm and the flaps are long. Rawlani et al found that periareolar incisions are associated with more nipple necrosis than lateral or inferior incisions (31% vs. 6%) (27).

At the time of surgery, the breast tissue is removed and reconstruction can then be accomplished by any method. While the cosmetic result can be excellent, there is controversy about the oncologic principles. Occult cancer can be present at the nipple ducts in 0% to 30% of nipples of mastectomies. Larger tumors and tumors closer to the areola are found to have higher incidence of nipple involvement (28). If the frozen section is positive at surgery, the NAC is removed. The longest follow-up of NAC preservation comes from Sakurai in Japan. He followed 932 patients over 19 years. The median follow-up time was 78 months and the longest was 21 years.

No significant difference in the probability of local recurrence between the NSM cohort and the SSM cohort was found (8.2% vs. 7.6%; P = .81). The rate of NAC relapse was low (3.7%), and the entire nipple and/or areola recurrence cases were treated with NAC removal. Furthermore, nipple and/or areola recurrence was associated with a significantly better prognosis than that of skin flap recurrences and local lymph node recurrences. For the 21-year disease-free survival and the 21-year overall survival, no significant difference between the NSM and SSM cohorts was observed (29). Boneti et al followed 281 total skin-sparing mastectomies (TSSMs) and 227 SSMs. The overall complication rate (TSSM 7.1% and SSM 6.2%; P = .67) and local–regional recurrence rate (TSSM 6% [7 of 152] and SSM 5.0% [7 of 141]; P = .89) were comparable (30). A meta-analysis by De la Cruz et al found 20 studies comparing different mastectomies with 5,594 patients. He found a 3.4% risk difference between NSM and SSM in overall survival and a 0.4% risk difference between NSM and SSM in local recurrence. Studies with follow-up intervals of <3 years, 3 to 5 years, and >5 years had mean survival of 97.2%, 97.9%, and 86.8%; a local recurrence risk of 5.4%, 1.4%, and 11.4%; and nipple–areola cancer rates of 2.1%, 1.0%, and 3.4%, respectively (31). The risk seems to be low but present, and it increases with time. Further studies that evaluate these patients for longer time intervals are needed.

BALANCING PROCEDURES FOR THE CONTRALATERAL BREAST IN A UNILATERAL MASTECTOMY

Breasts come in pairs and symmetry is expected. It is important, however, to remind patients that perfect symmetry is not realistic. Studies show that 90% of normal women are asymmetric and that breasts are "sisters, not twins" (32). When performing a unilateral reconstruction, one should never assume that a patient desires to match her opposite breast. She may wish to enlarge, lift, reduce, or remove the noncancerous side. Patients should consider the breast they would like to have, not what is present. A reduction, lift, or augment can be performed on the nonreconstructed breast to match the reconstructed breast. Generally, patients with larger breasts are delighted to have a reduction, and are very pleased with the new look and lightness. The pathological examination of the contralateral side is also comforting to the patient if it is normal. We have found that 1.78% of reductions in the contralateral breast of women with cancer have a pathological finding of cancer, despite a normal mammogram (Figure 8.5) (33). It is important to orient and identify these contralateral specimens so that if something is found, the surgeon can locate the area in question for further resection if necessary.

FAT GRAFTING

A normal breast is tapered at the edges but an implant or flap has a distinct edge. Some lumpectomies cause dents or depressions, and some flaps do not fill the entire mastectomy defect. These deformities can be treated with adjunct fat grafting. Fat is harvested by liposuction and reinjected into the areas of depression. This provides increased thickness and uniformity of the breast. The fat is revascularized by the surrounding tissue and this provides long-term correction of problem areas. A few authors advocate total breast reconstruction by injected fat, but this requires multiple procedures and has a risk of fat necrosis.

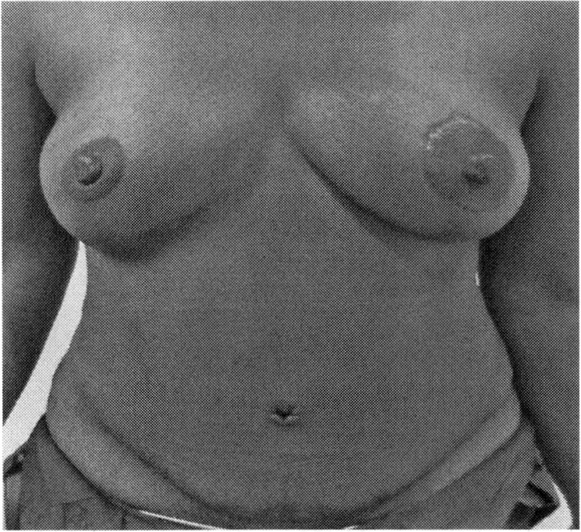

Figure 8.5 Right deep inferior epigastric perforator (DIEP) flap reconstruction and left mastopexy.

➤ MANAGEMENT PEARLS

1. Breast reconstruction is usually not a single operation but rather a process that is an integral part of holistic care of the breast cancer patient.
2. Every mastectomy patient should hear about reconstruction from both her oncologic surgeon and a plastic surgeon, but not all will choose reconstruction. Studies show that information given before surgery by both the oncologic surgeon and a plastic surgeon about reconstruction can mitigate some of the imagined fears of recurrence, pain, and out of pocket costs.
3. There are two ways to make a new breast: implants or autogenous tissue. A breast means different things to different women; therefore, different women pick different (or no) reconstructions—this is fine.
4. Breast reconstruction improves patients' ability to participate in desired activities, recover from cancer diagnosis, and ultimately achieve wholeness.
5. Treatment of breast cancer patients requires a multidisciplinary team approach; breast reconstruction is one aspect of that care and must be planned in conjunction with the patients' overall oncologic treatment and goals. Breast cancer reconstruction may occur immediately (at the time of mastectomy) or in a delayed fashion.
6. Although reconstruction is generally not needed for lumpectomy defects, new advances in oncoplastic surgery allow reconstruction of central breast lesions that require removal of the nipple/areola, large breasts that benefit from reduction, and balancing operations for the contralateral side.

REFERENCES

1. Morrow M, Li Y, Alderman AK, et al. Access to breast reconstruction after mastectomy and patient perspectives on reconstruction decision making. *JAMA Surg.* 2014;149(10):1015–1021. doi:10.1001/jamasurg.2014.548
2. Tarkowski R, Szmigiel K, Rubin A, et al. Patient's education before mastectomy influences the rate of reconstructive surgery. *J Cancer Educ.* 2016:1–16. doi:10.1007/s13187-016-0982-9
3. Sbitany H, Amalfi AN, Langstein HN. Preferences in choosing between breast reconstruction options: a survey of female plastic surgeons. *Plast Reconstr Surg.* 2009;124(6):1781–1789. doi:10.1097/PRS.0b013e3181bf8056
4. Ibrahim AM, Koolen PG, Ganor O, et al. Does acellular dermal matrix really improve aesthetic outcome in tissue expander/implant-based breast reconstruction? *Aesthetic Plas Surg.* 2015;39(3):359–368.
5. Lee K-T, Mun G-H. Updated evidence of acellular dermal matrix use for implant-based breast reconstruction: a meta-analysis. *Ann Surg Oncol.* 2016;23(2):600–610. doi:10.1245/s10434-015-4873-9
6. Alderman AK, Wilkins EG, Kim HM, Lowery JC. Complications in postmastectomy breast reconstruction: two-year results of the Michigan Breast Reconstruction Outcome Study. *Plast Reconstr Surg.* 2002;109(7):2265–2274.
7. McCarthy CM, Mehrara BJ, Riedel E, et al. Predicting complications following expander/implant breast reconstruction: an outcomes analysis based on preoperative clinical risk. *Plast Reconstr Surg.* 2008;121(6):1886–1892. doi:10.1097/PRS.0b013e31817151c4
8. Cunningham B. The mentor core study on silicone memorygel breast implants. *Plast Reconstr Surg.* 2007;120(7)(suppl 1):19S–29S; discussion 30S–32S. doi:10.1097/01.prs.0000286574.88752.04
9. Francis SH, Ruberg RL, Stevenson KB, et al. Independent risk factors for infection in tissue expander breast reconstruction. *Plast Reconstr Surg.* 2009;124(6):1790–1796. doi:10.1097/PRS.0b013e3181bf80aa
10. Spear SL, Seruya M. Management of the infected or exposed breast prosthesis: a single surgeon's 15-year experience with 69 patients. *Plast Reconstr Surg.* 2010;125(4):1074–1084. doi:10.1097/PRS.0b013e3181d17fff
11. Chun JK, Schulman MR. The infected breast prosthesis after mastectomy reconstruction: successful salvage of nine implants in eight consecutive patients. *Plast Reconstr Surg.* 2007;120(3):581–589. doi:10.1097/01.prs.0000270296.61765.28
12. Spear SL, Baker JL. Classification of capsular contracture after prosthetic breast reconstruction. *Plast Reconstr Surg.* 1995;96(5):1119–1123.
13. Del Pozo JL, Tran NV, Petty PM, et al. Pilot study of association of bacteria on breast implants with capsular contracture. *J Clin Microbiol.* 2009;47(5):1333–1337. doi:10.1128/JCM.00096-09
14. Schreml S, Heine N, Eisenmann-Klein M, Prantl L. Bacterial colonization is of major relevance for high-grade capsular contracture after augmentation mammaplasty. *Ann Plast Surg.* 2007;59(2):126–130. doi:10.1097/01.sap.0000252714.72161.4a
15. Lee K-T, Mun G-H. Comparison of one-stage vs two-stage prosthesis-based breast reconstruction: a systematic review and meta-analysis. *Am J Surg.* 2016;212(2):336–344. doi:10.1016/j.amjsurg.2015.07.015
16. Garvey PB, Buchel EW, Pockaj BA, et al. DIEP and pedicled TRAM flaps: a comparison of outcomes. *Plast Reconstr Surg.* 2006;117(6):1711–1719; discussion 1720–1721. doi:10.1097/01.prs.0000210679.77449.7d

17. Kronowitz SJ, Feledy JA, Hunt KK, et al. Determining the optimal approach to breast reconstruction after partial mastectomy. *Plast Reconstr Surg.* 2006;117(1):1–11; discussion 12–14.

18. Munhoz AM, Montag E, Gemperli R. Oncoplastic breast surgery: indications, techniques and perspectives. *Gland Surg.* 2013;2(3):143–157. doi:10.3978/j.issn.2227-684X .2013.08.02

19. Piper M, Peled AW, Sbitany H, et al. Comparison of mammographic findings following oncoplastic mammoplasty and lumpectomy without reconstruction. *Ann Surg Oncol.* 2016;23(1):65–71. doi:10.1245/s10434-015-4611-3

20. Losken A, Dugal CS, Styblo TM, Carlson GW. A meta-analysis comparing breast conservation therapy alone to the oncoplastic technique. *Ann Plast Surg.* 2014;72(2):145–149. doi:10.1097/SAP.0b013e3182605598

21. Silverstein MJ, Savalia N, Khan S, Ryan J. Extreme oncoplasty: breast conservation for patients who need mastectomy. *Breast J.* 2015;21(1):52–59. doi:10.1111/tbj.12356

22. Contant CME, Menke-Pluijmers MBE, Seynaeve C, et al. Clinical experience of prophylactic mastectomy followed by immediate breast reconstruction in women at hereditary risk of breast cancer (HB(O)C) or a proven BRCA1 and BRCA2 germ-line mutation. *Eur J Surg Oncol.* 2002;28(6):627–632.

23. Tokin C, Weiss A, Wang-Rodriguez J, Blair SL. Oncologic safety of skin-sparing and nipple-sparing mastectomy: a discussion and review of the literature. *Int J Surg Oncol.* 2012;2012(6):921821–921828. doi:10.1155/2012/921821

24. Atisha D, Alderman AK, Lowery JC, et al. Prospective analysis of long-term psychosocial outcomes in breast reconstruction: two-year postoperative results from the Michigan Breast Reconstruction Outcomes Study. *Ann Surg.* 2008;247(6):1019–1028. doi:10.1097/ SLA.0b013e3181728a5c

25. Metcalfe KA, Cil TD, Semple JL, et al. Long-term psychosocial functioning in women with bilateral prophylactic mastectomy: does preservation of the nipple-areolar complex make a difference? *Ann Surg Oncol.* 2015;22(10):3324–3330. doi:10.1245/s10434-015 -4761-3

26. Orzalesi L, Casella D, Santi C, et al. Nipple sparing mastectomy: surgical and oncological outcomes from a national multicentric registry with 913 patients (1006 cases) over a six year period. *Breast.* 2016;25:75–81. doi:10.1016/j.breast.2015.10.010

27. Rawlani V, Fiuk J, Johnson SA, et al. The effect of incision choice on outcomes of nipple-sparing mastectomy reconstruction. *Can J Plast Surg.* 2011;19(4):129–133.

28. Mallon P, Feron J-G, Couturaud B, et al. The role of nipple-sparing mastectomy in breast cancer: a comprehensive review of the literature. *Plast Reconstr Surg.* 2013;131(5): 969–984. doi:10.1097/PRS.0b013e3182865a3c

29. Sakurai T, Zhang N, Suzuma T, et al. Long-term follow-up of nipple-sparing mastectomy without radiotherapy: a single center study at a Japanese institution. *Med Oncol.* 2013;30(1):481. doi:10.1007/s12032-013-0481-3

30. Boneti C, Yuen J, Santiago C, et al. Oncologic safety of nipple skin-sparing or total skin-sparing mastectomies with immediate reconstruction. *J Am Coll Surg.* 2011;212(4):686–693; discussion 693–695. doi:10.1016/j.jamcollsurg.2010.12.039

31. La Cruz De L, Moody AM, Tappy EE, et al. Overall survival, disease-free survival, local recurrence, and nipple-areolar recurrence in the setting of nipple-sparing mastectomy: a meta-analysis and systematic review. *Ann Surg Oncol.* 2015;22(10):3241–3249. doi:10.1245/s10434-015-4739-1

32. Rohrich RJ, Hartley W, Brown S. Incidence of breast and chest wall asymmetry in breast augmentation: a retrospective analysis of 100 patients. *Plast Reconstr Surg.* 2006;118(suppl 7):7S–13S; discussion 14S–15S, 17S.

33. Slezak S, Bluebond-Langner R. Occult carcinoma in 866 reduction mammaplasties: preserving the choice of lumpectomy. *Plast Reconstr Surg.* 2011;127(2):525–530. doi:10.1097/PRS.0b013e3181fed5dc

Jessica Scott and Carolyn Rogers

HEREDITARY BREAST CANCER—GENERAL CHARACTERISTICS

- The majority of breast cancers, an estimated 90%, are sporadic and result from a combination of risk factors including environmental, hormonal, and stochastic events and are often related to natural aging. However, an estimated 10% of breast cancers are caused by underlying inherited cancer predisposition syndromes (1).
- Dr. Alfred Knudson proposed that hereditary cancer syndromes result from a "two-hit" process (2). In order for a tumor to develop, both copies of the same tumor suppressor gene must be inactivated by mutation. In sporadic cancers, this is caused by two separate sporadic events throughout a person's lifetime and results in the more common later-onset disease. However, in the case of an inherited cancer predisposition syndrome, a person is born with a germline mutation of one copy of the tumor suppressor gene, allowing for tumor development after only one sporadic event. This results in earlier ages of cancer onset and a significantly increased frequency of disease.
- Of the 10% of breast cancers that are due to an inherited cause, approximately half to two thirds are due to mutations within the *BRCA1* and *BRCA2* genes (3,4). The remainder are caused by mutations in various other high- and moderate-risk genes (5,6). Additional hereditary breast cancer syndromes may exist that have yet to be identified at this time.

BRCA1 AND *BRCA2*

Genetics

- The *BRCA1* gene is located at 17q21.31 and *BRCA2* is found at 13q31.1 (7,8). Mutations in the *BRCA* genes cause the hereditary breast/ovarian cancer syndrome (HBOC), which is inherited in an autosomal dominant fashion with reduced penetrance (9). These two genes are known to function in the DNA repair pathway by repairing double strand breaks and initiating homologous recombination. Loss of function germline mutations in these genes result in an inherited predisposition to cancer development because of increased genomic instability.
- *BRCA* gene mutations have been reported in all populations and are predicted to occur at a rate of approximately 1 in 400 people in the general population (9). However, certain populations are known to have higher *BRCA* mutation frequencies. Most notably are three mutations, two in the *BRCA1* gene and one in the *BRCA2* gene, which occur at a combined rate of 1 in 40 within the Ashkenazi Jewish population (9,10), placing this population at a significantly increased

risk for HBOC. Increased prevalence of HBOC has also been reported in the Icelandic and Dutch populations (9).

Features

- The lifetime risk for breast cancer (including invasive breast cancers and ductal carcinoma in situ [DCIS]) in female *BRCA* gene mutation carriers is significantly increased above that of the general population risk of approximately 12%, and is commonly early onset, defined as diagnosis before age 50 years (9). Mutations in *BRCA1* confer approximately a 50% to 80% risk for breast cancer for a woman's lifetime (9,11). In addition, the risk for a second breast primary is 6% to 17% within the first 5 years after the initial diagnosis, and 11% to 31% within the first 10 years after initial diagnosis (12,13). Mutations in *BRCA2* result in a lifetime breast cancer risk between 40% and 70%. The risk for contralateral cancer in the first 5 years is between 5% and 15%, and in the first 10 years is between 10% and 29% (12,13). Risk for contralateral cancer with a mutation in either gene reaches 50% to 60% over the woman's lifetime and varies based on initial age at diagnosis (14). Table 9.1 shows cancer risks by decade, which are separated by gene for quick reference.
- Breast cancers that develop in *BRCA* mutation carriers are most often invasive ductal adenocarcinoma with an aggressive phenotype, poorly differentiated (grade 3) with a high mitotic rate (17). Additionally, triple-negative (estrogen receptor [ER], progesterone receptor [PR], and HER2 neu negative) breast cancers have been shown to occur more frequently in *BRCA1* mutation carriers (17,18).
- The lifetime risk for the development of ovarian cancer is estimated to be 39% to 54% for *BRCA1* mutation carriers and up to 23% for *BRCA2* mutation carriers (11,19). Table 9.2 includes ovarian cancer risks by decade for reference. This cancer risk includes epithelial ovarian cancer, fallopian tube cancer, and primary peritoneal cancer (9).

Table 9.1 *BRCA* **Mutation Carrier Cancer Risks**

King et al (11)			Mavaddat et al (15)			Risch et al (16)	
Risks reported as percentages up to age listed			Risks reported per 1,000 person-years			Cumulative risk to age 80	
Age	*BRCA1*	*BRCA2*	Age	*BRCA1*	*BRCA2*	*BRCA1*	*BRCA2*
30	3%	0%	20–29	8.7	0		
40	21%	17%	30–39	16.9	11.9		
50	39%	34%	40–49	19.9	41.4		
60	58%	48%	50–59	36.1	15.2		
70	69%	74%	60–69	7.4	16.2		
80	81%	85%	≥70	0	0	90%	41%

Source: From Ref. (12). Molina-Montes E, Pérez-Nevot B, Pollán M, et al. Cumulative risk of second primary contralateral breast cancer in *BRCA1/BRCA2* mutation carriers with a first breast cancer: a systematic review and meta-analysis. *Breast.* 2014;23(6):721–742. doi:10.1016/j.breast.2014.10.005

Table 9.2 *BRCA* Mutation Carrier Ovarian Cancer Risks

| King et al (11) | | | Mavaddat et al (15) | | | Risch et al (16) | | Finch et al (20) | | |
| Risks reported as percentages up to age listed | | | Risks reported per 1,000 person-years | | | Cumulative risk to age 80 | | Risks reported per 100,000 per year | | |
Age	BRCA1	BRCA2	Age	BRCA1	BRCA2	BRCA1	BRCA2	Age	BRCA1	BRCA2
30	0%	0%	20–29	0	0					
40	3%	2%	30–39	1.1	1.7			30–39	206	
50	21%	2%	40–49	7.4	0			40–49	1918	0
60	40%	6%	50–59	20.3	2.4			50–59	3030	986.6
70	46%	12%	60–69	55.9	15.0			60–69	3505	927.1
80	54%	23%	≥70	23.9	11.2	24%	8.4%	70–74	1685	0

- Other associated cancers include male breast cancer (1%–2% lifetime risk for *BRCA1* carriers and 5%–10% lifetime risk for *BRCA2* carriers) and prostate cancer (30% in *BRCA1* carriers and up to 39% in *BRCA2* carriers) in male carriers as well as melanoma and pancreatic cancer (lifetime risk 1%–3% in *BRCA1* carriers and 2%–7% in *BRCA2* carriers) (9).

Several studies have been completed to estimate the risks for breast and ovarian cancer in *BRCA* mutation carriers by age. The risk estimates from several of these articles are included in Tables 9.1 and 9.2.

Medical Management for BRCA Positive Patients

- We generally adhere to NCCN guidelines in our medical management recommendations of BRCA positive patients and patients with other mutations (21):
  - Regarding breast cancer risk, several options for women who are known to carry deleterious *BRCA* gene mutations are available and include increased breast cancer surveillance by annual digital mammography and contrast enhanced breast MRI screening beginning at age 25 years, use of chemopreventive agents, or risk-reducing mastectomy.
  - Regarding the ovarian cancer risk, we recommend risk reducing bilateral salpingo-oophorectomy, typically between the ages of 35 and 40 years and after childbearing. Until the time of completion of oophorectomy, consideration could be given to screening; however, the efficacy of transvaginal ultrasound (US) and CA-125 testing in the early detection of ovarian cancer has not been proven.
  - We believe that in addition to annual GYN follow-up with pelvic examination, it is reasonable to offer CA-125 testing annually with completion of transvaginal US, if recommended by the GYN based on the pelvic exam findings or if any other clinical symptoms are noted.
  - For male carriers, we recommend annual clinical breast exam starting at age 35 years. Annual prostate cancer screening is recommended for all male *BRCA2* mutation carriers beginning at age 40 years with consideration of this screening for all male *BRCA1* mutation carriers.

OTHER HEREDITARY BREAST CANCER SYNDROMES

In addition to the *BRCA* genes, there are three other genes currently known that are considered to cause high-risk breast cancer syndromes. These genes are *CDH1*, *PTEN*, and *TP53*.

Hereditary Diffuse Gastric Cancer Syndrome

- The hereditary diffuse gastric cancer syndrome (HDGC) is an autosomal dominant condition caused by mutations in the *CDH1* gene. This syndrome is characterized by an 80% lifetime risk for the development of diffuse gastric cancer and an approximately 40% to 50% risk for lobular breast cancer in female mutation carriers (22).
  - Genetics—The *CDH1* gene is located at 16q22.1 and codes for epithelial (e-) cadherin, which is a member of a large family of transmembrane proteins (23). These proteins mediate cell–cell adhesion in a Ca^{2+} dependent manner

and play a key role in organ development (24). Loss of functional e-cadherin results in a phenomenon known as cadherin switching and a resultant upregulation of N-cadherin production. N-cadherin upregulation initiates a protein cascade that promotes cellular survival, migration, and invasion, which drives cancer development (24).

Cowden Syndrome

- Cowden syndrome, caused by mutations in the *PTEN* gene, is associated with an increased risk for breast, nonmedullary thyroid, and uterine cancers as well as various other noncancerous features. Other characteristics include benign disease such as fibrocystic breast disease, thyroid nodules, and leiomyomas, certain dermatological findings including facial trichilemmomas and papules, as well as subcutaneous lipomas, progressive macrocephaly, and, more rarely, learning disabilities (25).
  - Genetics—The *PTEN* gene is located at 10q23.31 and functions as a classic tumor suppressor (26). *PTEN* is involved in numerous functional processes in the body, the most salient being in regulation of the phosphoinositide 3-kinase (PI3K) pathway. In this pathway, *PTEN* negatively regulates PI3K and results in a decrease in cell cycle progression, induction of cell death, transcription, translation, stimulation of angiogenesis, and stem cell self-renewal. When *PTEN* function is lost, these cellular processes become less well regulated and can lead to cancer development.

Li–Fraumeni Syndrome

- Li–Fraumeni syndrome (LFS) is an autosomal dominant condition caused by mutations in the *TP53* gene that is characterized by a significantly increased risk for the development of breast cancer (potentially with very early onset), leukemia, bone and soft-tissue sarcomas, and brain tumors. Adrenocortical carcinoma and choroid plexus tumors are considered highly suggestive of LFS (27).
  - Genetics—The *TP53* gene is located at 17p13.1 and is involved in cell cycle regulation including inducing apoptosis or cell cycle arrest. Germline mutations in this gene result in LFS; however, somatic loss of p53 protein expression is almost universal in human cancer development regardless of the presence or absence of an underlying hereditary cancer syndrome (28).

In addition to these high-risk breast cancer syndromes, there are multiple known moderate-risk genes for which clinical genetic testing is also available. Of the known moderate-risk genes, only a portion currently have medical management guidelines published. The National Comprehensive Cancer Network (NCCN) currently recommends that carriers of mutations in various genes, including but not limited to the *ATM, CHEK2, PALB2,* and *STK11* genes, undergo increased breast cancer surveillance by annual mammography and breast MRI (21). Additionally, consideration could be given to risk-reducing bilateral mastectomy for *PALB2* mutation carriers but is not currently recommended for *ATM, CHEK2,* or *STK11* mutation carriers as they are understood to have lower breast cancer risks (22). Risk-reducing oophorectomy is currently recommended for *BRIP1, RAD51C,* and *RAD51D* mutation carriers in addition to *BRCA* mutation carriers (22). Other moderate-risk genes have been identified for which there is clinical genetic testing available. For some of these genes, increased surveillance is recommended and for others the medical management recommendations for carriers are still based on the known family history.

INDICATIONS FOR REFERRAL TO GENETIC COUNSELING AND TESTING

- Genetic counseling is recommended for all patients considering and undergoing genetic testing. The 2003 American Society of Clinical Oncology (ASCO) policy statement "strongly recommend(s) that genetic testing be done only in the setting of pre- and posttest counseling, which should include discussion of possible risks and benefits of cancer early detection and prevention modalities" (29). Therefore, referral for genetic counseling is critical in advance of testing to ensure the most appropriate testing is ordered and that full informed consent is obtained from the patient.
  - Patients who have completed genetic testing, with or without the benefit of pretest genetic counseling, and are found to carry a mutation in a cancer susceptibility gene should be provided in-depth posttest genetic counseling to discuss the implications of the mutation for their own medical management and to identify at-risk family members.
  - Posttest genetic counseling is of benefit to all patients undergoing testing to ensure accurate interpretation of results.

The NCCN Practice Guidelines in Oncology "Genetic/Familial High-Risk Assessment: Breast and Ovarian Cancer" provide the following indications for genetic risk evaluation (21):

- Any patient who has a family history of a known cancer susceptibility gene should be referred for genetic counseling, regardless of his or her personal cancer history.
- Personal history indications for genetic counseling include breast cancer before the age of 45, triple-negative (ER-, PR-, HER2-) breast cancer before the age of 60, multiple breast cancer primaries, Ashkenazi Jewish ancestry, invasive ovarian cancer diagnosis at any age, and breast cancer in a male patient.
- Indications for genetic counseling based on a combination of family history and personal history of breast cancer at any age include:
  - At least one close blood relative with breast cancer before age 50, at least one close blood relative with invasive ovarian cancer at any age, and two or more close relatives with breast and/or pancreatic cancer at any age.
  - Additionally, if the patient has breast cancer and a family history of three or more of the following cancers, he or she should be referred: pancreatic cancer, prostate cancer (Gleason score ≥ 7), sarcoma, adrenocortical carcinoma, brain tumors, endometrial cancer, thyroid cancer, kidney cancer, dermatologic manifestations and/or macrocephaly, hamartomatous polyps of the gastrointestinal (GI) tract, and diffuse gastric cancer (can include multiple primary cancers in the same individual).

Genetic counseling is indicated for patients based on family history alone, with no personal history of cancer, under these conditions:

- A known mutation in a cancer susceptibility gene in the family.
- Two or more breast cancer primaries in a single individual, two or more breast cancer diagnoses on one side of the family, a diagnosis of invasive ovarian cancer, a first or second degree relative with breast cancer diagnosed before age 45, or male breast cancer.
- Additionally, if the family history includes three or more of the following cancer diagnoses, the patient meets referral criteria: pancreatic cancer, prostate cancer (Gleason score ≥ 7), sarcoma, adrenocortical carcinoma, brain tumors, endometrial cancer, thyroid cancer, kidney cancer, dermatologic manifestations and/or macrocephaly, hamartomatous polyps of the GI tract, and diffuse gastric cancer (can include multiple primary cancers in the same individual).

"A Practice Guideline From the American College of Medical Genetics and Genomics and the National Society of Genetic Counselors: Referral Indications for Cancer Predisposition Assessment" states that the following criteria warrant assessment for cancer predisposition (30):

- For patients with a personal history of breast cancer diagnosed at age ≤50, triple-negative breast cancer diagnosed at age ≤60, ≥2 primary breast cancers in the same person, Ashkenazi Jewish ancestry and breast cancer at any age, or ≥3 cases of breast, ovarian, pancreatic, and/or aggressive prostate cancer in close relatives, including the patient.
- Considering the possibility of a hereditary cancer syndrome other than HBOC, the recommendations also include breast cancer and one additional LFS tumor (soft-tissue sarcoma, osteosarcoma, brain tumor, breast cancer, adrenocortical tumor, leukemia, bronchoalveolar cancer, colorectal cancer) in the same person or in two relatives (one diagnosis at age ≤45), breast cancer and ≥1 Peutz–Jeghers syndrome polyp in the same person, lobular breast cancer and diffuse gastric cancer in the same person, lobular breast cancer in one relative and diffuse gastric cancer in another (one diagnosis at age <50), or breast cancer and two additional Cowden syndrome criteria in the same person.
- The recommendations also include any male breast cancer, regardless of additional family history.

GENETIC TESTING RESULTS

Positive

A variant within a gene is classified as pathogenic or deleterious when known to impair gene function. A positive test result indicates that a pathogenic variant has been identified and clinical decisions can reasonably be made based on this result. As the implications of a positive genetic test are significant, strict criteria must be met before a variant can be classified as pathogenic.

Negative

A negative result indicates that either no variants have been identified in the analyzed gene or only variants classified as benign are present.

- Negative results are considered to be informative in two scenarios:
  - When a pathogenic mutation has previously been identified in another family member and the tested patient is shown to not carry the familial mutation. In this scenario, the patient is considered to be at general population risk for the development of the associated cancer types and would be screened according to the recommendations of the general population.
  - When testing is completed in a patient whose personal history includes early-onset cancer and no mutations are detected. While the underlying cause of this patient's cancer is still not known, this result eliminates the tested hereditary cancer syndrome(s) as the cause for the patient's cancer history, to the best of the current technical ability.
- If a patient completes testing based solely on family history and is found not to carry a mutation, then the results are considered to be uninformative as this result could occur for two reasons:
  - There may be a pathogenic mutation within the family that the patient did not inherit. If this scenario can be proven with additional familial testing, then the result would be an informative, or "true" negative. For this reason, genetic testing is always recommended for the affected family member in advance of testing any unaffected family members to clearly inform which gene(s) should be analyzed and the interpretation of the results.
  - The patient's family history may have been due to a genetic cause not tested; therefore, the completed genetic testing does not impact the patient's cancer risk assessment. Because of this possible explanation, any patient who receives an uninformative negative genetic test result still requires increased breast cancer screening based on his or her unexplained family history of disease.

Variant of Unknown Significance

A genetic variant for which the clinical impact cannot be determined is classified as a variant of unknown significance (VUS). The medical recommendations for mutation carriers should *not* be used for patients who carry VUSs as a significant proportion are benign and the increased screening and preventive measures could increase morbidity. Instead, the medical management of a patient shown to carry a VUS should be based on his or her known personal and family history of cancer. Reclassification of VUSs to either benign or pathogenic variants can occur after further research and identification of the variant in other families. At that time other medical recommendations can appropriately be made based on the results.

GENETIC TESTING OPTIONS

Genetic Testing for Hereditary Cancer Syndromes

Genetic testing for hereditary cancer syndromes can be completed in various ways.

- If a known gene mutation has previously been identified in a family member, then all other family members should ideally be tested by targeted analysis for this familial pathogenic variant. This testing procedure allows for the clearest interpretation of results and avoids the possibility of identifying a VUS, which could add unnecessary confusion for patients in their understanding of the test results. A known hereditary cancer syndrome mutation should be addressed through appropriate testing and counseling, but does not preclude the presence of an additional syndrome in the family. If the identified syndrome does not explain the family and personal history, further extensive testing may be more informative for the patient.

- In families where a known mutation has not been identified, testing can be completed for a single syndrome using focused molecular analysis of only the genes assessed that are likely to be causative of the reported family history.

- Alternatively, if a specific syndrome is not clearly indicated based on the family history, various conditions can be tested for by multiplex (multigene panel) testing. Multiple genetic labs currently offer multiplex panels for hereditary cancer syndromes. Test options exist for cancer site-specific syndromes (such as conditions that include breast cancer as a primary feature) as well as for hereditary cancer syndromes in general but that are not focused on one particular cancer as the primary feature. The benefits and limitations of panel testing should be discussed with a patient in detail to allow for completion of the test that will most appropriately address the potential hereditary concerns of the family and that will provide the depth of hereditary information that is wanted by the patient.

OTHER ASSOCIATED CONCERNS

Insurance Protection

- The Genetic Information Nondiscrimination Act (GINA) of 2008 was enacted by Congress to protect patients undergoing genetic testing from health insurance and employment discrimination (31). Title 1 of GINA addresses insurance discrimination and states that group health insurance companies cannot use the results of a genetic test to increase a patient's premiums or to limit his or her covered benefits. Title 2 addresses employment discrimination and states that no employer can fire an employee or refuse to hire or promote an employee based on results of a genetic test. Both titles specifically state that group health insurances and employers cannot require that a patient/employee or his or her family members take a genetic test. Of note, GINA does not apply to other types of insurance such as life insurance or disability insurance and, as such, protections against discrimination in these areas are not in place.

- The Patient Protection and Affordable Care Act (PPACA) was signed into law in 2010 to improve health insurance coverage of the American people and decrease the uninsured rate as well as health care costs (32). As genetic testing can be an expensive endeavor for individuals to complete on their own, requiring genetic counseling, the actual testing, and possibly significant cancer screening or preventive surgeries based on results, the increased availability of health insurance afforded by the ACA may allow for more at-risk patients to take advantage of the available genetics services for hereditary breast cancer.

All of the hereditary cancer conditions summarized in Table 9.3 follow an autosomal dominant pattern of inheritance; therefore, all first degree relatives of known carriers are at 50% risk to also carry a mutation.

Table 9.3 Summary of High Risk Breast Cancer Genes

Gene	Syndrome	Cancers
BRCA1, BRCA2 (9)	Hereditary breast/ovarian cancer syndrome (HBOC)	Women have a 40% to 80% lifetime risk for breast cancer and a 23% to 54% lifetime risk for ovarian cancer. Additionally, prostate cancer, male breast cancer, and pancreatic cancer are at an elevated lifetime risk. *BRCA2* carriers are at an elevated risk for melanoma.
CDH1 (22)	Hereditary diffuse gastric cancer syndrome (HDGC)	Men and women have an 80% lifetime risk for diffuse gastric cancer and women have a 39% to 52% lifetime risk for lobular breast cancer.
PTEN (33)	Cowden syndrome	Women have an 85% lifetime risk for breast cancer, 35% risk for thyroid cancer, and 28% risk for endometrial cancer. Individuals also have an elevated risk for hamartomatous and mixed gastrointestinal polyps, which may progress to colon cancer, renal cell carcinoma, and melanoma. Benign findings include thyroid disease, uterine fibroids, macrocephaly, fibrocystic breast disease, and lipomas.
TP53 (27)	Li–Fraumeni syndrome	Individuals have a greatly elevated risk for cancers including soft tissue sarcoma, osteosarcoma, brain tumor, premenopausal breast cancer, adrenocortical carcinoma, leukemia, and lung bronchoalveolar cancer. Lifetime risk for cancer approaches 90% risk.
PALB2 (34,35)		The risk for breast cancer in female carriers by age 70 has been shown to be 33% to 58% depending upon additional family history. *PALB2* mutations have also been associated with an elevated risk for pancreatic cancer and have been identified in male breast cancer patients.
CHEK2 (36,37)		*CHEK2* mutations result in a three- to fivefold increased risk for breast cancer and has been noted in early-onset disease. *CHEK2* mutations have also been associated with increased risk for various cancer types, including colorectal cancer, prostate cancer, and male breast cancer, among others.
ATM (38,39)		Associated with a moderately increased risk for breast cancer, specifically for early-onset disease (up to 9% by age 50 and at least 17% by age 80) and familial pancreatic cancer.

➤ MANAGEMENT PEARLS

1. Ten percent of all breast cancer cases are due to an underlying inherited cause. The most common inherited cause for breast cancer is HBOC, caused by mutations in the *BRCA1* and *BRCA2* genes. Multiple other inherited causes for breast cancer are also known.
2. The NCCN has published medical management guidelines for *BRCA* mutation carriers. *BRCA* guidelines are in place for screening and prevention of breast, ovarian, male breast, and prostate cancers.
3. Genetic testing is also available for several additional high-risk breast cancer syndromes (ie, Cowden syndrome, LFS, and hereditary diffuse gastric cancer) as well as multiple moderate-risk breast cancer conditions (ie, *ATM, PALB2, CHEK2*)
4. Published guidelines also exist for cases where hereditary breast cancer genetic testing is indicated. Genetic testing should always be precipitated by full genetic counseling to allow for completion of the most appropriate gene analyses and for collection of patient informed consent to testing.
5. For medical management of high-risk breast cancer syndromes options include increased surveillance by annual mammography and breast MRI, consideration of chemopreventive agents, or consideration of the option of bilateral risk reducing mastectomy. As these syndromes typically include risks for other cancers in addition to breast, screening or preventive options related to other risks may also be reasonable. For example, with respect to ovarian cancer, the recommendation is for risk reducing bilateral salpingo-oophorectomy after completion of childbearing.

REFERENCES

1. Claus EB, Schildkraut JM, Thompson WD, Risch NJ. The genetic attributable risk of breast and ovarian cancer. *Cancer*. 1996;77(11):2318–2324.
2. Knudson AG. Mutation and cancer: statistical study of retinoblastoma. *Proc Natl Acad Sci U S A*. 1971;68(4):820–823.
3. Tung N, Battelli C, Allen B, et al. Frequency of mutations in individuals with breast cancer referred for *BRCA1* and *BRCA2* testing using next-generation sequencing with a 25-gene panel. *Cancer*. 2015;121(1):25–33. doi:10.1002/cncr.29010
4. Walsh T, Casadei S, Lee MK, et al. Mutations in 12 genes for inherited ovarian, fallopian tube, and peritoneal carcinoma identified by massively parallel sequencing. *Proc Natl Acad Sci U S A*. 2011;108(44):18032–18037. doi:10.1073/pnas.1115052108
5. Antoniou AC, Pharoah PDP, Mcmullan G, et al. Evidence for further breast cancer susceptibility genes in addition to *BRCA1* and *BRCA2* in a population-based study. *Genet Epidemiol*. 2001;21:1–18.
6. Sharma L, Evans B, Abernethy J, et al. Spectrum of mutations identified in a 25-gene hereditary cancer panel for patients with breast cancer. *Myriad Genet*. 2015;75(9)(Suppl):P4-12-02.
7. Online Mendelian Inheritance in Man. Breast cancer 1 gene; *BRCA1*. http://www.omim.org/entry/113705. Updated February 4, 2016.

8. Online Mendelian Inheritance in Man. *BRCA2* Gene; *BRCA2*. http://www.omim.org/entry/600185. Updated February 4, 2016.

9. Petrucelli N, Daly MB, Feldman GL. *BRCA1* and *BRCA2* hereditary breast and ovarian cancer. *GeneReviews*. 2015;1–52. http://www.ncbi.nlm.nih.gov/books/NBK1247

10. Struewing JP, Hartge P, Wacholder S, et al. The risk of cancer associated with specific mutations of *BRCA1* and *BRCA2* among Ashkenazi Jews. *N Engl J Med*. 1997;336(20): 1401–1408. doi:10.1056/NEJM199705153362001

11. King MC, Marks JH, Mandell JB. Breast and ovarian cancer risks due to inherited mutations in *BRCA1* and *BRCA2*. *Science*. 2003;302:643–646.

12. Molina-Montes E, Pérez-Nevot B, Pollán M, et al. Cumulative risk of second primary contralateral breast cancer in *BRCA1/BRCA2* mutation carriers with a first breast cancer: a systematic review and meta-analysis. *Breast*. 2014;23(6):721–742. doi:10.1016/j .breast.2014.10.005

13. Malone KE, Begg CB, Haile RW, et al. Population-based study of the risk of second primary contralateral breast cancer associated with carrying a mutation in *BRCA1* or *BRCA2*. *J Clin Oncol*. 2010;28(14):2404–2410. doi:10.1200/JCO.2009.24.2495

14. Metcalfe K, Lynch HT, Ghadirian P, et al. Contralateral breast cancer in *BRCA1* and *BRCA2* mutation carriers. *J Clin Oncol*. 2004;22(12):2328–2335. doi:10.1200/JCO.2004 .04.033

15. Mavaddat N, Peock S, Frost D, et al. Cancer risks for *BRCA1* and *BRCA2* mutation carriers: results from prospective analysis of EMBRACE. *J Natl Cancer Inst*. 2013;105(11): 812–822. doi:10.1093/jnci/djt095

16. Risch H, McLaughlin JR, Cole DEC, et al. Population *BRCA1* and *BRCA2* mutation frequencies and cancer penetrances: a kin-cohort study in Ontario, Canada. *J Natl Cancer Inst*. 2006;98(23):1694–1706. doi:10.1093/jnci/djj465

17. Van der Groep P, van der Wall E, van Diest PJ. Pathology of hereditary breast cancer. *Cell Oncol*. 2011;34(2):71–88. doi:10.1007/s13402-011-0010-3

18. Verhoog LC, Brekelmans CTM, Seynaeve C, et al. Survival and tumour characteristics of breast-cancer patients with germline mutations of *BRCA1*. *Lancet*. 1998;351:17–20.

19. Antoniou A, Pharoah PDP, Narod S, et al. Average risks of breast and ovarian cancer associated with *BRCA1* or *BRCA2* mutations detected in case series unselected for family history: a combined analysis of 22 studies. *Am J Hum Genet*. 2003;72:1117–1130.

20. Finch A, Beiner M, Lubinski J, et al. Salpingo-oophorectomy and the risk of ovarian, fallopian tube, and peritoneal cancers in women with a *BRCA1* or *BRCA2* mutation. *JAMA*. 2006;296(2):185–192.

21. Genetic/familial high-risk assessment: breast and ovarian. *NCCN Clinical Practice Guidelines in Oncology (NCCN Guidelines)*. 2016:93.

22. Kaurah P, Huntsman DG. Hereditary diffuse gastric cancer. *GeneReviews*. 2015:1–25.

23. Online Mendelian Inheritance in Man. Cadherin 1; CDH1. http://www.omim.org/entry/192090. Updated January 7, 2015.

24. Van Roy F, Berx G. The cell-cell adhesion molecule E-cadherin. *Cell Mol Life Sci*. 2008;65(23):3756–3788. doi:10.1007/s00018-008-8281-1

25. Online Mendelian Inheritance in Man. Cowden Syndrome 1; CWS1. http://www.omim .org/entry/158350. Updated March 14, 2016.

26. Online Mendelian Inheritance in Man. Phosphatase and Tensin Homolog; PTEN. http://www.omim.org/entry/601728. Updated July 18, 2016.

27. Schneider K, Zelley K, Nichols KE, Garber J. Li-Fraumeni syndrome. *GeneReviews*. 2015:1–24.

28. Online Mendelian Inheritance in Man. Tumor Protein p53; TP53. http://omim.org/entry/191170. Updated August 30, 2016.

29. American Society of Clinical Oncology. American Society of Clinical Oncology policy statement update: genetic testing for cancer susceptibility. *J Clin Oncol*. 2003;21(12):2397–2406. doi:10.1200/JCO.2003.03.189

30. Hampel H, Bennett RL, Buchanan A, et al. A practice guideline from the American College of Medical Genetics and Genomics and the National Society of Genetic Counselors: referral indications for cancer predisposition assessment. *Genet Med*. 2014;17(1):70–87. doi:10.1038/gim.2014.147

31. Public Law 110-233. *Genetic Information Nondiscrimmination Act of 2008*. 2008:881–922.

32. U.S. House of Representatives. *Compilation of Patient Protection and Affordable Care Act*. 2010:1–955.

33. Eng C. PTEN hamartoma tumor syndrome (PHTS). *GeneReviews*. 2014:1–25.

34. Antoniou AC, Casadei S, Heikkinen T, et al. Breast-cancer risk in families with mutations in PALB2. *N Engl J Med*. 2014;371(6):497–506. doi:10.1056/NEJMoa1400382

35. Slater EP, Langer P, Niemczyk E, et al. PALB2 mutations in European familial pancreatic cancer families. *Clin Genet*. 2010;78(5):490–494. doi:10.1111/j.1399-0004.2010.01425.x

36. Weischer M, Bojesen SE, Ellervik C, et al. CHEK2*1100delC genotyping for clinical assessment of breast cancer risk: meta-analyses of 26,000 patient cases and 27,000 controls. *J Clin Oncol*. 2008;26(4):542–548. doi:10.1200/JCO.2007.12.5922

37. Cybulski C, Gorski B, Huzarski T, et al. CHEK2 is a multiorgan cancer susceptibility gene. *Am J Hum Genet*. 2004;75(6):1131–1135.

38. Roberts NJ, Jiao Y, Yu J, et al. ATM mutations in patients with hereditary pancreatic cancer. *Cancer Discov*. 2012;2(1):41–46. doi:10.1158/2159-8290.CD-11-0194

39. Thompson D, Duedal S, Kirner J, et al. Cancer risks and mortality in heterozygous ATM mutation carriers. *J Natl Cancer Inst*. 2005;97(11):813–822. doi:10.1093/jnci/dji141

<table><tr><td style="font-size:3em">10</td><td>Integrative Approaches to Symptom
Management in Breast Cancer Patients</td></tr></table>

Ting Bao

INTRODUCTION

An increasing number of breast cancer patients are using integrative medicine approaches to manage symptoms associated with cancer or its treatment. Studies indicate that there is a high prevalence of complementary and integrative medicine (CIM) use among cancer survivors. A population-based study of 1,471 patients showed that 66% of cancer survivors used CIM in their lifetime, and 43% used CIM in the last 12 months (1). General disease prevention, immune enhancement, and pain were identified as the top three reasons for CIM use. Compared to the general population, cancer survivors were more likely to use a CIM therapy if it was recommended by their provider and were also more likely to disclose CIM use to their providers (1). While patients seek informed advice and communication from their physician on this subject, at the same time they believe that physicians have limited knowledge on the topic and no interest in discussing its use (2). Cancer patients who experience unmet needs from their health care team throughout survivorship are more likely to seek out CIM to address those needs (3). From a clinical perspective, symptom management is also integral to the successful implementation of cancer care: addressing symptoms supports patient adherence to prescribed treatments and follow-up plans, and fosters a patient's return to a state of well-being, whereas failure to address these issues can lessen the impact of mainstream therapies due to decreased compliance, leading to worse outcomes (4,5).

Therefore, it is important for health care providers to have some basic knowledge of CIM to facilitate an open dialog about what patients may be using and to offer appropriate guidance. This chapter provides an overview of the integrative therapies clinically used for symptom management in patients with breast cancer.

THE ROLES OF INTEGRATIVE MEDICINE IN CANCER SUPPORTIVE CARE

Cancer treatments often produce difficult physical and emotional symptoms, and late or long-term effects are common (5,6). Symptoms can also be related to age, comorbidities, or the cancer diagnosis itself, and have multifactorial etiologies (7). Symptom relief is therefore commonly sought both during treatment and throughout survivorship.

Complementary and integrative medicine has grown to replace the term "complementary and alternative medicine" (CAM) to reflect the incorporation of evidence-based complementary modalities into mainstream cancer care (4,8). Integrative medicine uses nonpharmacologic therapies adjunctively to address symptoms safely and effectively, improve quality of life (QoL), and facilitate lifestyle changes. A number of symptoms can be controlled or improved with integrative therapies including anxiety, depression, stress, fatigue, feelings of isolation, hot flashes, lymphedema, nausea, neuropathy, pain, perioperative symptoms, sexual dysfunction, physical deconditioning, dyspnea, urinary problems, and xerostomia.

Four main types of integrative approaches are clinically used to help breast cancer patients manage symptoms associated with the disease and its treatment: diet and exercise recommendations, mind–body techniques such as yoga and meditation, individualized therapies such as acupuncture and massage, and the use of dietary supplements.

Diet

The World Cancer Research Foundation describes diets linked to increased cancer risk as those that include the regular consumption of red and/or processed meats, alcoholic drinks, and foods containing refined sugars (9). Diets linked to decreases in cancer risk include foods containing dietary fiber, fruits, nonstarchy vegetables, and those containing vitamin D such as salmon, sardines, and some fortified foods. As such, the recommended diet for cancer patients and survivors includes a diverse and balanced diet, with an emphasis on plant-based foods from natural sources. For breast cancer survivors, we usually encourage eating 3 to 5 servings of non-starchy vegetables per day and 2 to 4 servings of nonsweet fruits a day. It is also important to ask the patient to eat a variety of foods: plant-based proteins such as beans, peas, lentils, and nuts; animal proteins such as lean poultry, fatty fish including salmon and sardines, and low-fat dairy; and whole grains such as oats, bulgur, and high-fiber breads and cereals (10). We usually recommend that patients limit red meat to 1 to 2 servings per week, with each serving being fist size (approximately 3 ounces). We also recommend that patients avoid processed meats, limit alcohol intake, and eliminate white sugar, high-fructose corn syrup, and artificial sweeteners as much as possible.

Most of these dietary recommendations stem from epidemiological studies. A randomized controlled trial (RCT) known as PREDIMED showed that a heart-healthy Mediterranean diet may reduce breast cancer risk (11). In this study, 4,282 women aged 60 to 80 years who were at high risk for cardiovascular disease were randomized to either a Mediterranean diet supplemented with extra-virgin olive oil (EVOO), a Mediterranean diet supplemented with mixed nuts, or a low-fat diet serving as the control group. After a median follow-up of 4.8 years, 35 patients were diagnosed with breast cancer. Participants in the Mediterranean diet/EVOO group had the lowest incidence of breast cancer (1.1 per 1,000 person-years), compared to the nut-supplemented Mediterranean diet, or low-fat control group (1.8 and 2.9 per 1,000 person-years, respectively) (11). This is the first RCT to demonstrate an effect on breast cancer incidence from the implementation of a long-term diet, suggesting benefits from following a Mediterranean/EVOO-supplemented diet for the primary prevention of breast cancer. The Mediterranean diet consists of a variety of fruits, vegetables, cereals, legumes, poultry, fish, nuts, seeds, olive oil, moderate intake of red wine with meals, and low consumption of meat and dairy products.

In addition, several prospective cohort studies conducted in women after breast cancer diagnosis and treatment showed that a diet high in fruits, vegetables, whole

Table 10.1 Dietary Guidance for Cancer Survivors

Eat	Limit

• *Whole foods*: emphasize plant-based foods
• *Nonstarchy vegetables*: 3–5 servings daily*
• *Nonsweet fruits*: 2–4 servings daily*
• *Vary protein sources*
 ○ *Plant-based*
  ▪ Beans, peas, lentils, and nuts
 ○ *Animal-based*
  ▪ Lean poultry, fatty fish including salmon and sardines, and low-fat dairy
• *Choose whole grains*
 ○ Oats, bulgur, whole wheat, high-fiber breads and cereals
• *Rinse all produce thoroughly with clean water*
 ○ Whether organic or conventional
	• *Red meat*: 1–2 fist-size servings weekly (approximately 3 oz)
	• *Alcohol:* less than 1 drink daily
	
	Avoid when possible
	• *Processed meats*
	• *Refined sugars*: white sugar, high-fructose corn syrup
	• *Artificial sweeteners*

*1 serving = 1 cup of dark leafy greens or berries, 1 medium fruit, or 1/2 cup of other colorful fruits and vegetables.
Source: From Ref. (10). National Comprehensive Cancer Network. Nutrition for cancer survivors. http://www.nccn.org/patients/resources/life_aft er_cancer/nutrition.aspx

grains, poultry, and fish was associated with better survival when compared to a diet high in refined grains, red and processed meats, desserts, high-fat dairy, and French fries (12,13). Table 10.1 highlights important recommendations for cancer patients both during treatment and throughout survivorship (10).

ORGANIC VERSUS CONVENTIONAL

A common question among cancer patients is whether or not organic foods are better than conventional sources. Current research on this subject has been mixed (14–19), and not without polarizing debate. Recently, a large prospective study indicated that the consumption of organic food had either little or no effect on cancer incidence, with the possible exception of non-Hodgkin's lymphoma (20). However, organic choices may reduce exposure to pesticide residues and antibiotic-resistant bacteria (15). Still, given that (a) the more likely issue for many cancer patients is the adoption of a diet emphasizing a variety of whole foods in the first place, (b) the evidence on organic versus conventional foods is fluid, and (c) accessibility is confounded by marketing practices, regions, price points, and availability, patients should rather be encouraged to focus on incorporating the best possible sources of whole foods available to them, and to rinse produce thoroughly with clean water before eating, whether organic or conventional.

REFINED SUGARS

Although there are currently no clinical trials to suggest that sugar helps cancer grow and progress, one study does suggest associations between high sugar intake and breast cancer risk (21). In recent animal studies that mimicked conditions of the human Western diet, a clear risk between increased sugar consumption and breast cancer occurrence, tumor growth, and metastasis was also demonstrated (22). Investigators determined that fructose in particular, as available in table sugar and high-fructose corn syrup, appeared to be responsible for facilitating lung metastasis and 12-hydroxyeicosatetraenoic acid (12-HETE) production in breast tumors. Added sugars also contribute significant amounts of calories, which can cause weight gain, a risk factor for breast (23,24) and other cancers (25), diabetes and Alzheimer's disease (26), and mortality from cardiovascular disease (27). The American Heart Association currently recommends that women with moderate activity levels consume no more than five teaspoons of added sugar daily, and that sedentary women limit their intake even more, to the equivalent of three teaspoons daily (28).

ALCOHOL

Research has also shown a direct correlation between alcohol intake and risk of breast cancer. Reanalysis of data on 58,515 women with breast cancer and 95,067 women without the disease from 53 epidemiological studies showed that the relative risk of breast cancer was 1.32 (1.19–1.45; $P < .00001$) for an intake of 35 to 44 g (2.2–3.2 drinks) per day, and 1.46 (1.33–1.61; $P < .00001$) for $\geq$45 g per day compared to women who reported drinking no alcohol. Relative risk increased by 7.1% (95% CI 5.5%–8.7%; $P < .00001$) for each additional 10 g intake per day (ie, for each extra unit or drink of alcohol consumed daily) (29). Therefore, and also in accordance with National Comprehensive Cancer Network risk reduction guidelines (30), we usually recommend that breast cancer survivors limit their alcohol intake to less than 1 drink per day (equivalent to 1 oz of liquor, 6 oz wine, or 8 oz beer).

SOY ISOFLAVONES

Isoflavones, a type of phytoestrogen, are found in some foods, most notably soy products. These naturally occurring compounds have been shown to have antioxidant and free-radical scavenging activities, but such properties may be altered by their metabolism in the human body (31,32). In addition, there are many questions about whether soy products actually increase or decrease breast cancer risk. A 2014 meta-analysis of 35 studies on the association between soy isoflavone intake and breast cancer risk suggests a lower risk for both pre- and postmenopausal women in Asian countries, but no influence on risk for women in Western countries (33). Consequently in general, we do not instruct patients to "avoid soy" or reduce whole soy foods (eg, tofu, edamame, miso, soymilk) as there is no evidence to suggest that eating them at practical levels increases breast cancer risk or recurrence in humans.

Exercise and Physical Activity

Sitting for many hours daily is a known independent risk factor for cancers of the colon, endometrium, and lung (34). In addition, sedentary lifestyle contributes to obesity, and there are well-established links between obesity and many types of cancer (35,36). Even more specifically, weight gain and obesity are risk factors for the development of postmenopausal breast cancer (37,38), while physical activity is associated with improvements in cancer-related survival (39–41).

Publications in the oncology literature, therefore, recommend exercise as part of survivorship self-care (30,42–44). In addition, exercise and physical activity can help to relieve or reduce symptoms that are often of multifactorial etiology, including pain (45,46), such as aromatase inhibitor (AI) induced arthralgia (47), fatigue (46,48–50), physical deconditioning (48,51–55), and nausea/vomiting (45), any of which may contribute to the interruption or even cessation of cancer treatment regimens (56). For breast cancer patients, additional side effects from treatment such as bone loss (57,58), weight gain (57,59), and hot flashes (60) may also be decreased with established exercise regimens.

Table 10.2 highlights important recommendations for cancer patients both during treatment and throughout survivorship (61). At our institution, we usually recommend that breast cancer survivors do some type of moderate exercise for at least 30 minutes daily, with the goal of at least 300 minutes per week.

Mind–Body Therapies

Mind–body modalities recognize the inherent and reciprocal relationship between physical and psychological states, and that physical well-being may be modulated via neurohormonal and immunological pathways. Along with diet and exercise, they are among the most effective therapies to affect positive change in emotional and psychological profiles among cancer patients.

The most commonly practiced and scientifically studied among breast cancer survivors are meditation, yoga, and tai chi/qigong, which are used to address emotional self-regulation, anxiety, and depression, as well as cognitive impairment, sleep disturbance, and balance issues. Broadly speaking, there is more overlap than distinction among these practices as adopted attitudes of relaxed, open awareness without goal orientation, both in movement and stillness, lead to reclaimed states of physical, emotional, and mental well-being. In the case of yoga, tai chi, and qigong as movement arts and depending on the level of activity, there are also benefits similar to exercise.

Several approaches to meditation have been described (62–64). Methods of focused attention meditation include voluntary mental immersion on a chosen

---

Table 10.2 Physical Activity Recommendations for Cancer Survivors

- *Avoid inactivity*
- *Exercise*: can include daily routines and recreational activities that would also be described as physical activity
- *Tailor activities* to individual:
  - Abilities → reduces injury
  - Preferences → increases compliance
- Incorporate activity of *at least*:
  - 150 min of *moderate intensity*
  - 75 min of *vigorous intensity*, if possible
- *Strength training*:
  - 2–3 times weekly
  - Include major muscle groups
- Stretch major muscle groups regularly

Source: From Ref. (61). National Comprehensive Cancer Network. NCCN guidelines: survivorship, Version 2.2015. http://www.nccn.org/professionals/physician_gls/pdf/survivorship.pdf

object, with nonjudgmental detection and disengagement from distraction, and a gentle return or redirection to the intended object. Another style, open monitoring meditation, involves nonreactive observation of the content of one's experience and how that may change from moment to moment. The potential regulatory functions of these practices on attention and emotion processes could have a long-term impact on the brain and behavior.

Mindfulness-based stress reduction (MBSR) is a form of meditation that has been rapidly adopted in cancer clinical practice. It uses a combination of mindfulness meditation, yoga, and body awareness to help people become more mindful and reduce stress. Studies of MBSR in breast cancer patients indicate those who practice regularly experience significantly lower depression, anxiety, and fear of recurrence, as well as higher energy and physical functioning compared to usual care (65). Further, the benefits of MBSR on psychosocial adjustment go beyond that of credible controls and are universal across levels of expectation to its efficacy (66). Clinically meaningful, statistically significant effects on depression and anxiety have also been demonstrated after 12 months of follow-up, with medium-to-large effect sizes (67). Improvements in endocrine-treatment-related side effects (68), sleep quality immediately postintervention (69), cortisol profiles, and hypothalamic–pituitary–adrenal (HPA) axis functioning, as well as maintenance of telomere length, have also been noted (70–72). Similarly, studies evaluating a mindfulness-based cancer recovery (MBCR) program indicate this intervention is better for treating distress and stress, and improving QoL, in breast cancer survivors compared to supportive–expressive group therapy (73). It also demonstrated noninferiority in some measures for treatment of insomnia compared to cognitive behavioral therapy (63). A brief, mindfulness-based intervention for younger breast cancer survivors also suggests efficacy for the reduction of behavioral symptoms and proinflammatory signaling (74).

Yoga is a traditional Indian practice that incorporates breathing exercises (pranayama) and movement through postures or holding of postures (asanas). It has been shown to reduce stress and improve QoL, memory, and sleep quality in cancer survivors (75–79). In breast cancer patients, yoga improves range of motion (80) and social functioning and mood, as well as reduces stress (81–83), anxiety (84), and a range of other psychological symptoms (73). In survivors with persistent fatigue and treatment-induced or exacerbated menopausal symptoms, yoga reduces fatigue, joint pain, and number of hot flashes while increasing vigor, with benefits persisting at 3-month follow-up (85,86).

Both qigong and tai chi are based on traditional Chinese medicine (TCM) theory. They use precise movement sequences, meditation, and synchronized breathing to restore the flow of qi (*chi*, internal energy). These practices have significant impact on sleep dysfunction, anxiety, depression, mood, fear of falling, and QoL (87–90). Improvements in aerobic capacity, muscular strength, and flexibility (91); balance, cognitive functioning, cancer pain, fatigue, numbness, and dizziness (87,92,93); and reduced markers of inflammation (93,94) have also been demonstrated. As a moderate weight-bearing exercise, preliminary data indicate that tai chi may also exert positive effects on markers of bone metabolism (95), as well as insulin and cytokine levels associated with lean body mass (96).

Although initial instruction is required, mind–body approaches are largely self-administered, low-cost, effective, and safe, with minimal to no side effects, and are therefore highly recommended for cancer patients.

Acupuncture

Acupuncture is a TCM technique that involves inserting and manipulating filiform needles into specific points on the body to alleviate symptoms. Although its mechanisms are not fully established, acupuncture appears to interact with and modulate the functioning of nerves, neurotransmitters, and neurohormones (97–100). Two methods of acupuncture stimulation are clinically used. In manual acupuncture, needles are inserted and rotated by the practitioner to achieve a de qui sensation (*duh chee*; soreness, fullness, heaviness, or local area distension) (101,102), while electroacupuncture (EA) refers to the added use of mild to moderate electrical current through inserted needles to stimulate acupuncture points.

Acupuncture has been used as a complementary therapy to treat a wide range of conditions experienced by breast cancer survivors. Growing evidence suggests that acupuncture may be beneficial for cancer-treatment-induced symptoms including musculoskeletal symptoms, hot flashes, lymphedema, peripheral neuropathy (PN), fatigue, anxiety, and depression.

MANAGEMENT OF AROMATASE INHIBITOR-INDUCED MUSCULOSKELETAL SYMPTOMS (AIMSS)

AIs are the recommended first-line adjuvant endocrine therapy in postmenopausal women with hormone-receptor-positive breast cancer, either as monotherapy or in sequence with tamoxifen (103). AIMSS are reported in up to 50% of women, leading to drug discontinuation in approximately 13% of users (104,105). Maximum benefit is observed with 5 years of adjuvant endocrine therapy and is therefore the recommended duration of treatment for breast cancer survivors. Current interventions for AIMSS including oral analgesics and exercise have limited efficacy (106,107), in addition to the fact that long-term use of the former is challenging.

To date there have been four RCTs comparing the effects of real acupuncture (RA) and sham acupuncture (SA) in reducing AIMSS symptoms, with no significant adverse reactions to either treatment (108–111). Although one of the trials (108) indicates that RA may be significantly better for joint muscle pain than SA, this finding was not confirmed by the other three. Mao et al (111) is the only study among these with an added waitlist control arm showing statistically significant greater pain reductions with RA. An ongoing three-arm Southwest Oncology Group study (112) with a sample size of 228 patients may further clarify the role of acupuncture in helping breast cancer survivors with AIMSS (112). For now, it may be reasonable to suggest that breast cancer patients try acupuncture for AIMSS, as it has minimal risk and potentially carries significant benefits.

CONTROL OF VASOMOTOR SYMPTOMS

Vasomotor symptoms such as hot flashes and night sweats are other common symptoms that result from breast-cancer-related treatments including chemotherapy or estrogen deprivation therapy-induced menopause. The management of hot flashes among breast cancer survivors is challenging, as the most effective treatment, estrogen therapy, is associated with increased risk of breast cancer recurrence and development of new breast cancers. Acupuncture shows promise as a therapeutic approach for hot flashes with minimal side effects in women with breast cancer across several RCTs (113–116). A recent systematic review of acupuncture to control hot flashes in cancer patients showed significant improvements from baseline in all eight studies evaluated, and that RA was significantly better than SA for different aspects of hot flashes in three studies (117). However, none of the studies were rated with a low risk of bias, making the current evidence insufficient to either support or refute the use of acupuncture for hot flashes.

LYMPHEDEMA MANAGEMENT

Treatment-induced lymphedema may be a lifelong concern for some breast cancer survivors. Up to 22% of patients suffer from this complication even with conservative surgical approaches, while it occurs more commonly in patients who undergo more extensive surgical procedures and radiation therapy (118–120). Lymphedema presents as chronic, persistent swelling in the affected extremity, causing increased risk of infection, pain, immobility, and worsened body image and QoL. The mainstay of treatment is a nonpharmacologic intervention known as complete decongestive therapy (CDT), which has four major components: manual lymph drainage, compression bandaging, compression garments, and exercise. Manual lymph drainage involves the movement of lymphatic fluid from the nonfunctioning region to a nearby region that drains effectively. Compression bandaging involves applying multiple layers of short stretch bandages from distal to proximal regions in order to promote lymphatic fluid movement. Compression garments are then applied with a steady pressure of 20 to 60 mmHg to prevent lymphedema recurrence. Upper body exercises may also reduce risk and severity (121). These treatments are labor-intensive, have limited efficacy, and are estimated to cost $10,000 per year per patient (122).

Previous case reports, retrospective chart reviews, and pilot studies have demonstrated acupuncture to be safe and potentially effective in reducing swelling and improving both upper and lower extremity edema (123–126). Among them, a 2013 study was the largest (n = 33), well-designed single-arm trial to evaluate acupuncture safety and efficacy in patients with moderate to severe chronic breast-cancer-related lymphedema (BCRL) (126). No serious adverse events were reported after a total of 255 acupuncture sessions. Twelve of thirty-three evaluable patients reported mild bruising or minor pain/tingling in the arm, shoulder, or acupuncture site at least once. Importantly, no infections were reported even though the standard acupuncture treatment protocol involves inserting four acupuncture needles in the limb with lymphedema. In addition, even though this was not an RCT, a mean reduction of 0.90 cm in arm circumference was demonstrated, and 11 patients (33%) experienced a ≥30% relative reduction in the difference between arm circumferences from baseline to postintervention. The same research group is conducting an RCT to further determine the efficacy of acupuncture in reducing BCRL symptoms.

The use of acupuncture to treat lymphedema is controversial as placing needles in the affected area is considered contraindicated by most breast oncologists and lymphedema experts due to concerns about infection and worsening the condition. To date, these negative outcomes have not been reported in pilot studies, which is encouraging, but may also be due to small sample size. Therefore, the recommendation is still to avoid placing acupuncture needles in the extremity with lymphedema outside of clinical trial settings.

NEUROPATHIC PAIN

Several clinical trials demonstrate benefits with acupuncture in reducing neuropathic pain in cancer patients (127–130). Among them, one clinical trial showed the effectiveness of auricular acupuncture for cancer-treatment-induced neuropathic pain (128). Patients were randomized to either real auricular acupuncture at active points or one of two placebo arms (real auricular acupuncture at placebo points, or SA through auricular seeds at placebo points). Pain intensity decreased by 36% in the active intervention group at the end of 2 months compared to baseline, whereas both placebo groups experienced only a 2% decrease in pain intensity ($P < .0001$) (128). In a study of acupuncture versus best medical care (BMC) for PN, a majority of patients in the acupuncture group (76%) had improvement in symptoms and nerve conduction studies compared to only 15% in the BMC group (131). In addition, investigators found full correlation between symptom improvement and nerve conduction studies (131). Although PN etiology was either unknown or due to diabetes, investigators found comparable results for patients with chemotherapy-induced PN (132).

FATIGUE

Another debilitating side effect of radiation and/or chemotherapy with no effective treatment options is fatigue. To address this problem, a large RCT was conducted to evaluate the effects of acupuncture plus usual care versus usual care alone for breast-cancer-related fatigue in 302 patients (133). The mean general fatigue score was significantly lower in those who received six weekly acupuncture treatments compared to those who did not (−3.11 on a 0–20 scale). In addition, acupuncture improved specific aspects of fatigue such as physical and mental fatigue, anxiety, and depression, and improved patients' QoL (133). Although mechanisms were not elucidated and the study design lacked a placebo control, the results are consistent with existing literature (134,135). Another well-designed but smaller RCT that evaluated EA for fatigue, sleep, and psychological distress in breast cancer patients with AI-related arthralgia did include both wait-listed controls (WLCs) and an SA arm. Compared to usual care, EA produced significantly and clinically relevant improvements in fatigue, anxiety, and depression, while SA improved only depression (136).

Taken together, current research suggests that acupuncture may be a valuable and safe nonpharmacological modality to treat various symptoms and improve QoL in breast cancer survivors, but these preliminary findings should be confirmed in larger trials with longer follow-up.

Touch Therapy

A number of studies have evaluated the effects of massage on cancer patients. Although many have been preliminary or of mixed quality, there are recurring themes of improved QoL and clinically meaningful reductions in pain, anxiety, and stress. A recent meta-analysis suggests there is mild evidence that massage may help to address negative emotions and fatigue in patients with breast cancer (137). Another meta-analysis found massage to be effective in relieving cancer pain, and especially surgery-related pain, with foot reflexology more effective than body or aroma massage (138). A multidimensional program that included strengthening exercises and massage as major components improved neck and shoulder pain and reduced widespread pressure hyperalgesia in breast cancer survivors compared to usual care treatment (139).

In a large sample of women with advanced-stage breast cancer receiving chemotherapy and/or hormonal therapy, investigators determined there were significant improvements in physical functioning and dyspnea severity with reflexology when compared to both a lay foot manipulation group and conventional care (140). Studies have also found benefit for patients with terminal cancer to improve pain, mood, and sleep quality (141,142). A study evaluating an abdominal massage intervention for end-stage cancer patients also found a significant group-by-time interaction on depression, anxiety, poor well-being, and perceived abdominal bloating (143).

Given that survivors have unique needs at different stages of disease, it is important for patients to have access to massage therapists who are specially trained in working with cancer patients. At the same time, certain types of massage may be safely given by caregivers who are specially trained on safe therapeutic touch. A recent study found a model of massage intervention using a multimedia caregiver education program to be feasible while decreasing patient pain, depression, and other symptoms (144). For many patients, massage therapy is a useful therapeutic tool to manage cancer symptoms, and is included among the services available at our institution both on an inpatient and outpatient basis. We also offer online and monthly demonstrations to provide caregivers with the knowledge and confidence to provide safe and effective touch therapy at home.

Supplements and Botanical Products

The issue of supplement use, especially among those who are undergoing treatment, is an important topic to address with patients. Supplement manufacturers are not required to have standards for the safety, content, and quality of their products, and possible side effects are not included in labeling. One of the most important messages to patients should be the encouragement of a well-balanced diet as previously described to obtain the right amounts of vitamins, minerals, and antioxidants, as well as micronutrients, which are lost when one relies on supplements. Further, supplement use during cancer treatments may result in perioperative complications, or interact with chemotherapy or radiation to cause serious side effects or reduce treatment efficacy.

A popular example is turmeric, a plant that is native to South Asia but cultivated around the world and used in traditional medicine for improving circulation and digestion. Turmeric extracts have been marketed for memory problems, arthritis, and cancer prevention. Because the active ingredient of turmeric, curcumin, is known to interfere with cytochrome P450 enzymes (145,146) and may interact with chemotherapy drugs like cyclophosphamide and doxorubicin (147), we advise patients not to take turmeric or curcumin during chemotherapy or hormonal therapy due to herb–drug interaction concerns. Many other herbal supplements can fall under this category, including St. John's wort, green tea extract, and astragalus. *AboutHerbs.com* (148) is a free resource for both health care professionals and consumers provided by Memorial Sloan Kettering, which outlines the current evidence for various supplements that are of interest to cancer patients including potential interactions and side effects.

In some instances, however, it can be difficult to obtain a nutrient from diet alone. Such is the case with vitamin D, which in addition to helping bone formation has been reported to be a pro-differentiation hormone (149) with antiproliferative (150), anti-inflammatory, and immune-regulatory effects (151). Epidemiological studies show that vitamin D from sunlight exposure and dietary intake may have protective effects against breast cancer (152,153), and data correlate with observations that many breast cancer survivors are vitamin-D-deficient (154). As such, we monitor patients' vitamin D levels and recommend supplementation in patients with low serum levels accordingly.

CONCLUSIONS

Diet and exercise recommendations are important components to integrate into mainstream cancer care. A majority of breast cancer survivors may be obese or overweight, with greater risks for recurrence, cardiovascular disease, diabetes, and overall poorer QoL (155), and many women report initiating dietary changes during active treatment (156). A number of cancer-treatment-related side effects can also be addressed with integrative therapies such as acupuncture, massage, and mind–body therapies, and cancer patients often seek advice from their health care providers on which modalities may be most effective for them. Table 10.3 provides a general overview of integrative modalities that are clinically practiced in breast cancer symptom management, and Table 10.4 provides links to trusted online sources on integrative therapies for health care professionals and consumers.

A referral system to integrative therapy programs such as exists at our institution is vital to ensure continuity of care for patients with unique and changing issues in their health status. Indeed, the provision of such structure, guidance, support, and feedback is an important aspect for many patients who have just undergone medical treatment, may be unsure of their capacity to safely reclaim levels of physical fitness, struggle with corresponding psychosocial issues, and to support their natural healing process. Themes articulated among cancer patients who use integrative modalities include empowerment, camaraderie, and community with those facing similar challenges, pain relief, increased fitness, relief or transferability of anxiety and stress through the use of various techniques learned, enhanced future perspective, and higher levels of motivation to continue improvements in fitness levels and pain reduction (46,157–159).

Of equal importance is the engaged dialog of health care professionals with patients on interventions such as dietary supplements, which may help or harm, particularly during active treatment, and rather steering patients toward modalities that have demonstrated levels of efficacy, are cost-effective, and with minimal or no side effects.

Table 10.3 Strategies for Symptom Management in Breast Cancer Patients

Recommended/encouraged

Diet Mediterranean diet or varied diet focusing on whole foods	**In addition to Table 10.1** Discuss/manage areas of deficiency such as vitamin D insufficiency	
Exercise/physical activity Aerobic exercise Moderate to vigorous ADL Weight-bearing Resistance training Tai chi Walking Yoga	**See Table 10.2; helpful for** • Balance issues • Bone loss • Fatigue • Hot flashes • Pain • Physical deconditioning • Weight gain	**May also address/affect** • Feelings of alienation • Motivation to continue • Corresponding biomarkers
Mind–body therapies Meditation Mindfulness training (MBSR, MBCR) Qigong Stress reduction Tai chi Yoga	**Helpful for** • Anxiety • Balance issues • Cognitive impairment • Depression • Emotional self-regulation • Fear of recurrence • Sleep disturbance	**May also address/affect** • Feelings of alienation • Motivation to continue • Corresponding biomarkers

Potentially helpful

Massage	• Abdominal bloating • Anxiety • Depression • Dyspnea • Fatigue • Hyperalgesia • Mood, negative emotions	• Pain, including surgery-related pain • Physical functioning • Sleep quality • Stress • Well-being
Acupuncture	• AI-induced musculoskeletal symptoms • Anxiety • Depression • Fatigue • Hot flashes, vasomotor symptoms • Peripheral neuropathy, including CIPN	

Only in clinical trials

Acupuncture	• Lymphedema

ADL, activities of daily living; AI, aromatase inhibitor; CIPN, chemotherapy-induced peripheral neuropathy; MBCR, mindfulness-based cancer recovery; MBSR, mindfulness-based stress reduction.

Table 10.4 Online Resources on Integrative Therapies for Health Care Professionals and Consumers

About Herbs, Botanicals & Other Products (also known as AboutHerbs.com)
https://www.mskcc.org/cancer-care/treatments/symptom-management/integrative-medicine/herbs

This free online resource from MSK presents the current evidence on herbal dietary supplements as well as integrative modalities such as acupuncture, tai chi, yoga, and massage for both health care professionals and consumers.

Online Integrative Medicine Modality Videos
https://www.mskcc.org/cancer-care/treatments/symptom-management/integrative-medicine/videos

Another free online resource from MSK provides demonstrations of exercises to improve physical conditioning that are appropriate and safe for cancer patients, as well as various stress reduction and meditation techniques.

National Center for Complementary and Integrative Health (NCCIH)
https://nccih.nih.gov/health/decisions

Provides useful articles to consumers on complementary and integrative health care approaches, choosing a practitioner, and issues regarding insurance coverage and out of pocket payments.

NCCN Patient and Caregiver Resources
Nutrition for Cancer Survivors
www.nccn.org/patients/resources/life_after_cancer/nutrition.aspx

Exercise for Life
www.nccn.org/patients/resources/life_after_cancer/exercise.aspx

These resources provide practical guidance to patients on diet and exercise.

University of Maryland Complementary and Alternative Medicine Guide
http://umm.edu/health/medical/altmed/

This free online resource from the University of Maryland presents the current information on herbs for consumers.

MSK, Memorial Sloan Kettering Cancer Center; NCCN, National Comprehensive Cancer Network.

➤ MANAGEMENT PEARLS

1. Integrative medicine uses nonpharmacologic therapies adjunctively to treat symptoms safely and effectively, improve QoL, and facilitate lifestyle changes.

2. Integrative therapies should be considered in management of cancer symptoms such as anxiety, depression, stress, fatigue, feelings of isolation, hot flashes, lymphedema, nausea, neuropathy, pain, perioperative symptoms, sexual dysfunction, physical deconditioning, dyspnea, urinary problems, and xerostomia.
3. Cancer- and cancer-treatment-related side effects can be controlled with integrative therapies such as acupuncture, massage, and mind–body therapies.
   - Of equal importance is the engaged dialog of health care professionals with patients on interventions such as dietary supplements.
4. Institutional guidelines and referral system to integrative therapy programs are vital to ensure continuity of care for cancer patients with unique and changing issues in their health status.

ACKNOWLEDGMENT

The author thanks Ing Haviland for contributing her invaluable writing and editing skills that helped to shape this manuscript.

REFERENCES

1. Mao JJ, Palmer CS, Healy KE, et al. Complementary and alternative medicine use among cancer survivors: a population-based study. *J Cancer Surviv.* 2011;5:8–17.
2. Frenkel M, Cohen L. Effective communication about the use of complementary and integrative medicine in cancer care. *J Altern Complement Med.* 2014;20:12–18.
3. Mao JJ, Palmer SC, Straton JB, et al. Cancer survivors with unmet needs were more likely to use complementary and alternative medicine. *J Cancer Surviv.* 2008;2:116–124.
4. Frenkel M, Sierpina V, Sapire K. Effects of complementary and integrative medicine on cancer survivorship. *Curr Oncol Rep.* 2015;17:445.
5. Cardoso F, Bese N, Distelhorst SR, et al. Supportive care during treatment for breast cancer: resource allocations in low- and middle-income countries. A breast health global initiative 2013 consensus statement. *Breast.* 2013;22:593–605.
6. Gosain R, Miller K. Symptoms and symptom management in long-term cancer survivors. *Cancer J.* 2013;19:405–409.
7. Klepin H, Mohile S, Hurria A. Geriatric assessment in older patients with breast cancer. *J Natl Compr Canc Netw.* 2009;7:226–236.
8. Greenlee H, Balneaves LG, Carlson LE, et al. Clinical practice guidelines on the use of integrative therapies as supportive care in patients treated for breast cancer. *J Natl Cancer Inst Monogr.* 2014;2014:346–358.
9. World Cancer Research Fund International, American Institute for Cancer Research. *Summary: Food, Nutrition, Physical Activity, and the Prevention of Cancer: A Global Perspective.* Washington, DC: AICR; 2007. http://www.aicr.org/assets/docs/pdf/reports/Second_Expert_Report.pdf
10. National Comprehensive Cancer Network. Nutrition for cancer survivors. http://www.nccn.org/patients/resources/life_after_cancer/nutrition.aspx

11. Toledo E, Salas-Salvado J, Donat-Vargas C, et al. Mediterranean diet and invasive breast cancer risk among women at high cardiovascular risk in the PREDIMED trial: a randomized clinical trial. *JAMA Intern Med.* 2015;175:1752–1760.

12. Kwan ML, Weltzien E, Kushi LH, et al. Dietary patterns and breast cancer recurrence and survival among women with early-stage breast cancer. *J Clin Oncol.* 2009;27:919–926.

13. Kroenke CH, Fung TT, Hu FB, et al. Dietary patterns and survival after breast cancer diagnosis. *J Clin Oncol.* 2005;23:9295–9303.

14. Baranski M, Srednicka-Tober D, Volakakis N, et al. Higher antioxidant and lower cadmium concentrations and lower incidence of pesticide residues in organically grown crops: a systematic literature review and meta-analyses. *Br J Nutr.* 2014;112:794–811.

15. Smith-Spangler C, Brandeau ML, Hunter GE, et al. Are organic foods safer or healthier than conventional alternatives? A systematic review. *Ann Intern Med.* 2012;157:348–366.

16. Dangour AD, Lock K, Hayter A, et al. Nutrition-related health effects of organic foods: a systematic review. *Am J Clin Nutr.* 2010;92:203–210.

17. Palupi E, Jayanegara A, Ploeger A, et al. Comparison of nutritional quality between conventional and organic dairy products: a meta-analysis. *J Sci Food Agric.* 2012;92:2774–2781.

18. Crinnion WJ. Organic foods contain higher levels of certain nutrients, lower levels of pesticides, and may provide health benefits for the consumer. *Altern Med Rev.* 2010;15:4–12.

19. Stracke BA, Rufer CE, Bub A, et al. Bioavailability and nutritional effects of carotenoids from organically and conventionally produced carrots in healthy men. *Br J Nutr.* 2009;101:1664–1672.

20. Bradbury KE, Balkwill A, Spencer EA, et al. Organic food consumption and the incidence of cancer in a large prospective study of women in the United Kingdom. *Br J Cancer.* 2014;110:2321–2326.

21. Sulaiman S, Shahril MR, Wafa SW, et al. Dietary carbohydrate, fiber and sugar and risk of breast cancer according to menopausal status in Malaysia. *Asian Pac J Cancer Prev.* 2014;15:5959–5964.

22. Jiang Y, Pan Y, Rhea PR, et al. Abstract 3735: dietary sugar induces tumorigenesis in mammary gland partially through 12 lipoxygenase pathway. *Cancer Res.* 2015;75(suppl 15):3735. doi:10.1158/1538-7445.AM2015-3735

23. Suzuki S, Kojima M, Tokudome S, et al. Obesity/weight gain and breast cancer risk: findings from the Japan collaborative cohort study for the evaluation of cancer risk. *J Epidemiol.* 2013;23:139–145.

24. Cleveland RJ, Eng SM, Abrahamson PE, et al. Weight gain prior to diagnosis and survival from breast cancer. *Cancer Epidemiol Biomarkers Prev.* 2007;16:1803–1811.

25. Vucenik I, Stains JP. Obesity and cancer risk: evidence, mechanisms, and recommendations. *Ann N Y Acad Sci.* 2012;1271:37–43.

26. Moreira PI. High-sugar diets, type 2 diabetes and Alzheimer's disease. *Curr Opin Clin Nutr Metab Care.* 2013;16:440–445.

27. Yang Q, Zhang Z, Gregg EW, et al. Added sugar intake and cardiovascular diseases mortality among US adults. *JAMA Intern Med.* 2014;174:516–524.

28. Johnson RK, Appel LJ, Brands M, et al. Dietary sugars intake and cardiovascular health: a scientific statement from the American Heart Association. *Circulation.* 2009;120:1011–1020.

29. Hamajima N, Hirose K, Tajima K, et al. Alcohol, tobacco and breast cancer—collaborative reanalysis of individual data from 53 epidemiological studies, including 58,515 women with breast cancer and 95,067 women without the disease. *Br J Cancer.* 2002;87:1234–1245.

30. National Comprehensive Cancer Network. NCCN guidelines: breast cancer risk reduction, Version 2.2015. http://www.nccn.org/professionals/physician_gls/pdf/breast_risk.pdf

31. Rufer CE, Kulling SE. Antioxidant activity of isoflavones and their major metabolites using different in vitro assays. *J Agric Food Chem*. 2006;54:2926–2931.

32. Rimbach G, De Pascual-Teresa S, Ewins BA, et al. Antioxidant and free radical scavenging activity of isoflavone metabolites. *Xenobiotica*. 2003;33:913–925.

33. Chen M, Rao Y, Zheng Y, et al. Association between soy isoflavone intake and breast cancer risk for pre- and post-menopausal women: a meta-analysis of epidemiological studies. *PLOS ONE*. 2014;9:e89288.

34. Schmid D, Leitzmann MF. Television viewing and time spent sedentary in relation to cancer risk: a meta-analysis. *J Natl Cancer Inst*. 2014;106.

35. Calle EE, Kaaks R. Overweight, obesity and cancer: epidemiological evidence and proposed mechanisms. *Nat Rev Cancer*. 2004;4:579–591.

36. National Cancer Institute. Obesity and cancer risk fact sheet. http://www.cancer.gov/cancertopics/factsheet/Risk/obesity

37. Eliassen AH, Colditz GA, Rosner B, et al. Adult weight change and risk of postmenopausal breast cancer. *JAMA*. 2006;296:193–201.

38. Mahoney MC, Bevers T, Linos E, et al. Opportunities and strategies for breast cancer prevention through risk reduction. *CA Cancer J Clin*. 2008;58:347–371.

39. Irwin ML, Smith AW, McTiernan A, et al. Influence of pre- and postdiagnosis physical activity on mortality in breast cancer survivors: the health, eating, activity, and lifestyle study. *J Clin Oncol*. 2008;26:3958–3964.

40. Holick CN, Newcomb PA, Trentham-Dietz A, et al. Physical activity and survival after diagnosis of invasive breast cancer. *Cancer Epidemiol Biomarkers Prev*. 2008;17:379–386.

41. Holmes MD, Chen WY, Feskanich D, et al. Physical activity and survival after breast cancer diagnosis. *JAMA*. 2005;293:2479–2486.

42. Deng GE, Rausch SM, Jones LW, et al. Complementary therapies and integrative medicine in lung cancer, Diagnosis and management of lung cancer, 3rd ed, American College of Chest Physicians evidence-based clinical practice guidelines. *Chest*. 2013;143:e420S–436S.

43. Schmitz KH, Courneya KS, Matthews C, et al. American College of Sports Medicine roundtable on exercise guidelines for cancer survivors. *Med Sci Sports Exerc*. 2010;42:1409–1426.

44. Deng GE, Frenkel M, Cohen L, et al. Evidence-based clinical practice guidelines for integrative oncology: complementary therapies and botanicals. *J Soc Integr Oncol*. 2009;7:85–120.

45. van Waart H, Stuiver MM, van Harten WH, et al. Effect of low-intensity physical activity and moderate- to high-intensity physical exercise during adjuvant chemotherapy on physical fitness, fatigue, and chemotherapy completion rates: results of the PACES randomized clinical trial. *J Clin Oncol*. 2015;33:1918–1927.

46. Steindorf K, Schmidt ME, Klassen O, et al. Randomized, controlled trial of resistance training in breast cancer patients receiving adjuvant radiotherapy: results on cancer-related fatigue and quality of life. *Ann Oncol*. 2014;25:2237–2243.

47. Irwin ML, Cartmel B, Gross CP, et al. Randomized exercise trial of aromatase inhibitor-induced arthralgia in breast cancer survivors. *J Clin Oncol*. 2015;33:1104–1111.

48. Travier N, Velthuis MJ, Steins Bisschop CN, et al. Effects of an 18-week exercise programme started early during breast cancer treatment: a randomised controlled trial. *BMC Med*. 2015;13:121.

49. Schmidt ME, Wiskemann J, Armbrust P, et al. Effects of resistance exercise on fatigue and quality of life in breast cancer patients undergoing adjuvant chemotherapy: a randomized controlled trial. *Int J Cancer*. 2015;137:471–480.

50. Taso CJ, Lin HS, Lin WL, et al. The effect of yoga exercise on improving depression, anxiety, and fatigue in women with breast cancer: a randomized controlled trial. *J Nurs Res.* 2014;22:155–164.

51. Schmidt T, Weisser B, Durkop J, et al. Comparing endurance and resistance training with standard care during chemotherapy for patients with primary breast cancer. *Anticancer Res.* 2015;35:5623–5629.

52. Rogers LQ, Courneya KS, Anton PM, et al. Effects of the BEAT Cancer physical activity behavior change intervention on physical activity, aerobic fitness, and quality of life in breast cancer survivors: a multicenter randomized controlled trial. *Breast Cancer Res Treat.* 2015;149:109–119.

53. Beidas RS, Paciotti B, Barg F, et al. A hybrid effectiveness-implementation trial of an evidence-based exercise intervention for breast cancer survivors. *J Natl Cancer Inst Monogr.* 2014;2014:338–345.

54. Murtezani A, Ibraimi Z, Bakalli A, et al. The effect of aerobic exercise on quality of life among breast cancer survivors: a randomized controlled trial. *J Cancer Res Ther.* 2014;10:658–664.

55. Brown JC, Schmitz KH. Weight lifting and physical function among survivors of breast cancer: a post hoc analysis of a randomized controlled trial. *J Clin Oncol.* 2015;33:2184–2189.

56. Borneman T, Koczywas M, Sun VC, et al. Reducing patient barriers to pain and fatigue management. *J Pain Symptom Manage.* 2010;39:486–501.

57. Winters-Stone KM, Dobek J, Nail LM, et al. Impact + resistance training improves bone health and body composition in prematurely menopausal breast cancer survivors: a randomized controlled trial. *Osteoporos Int.* 2013;24:1637–1646.

58. Dobek J, Winters-Stone KM, Bennett JA, et al. Musculoskeletal changes after 1 year of exercise in older breast cancer survivors. *J Cancer Surviv.* 2014;8:304–311.

59. Rock CL, Flatt SW, Byers TE, et al. Results of the exercise and nutrition to enhance recovery and good health for you (ENERGY) trial: a behavioral weight loss intervention in overweight or obese breast cancer survivors. *J Clin Oncol.* 2015;33:3169–3176.

60. Duijts SF, van Beurden M, Oldenburg HS, et al. Efficacy of cognitive behavioral therapy and physical exercise in alleviating treatment-induced menopausal symptoms in patients with breast cancer: results of a randomized, controlled, multicenter trial. *J Clin Oncol.* 2012;30:4124–4133.

61. National Comprehensive Cancer Network. NCCN guidelines: survivorship, Version 2.2015. http://www.nccn.org/professionals/physician_gls/pdf/survivorship.pdf

62. Lutz A, Slagter HA, Dunne JD, et al. Attention regulation and monitoring in meditation. *Trends Cogn Sci.* 2008;12:163–169.

63. Garland SN, Carlson LE, Stephens AJ, et al. Mindfulness-based stress reduction compared with cognitive behavioral therapy for the treatment of insomnia comorbid with cancer: a randomized, partially blinded, noninferiority trial. *J Clin Oncol.* 2014;32:449–457.

64. Nidich SI, Fields JZ, Rainforth MV, et al. A randomized controlled trial of the effects of transcendental meditation on quality of life in older breast cancer patients. *Integr Cancer Ther.* 2009;8:228–234.

65. Lengacher CA, Johnson-Mallard V, Post-White J, et al. Randomized controlled trial of mindfulness-based stress reduction (MBSR) for survivors of breast cancer. *Psychooncology.* 2009;18:1261–1272.

66. Henderson VP, Clemow L, Massion AO, et al. The effects of mindfulness-based stress reduction on psychosocial outcomes and quality of life in early-stage breast cancer patients: a randomized trial. *Breast Cancer Res Treat.* 2012;131:99–109.

67. Wurtzen H, Dalton SO, Elsass P, et al. Mindfulness significantly reduces self-reported levels of anxiety and depression: results of a randomised controlled trial among 336 Danish women treated for stage I-III breast cancer. *Eur J Cancer.* 2013;49:1365–1373.

68. Hoffman CJ, Ersser SJ, Hopkinson JB, et al. Effectiveness of mindfulness-based stress reduction in mood, breast- and endocrine-related quality of life, and well-being in stage 0 to III breast cancer: a randomized, controlled trial. *J Clin Oncol.* 2012;30:1335–1342.

69. Andersen SR, Wurtzen H, Steding-Jessen M, et al. Effect of mindfulness-based stress reduction on sleep quality: results of a randomized trial among Danish breast cancer patients. *Acta Oncol.* 2013;52:336–344.

70. Matousek RH, Pruessner JC, Dobkin PL. Changes in the cortisol awakening response (CAR) following participation in mindfulness-based stress reduction in women who completed treatment for breast cancer. *Complement Ther Clin Pract.* 2011;17:65–70.

71. Carlson LE, Beattie TL, Giese-Davis J, et al. Mindfulness-based cancer recovery and supportive-expressive therapy maintain telomere length relative to controls in distressed breast cancer survivors. *Cancer.* 2015;121:476–484.

72. Carlson LE, Speca M, Patel KD, et al. Mindfulness-based stress reduction in relation to quality of life, mood, symptoms of stress and levels of cortisol, dehydroepiandrosterone sulfate (DHEAS) and melatonin in breast and prostate cancer outpatients. *Psychoneuroendocrinology.* 2004;29:448–474.

73. Carlson LE, Doll R, Stephen J, et al. Randomized controlled trial of mindfulness-based cancer recovery versus supportive expressive group therapy for distressed survivors of breast cancer. *J Clin Oncol.* 2013;31:3119–3126.

74. Bower JE, Crosswell AD, Stanton AL, et al. Mindfulness meditation for younger breast cancer survivors: a randomized controlled trial. *Cancer.* 2015;121:1231–1240.

75. Mustian KM, Sprod LK, Janelsins M, et al. Multicenter, randomized controlled trial of yoga for sleep quality among cancer survivors. *J Clin Oncol.* 2013;31:3233–3241.

76. Mustian KM, Sprod LK, Janelsins M, et al. Exercise recommendations for cancer-related fatigue, cognitive impairment, sleep problems, depression, pain, anxiety, and physical dysfunction: a review. *Oncol Hematol Rev.* 2012;8:81–88.

77. Bower JE, Woolery A, Sternlieb B, et al. Yoga for cancer patients and survivors. *Cancer Control.* 2005;12:165–171.

78. Rosenbaum E, Gautier H, Fobair P, et al. Cancer supportive care, improving the quality of life for cancer patients. A program evaluation report. *Support Care Cancer.* 2004;12:293–301.

79. Janelsins MC, Peppone LJ, Heckler CE, et al. YOCAS(c)(R) Yoga reduces self-reported memory difficulty in cancer survivors in a nationwide randomized clinical trial: investigating relationships between memory and sleep. *Integr Cancer Ther.* 2015;15(3):263–271.

80. Sudarshan M, Petrucci A, Dumitra S, et al. Yoga therapy for breast cancer patients: a prospective cohort study. *Complement Ther Clin Pract.* 2013;19:227–229.

81. Moadel AB, Shah C, Wylie-Rosett J, et al. Randomized controlled trial of yoga among a multiethnic sample of breast cancer patients: effects on quality of life. *J Clin Oncol.* 2007;25:4387–4395.

82. Culos-Reed SN, Carlson LE, Daroux LM, et al. A pilot study of yoga for breast cancer survivors: physical and psychological benefits. *Psychooncology.* 2006;15:891–897.

83. Vadiraja HS, Raghavendra RM, Nagarathna R, et al. Effects of a yoga program on cortisol rhythm and mood states in early breast cancer patients undergoing adjuvant radiotherapy: a randomized controlled trial. *Integr Cancer Ther.* 2009;8:37–46.

84. Rao MR, Raghuram N, Nagendra HR, et al. Anxiolytic effects of a yoga program in early breast cancer patients undergoing conventional treatment: a randomized controlled trial. *Complement Ther Med.* 2009;17:1–8.

85. Bower JE, Garet D, Sternlieb B, et al. Yoga for persistent fatigue in breast cancer survivors: a randomized controlled trial. *Cancer.* 2012;118:3766–3775.

86. Carson JW, Carson KM, Porter LS, et al. Yoga of Awareness program for menopausal symptoms in breast cancer survivors: results from a randomized trial. *Support Care Cancer.* 2009;17:1301–1309.

87. Oh B, Butow P, Mullan B, et al. Impact of medical qigong on quality of life, fatigue, mood and inflammation in cancer patients: a randomized controlled trial. *Ann Oncol.* 2010;21:608–614.

88. Navarro M. Qigong improves quality of life in cancer patients. Presented at: 9th International Conference of the Society for Integrative Oncology; Albuquerque, NM, October 8, 2012.

89. Larkey LK, Roe DJ, Weihs KL, et al. Randomized controlled trial of qigong/tai chi easy on cancer-related fatigue in breast cancer survivors. *Ann Behav Med.* 2015;49:165–176.

90. Li F, Harmer P, Fisher KJ, et al. Tai chi and fall reductions in older adults: a randomized controlled trial. *J Gerontol A Biol Sci Med Sci.* 2005;60:187–194.

91. Mustian KM, Palesh OG, Flecksteiner SA. Tai chi chuan for breast cancer survivors. *Med Sport Sci.* 2008;52:209–217.

92. Lee TI, Chen HH, Yeh ML. Effects of chan-chuang qigong on improving symptom and psychological distress in chemotherapy patients. *Am J Chin Med.* 2006;34:37–46.

93. Oh B, Butow PN, Mullan BA, et al. Effect of medical qigong on cognitive function, quality of life, and a biomarker of inflammation in cancer patients: a randomized controlled trial. *Support Care Cancer.* 2012;20:1235–1242.

94. Irwin MR, Olmstead R, Breen EC, et al. Tai chi, cellular inflammation, and transcriptome dynamics in breast cancer survivors with insomnia: a randomized controlled trial. *J Natl Cancer Inst Monogr.* 2014;2014:295–301.

95. Peppone LJ, Mustian KM, Janelsins MC, et al. Effects of a structured weight-bearing exercise program on bone metabolism among breast cancer survivors: a feasibility trial. *Clin Breast Cancer.* 2010;10:224–229.

96. Janelsins MC, Davis PG, Wideman L, et al. Effects of tai chi chuan on insulin and cytokine levels in a randomized controlled pilot study on breast cancer survivors. *Clin Breast Cancer.* 2011;11:161–170.

97. Zhang R, Lao L, Ren K, et al. Mechanisms of acupuncture-electroacupuncture on persistent pain. *Anesthesiology.* 2014;120:482–503.

98. Takeshige C. Mechanism of acupuncture analgesia based on animal experiments. In: Pomerantz BSG, ed. *Scientific Bases of Acupuncture.* Berlin, Germany: Springer-Verlag; 1989:53–78.

99. Lee BY, Newberg AB. Acupuncture in theory and practice. *Hospital Physician.* 2004;40:11–18.

100. Zhao ZQ. Neural mechanism underlying acupuncture analgesia. *Prog Neurobiol.* 2008;85:355–375.

101. Gottschling S, Reindl TK, Meyer S, et al. Acupuncture to alleviate chemotherapy-induced nausea and vomiting in pediatric oncology—a randomized multicenter crossover pilot trial. *Klin Padiatr.* 2008;220:365–370.

102. Rithirangsriroj K, Manchana T, Akkayagorn L. Efficacy of acupuncture in prevention of delayed chemotherapy induced nausea and vomiting in gynecologic cancer patients. *Gynecol Oncol.* 2015;136:82–86.

103. Burstein HJ, Prestrud AA, Seidenfeld J, et al. American Society of Clinical Oncology clinical practice guideline: update on adjuvant endocrine therapy for women with hormone receptor-positive breast cancer. *J Clin Oncol.* 2010;28:3784–3796.

104. Crew KD, Greenlee H, Capodice J, et al. Prevalence of joint symptoms in postmenopausal women taking aromatase inhibitors for early-stage breast cancer. *J Clin Oncol.* 2007;25:3877–3883.

105. Henry NL, Azzouz F, Desta Z, et al. Predictors of aromatase inhibitor discontinuation as a result of treatment-emergent symptoms in early-stage breast cancer. *J Clin Oncol.* 2012;30:936–942.

106. Burstein HJ. Aromatase inhibitor-associated arthralgia syndrome. *Breast.* 2007;16: 223–234.

107. Henry NL, Giles JT, Stearns V. Aromatase inhibitor-associated musculoskeletal symptoms: etiology and strategies for management. *Oncology (Williston Park).* 2008;22:1401–1408.

108. Crew KD, Capodice JL, Greenlee H, et al. Randomized, blinded, sham-controlled trial of acupuncture for the management of aromatase inhibitor-associated joint symptoms in women with early-stage breast cancer. *J Clin Oncol.* 2010;28:1154–1160.

109. Bao T, Cai L, Giles JT, et al. A dual-center randomized controlled double blind trial assessing the effect of acupuncture in reducing musculoskeletal symptoms in breast cancer patients taking aromatase inhibitors. *Breast Cancer Res Treat.* 2013;138:167–174.

110. Oh B, Kimble B, Costa DS, et al. Acupuncture for treatment of arthralgia secondary to aromatase inhibitor therapy in women with early breast cancer: pilot study. *Acupunct Med,* 2013;31:264–271.

111. Mao JJ, Xie SX, Farrar JT, et al. A randomised trial of electro-acupuncture for arthralgia related to aromatase inhibitor use. *Eur J Cancer.* 2014;50:267–276.

112. Greenlee H, Crew KD, Capodice J, et al. Methods to standardize a multicenter acupuncture trial protocol to reduce aromatase inhibitor-related joint symptoms in breast cancer patients. *J Acupunct Meridian Stud.* 2015;8:152–158.

113. Deng G, Vickers A, Yeung S, et al. Randomized, controlled trial of acupuncture for the treatment of hot flashes in breast cancer patients. *J Clin Oncol.* 2007;25:5584–5590.

114. Hervik J, Mjaland O. Acupuncture for the treatment of hot flashes in breast cancer patients, a randomized, controlled trial. *Breast Cancer Res Treat.* 2009;116:311–316.

115. Frisk J, Carlhall S, Kallstrom AC, et al. Long-term follow-up of acupuncture and hormone therapy on hot flushes in women with breast cancer: a prospective, randomized, controlled multicenter trial. *Climacteric.* 2008;11:166–174.

116. Walker EM, Rodriguez AI, Kohn B, et al. Acupuncture versus venlafaxine for the management of vasomotor symptoms in patients with hormone receptor-positive breast cancer: a randomized controlled trial. *J Clin Oncol.* 2010;28:634–640.

117. Garcia MK, Graham-Getty L, Haddad R, et al. Systematic review of acupuncture to control hot flashes in cancer patients. *Cancer.* 2015;121:3948–3958.

118. Warren LE, Miller CL, Horick N, et al. The impact of radiation therapy on the risk of lymphedema after treatment for breast cancer: a prospective cohort study. *Int J Radiat Oncol Biol Phys.* 2014;88:565–571.

119. Wernicke AG, Shamis M, Sidhu KK, et al. Complication rates in patients with negative axillary nodes 10 years after local breast radiotherapy after either sentinel lymph node dissection or axillary clearance. *Am J Clin Oncol.* 2013;36:12–19.

120. Letellier ME, Towers A, Shimony A, et al. Breast cancer-related lymphedema: a randomized controlled pilot and feasibility study. *Am J Phys Med Rehabil.* 2014;93:751–759;quiz 760–761.

121. Lawenda BD, Mondry TE, Johnstone PA. Lymphedema: a primer on the identification and management of a chronic condition in oncologic treatment. *CA Cancer J Clin.* 2009;59:8–24.

122. Shih YC, Xu Y, Cormier JN, et al. Incidence, treatment costs, and complications of lymphedema after breast cancer among women of working age: a 2-year follow-up study. *J Clin Oncol.* 2009;27:2007–2014.

123. Kanakura Y, Niwa K, Kometani K, et al. Effectiveness of acupuncture and moxibustion treatment for lymphedema following intrapelvic lymph node dissection: a preliminary report. *Am J Chin Med.* 2002;30:37–43.

124. Alem M, Gurgel MS. Acupuncture in the rehabilitation of women after breast cancer surgery–a case series. *Acupunct Med.* 2008;26:87–93.

125. Cassileth BR, Van Zee KJ, Chan Y, et al. A safety and efficacy pilot study of acupuncture for the treatment of chronic lymphoedema. *Acupunct Med.* 2011;29:170–172.

126. Cassileth BR, Van Zee KJ, Yeung KS, et al. Acupuncture in the treatment of upper-limb lymphedema: results of a pilot study. *Cancer.* 2013;119:2455–2461.

127. Minton O, Higginson IJ. Electroacupuncture as an adjunctive treatment to control neuropathic pain in patients with cancer. *J Pain Symptom Manage.* 2007;33:115–117.

128. Alimi D, Rubino C, Pichard-Leandri E, et al. Analgesic effect of auricular acupuncture for cancer pain: a randomized, blinded, controlled trial. *J Clin Oncol.* 2003;21:4120–4126.

129. Bao T, Goloubeva O, Pelser C, et al. A pilot study of acupuncture in treating bortezomib-induced peripheral neuropathy in patients with multiple myeloma. *Integr Cancer Ther.* 2014;13:396–404.

130. Garcia MK, Cohen L, Guo Y, et al. Electroacupuncture for thalidomide/bortezomib-induced peripheral neuropathy in multiple myeloma: a feasibility study. *J Hematol Oncol.* 2014;7:41.

131. Schroder S, Liepert J, Remppis A, et al. Acupuncture treatment improves nerve conduction in peripheral neuropathy. *Eur J Neurol.* 2007;14:276–281.

132. Schroeder S, Meyer-Hamme G, Epplee S. Acupuncture for chemotherapy-induced peripheral neuropathy (CIPN): a pilot study using neurography. *Acupunct Med,* 2012;30:4–7.

133. Molassiotis A, Bardy J, Finnegan-John J, et al. Acupuncture for cancer-related fatigue in patients with breast cancer: a pragmatic randomized controlled trial. *J Clin Oncol.* 2012;30:4470–4476.

134. Vickers AJ, Straus DJ, Fearon B, et al. Acupuncture for postchemotherapy fatigue: a phase II study. *J Clin Oncol.* 2004;22:1731–1735.

135. Molassiotis A, Sylt P, Diggins H. The management of cancer-related fatigue after chemotherapy with acupuncture and acupressure: a randomised controlled trial. *Complement Ther Med.* 2007;15:228–237.

136. Mao JJ, Farrar JT, Bruner D, et al. Electroacupuncture for fatigue, sleep, and psychological distress in breast cancer patients with aromatase inhibitor-related arthralgia: a randomized trial. *Cancer.* 2014;120:3744–3751.

137. Pan YQ, Yang KH, Wang YL, et al. Massage interventions and treatment-related side effects of breast cancer: a systematic review and meta-analysis. *Int J Clin Oncol.* 2014;19:829–841.

138. Lee SH, Kim JY, Yeo S, et al. Meta-analysis of massage therapy on cancer pain. *Integr Cancer Ther.* 2015;14:297–304.

139. Fernandez-Lao C, Cantarero-Villanueva I, Fernandez-de-Las-Penas C, et al. Effectiveness of a multidimensional physical therapy program on pain, pressure hypersensitivity, and trigger points in breast cancer survivors: a randomized controlled clinical trial. *Clin J Pain.* 2012;28:113–121.

140. Wyatt G, Sikorskii A, Rahbar MH, et al. Health-related quality-of-life outcomes: a reflexology trial with patients with advanced-stage breast cancer. *Oncol Nurs Forum.* 2012;39:568–577.

141. Toth M, Marcantonio ER, Davis RB, et al. Massage therapy for patients with metastatic cancer: a pilot randomized controlled trial. *J Altern Complement Med.* 2013;19:650–656.

142. Lopez-Sendin N, Alburquerque-Sendin F, Cleland JA, et al. Effects of physical therapy on pain and mood in patients with terminal cancer: a pilot randomized clinical trial. *J Altern Complement Med.* 2012;18:480–486.

143. Wang TJ, Wang HM, Yang TS, et al. The effect of abdominal massage in reducing malignant ascites symptoms. *Res Nurs Health.* 2015;38:51–59.

144. Collinge W, Kahn J, Walton T, et al. Touch, caring, and cancer: randomized controlled trial of a multimedia caregiver education program. *Support Care Cancer.* 2013;21:1405–1414.

145. Chen Y, Liu WH, Chen BL, et al. Plant polyphenol curcumin significantly affects CYP1A2 and CYP2A6 activity in healthy, male Chinese volunteers. *Ann Pharmacother.* 2010;44:1038–1045.

146. Zhang W, Lim LY. Effects of spice constituents on P-glycoprotein-mediated transport and CYP3A4-mediated metabolism in vitro. *Drug Metab Dispos.* 2008;36:1283–1290.

147. Somasundaram S, Edmund NA, Moore DT, et al. Dietary curcumin inhibits chemotherapy-induced apoptosis in models of human breast cancer. *Cancer Res.* 2002;62:3868–3875.

148. Memorial Sloan Kettering Cancer Center. *About Herbs, Botanicals & Other Products.* http://AboutHerbs.com

149. Holick MF. Sunlight and vitamin D for bone health and prevention of autoimmune diseases, cancers, and cardiovascular disease. *Am J Clin Nutr.* 2004;80:1678s–1688s.

150. Tanaka H, Abe E, Miyaura C, et al. 1 alpha,25-Dihydroxycholecalciferol and a human myeloid leukaemia cell line (HL-60). *Biochem J.* 1982;204:713–719.

151. Antico A, Tampoia M, Tozzoli R, et al. Can supplementation with vitamin D reduce the risk or modify the course of autoimmune diseases? A systematic review of the literature. *Autoimmun Rev.* 2012;12:127–136.

152. Blackmore KM, Lesosky M, Barnett H, et al. Vitamin D from dietary intake and sunlight exposure and the risk of hormone-receptor-defined breast cancer. *Am J Epidemiol.* 2008;168:915–924.

153. Robien K, Cutler GJ, Lazovich D. Vitamin D intake and breast cancer risk in postmenopausal women: the Iowa Women's Health Study. *Cancer Causes Control.* 2007;18:775–782.

154. Neuhouser ML, Sorensen B, Hollis BW, et al. Vitamin D insufficiency in a multiethnic cohort of breast cancer survivors. *Am J Clin Nutr.* 2008;88:133–139.

155. Paskett ED, Naughton MJ, McCoy TP, et al. The epidemiology of arm and hand swelling in premenopausal breast cancer survivors. *Cancer Epidemiol Biomarkers Prev.* 2007;16:775–782.

156. Vance V, Campbell S, McCargar L, et al. Dietary changes and food intake in the first year after breast cancer treatment. *Appl Physiol Nutr Metab.* 2014;39:707–714.

157. Galantino ML, Greene L, Archetto B, et al. A qualitative exploration of the impact of yoga on breast cancer survivors with aromatase inhibitor-associated arthralgias. *Explore (NY).* 2012;8:40–47.

158. Pinto BM, Ciccolo JT. Physical activity motivation and cancer survivorship. *Recent Results Cancer Res.* 2011;186:367–387.

159. Trinh L, Mutrie N, Campbell AM, et al. Effects of supervised exercise on motivational outcomes in breast cancer survivors at 5-year follow-up. *Eur J Oncol Nurs.* 2014;18:557–563.

Paula Rosenblatt, Ikumi Suzuki, Angela DeRidder, and Nilam Patel

The National Cancer Institute (NCI) defines a cancer survivor as the individual from the "time of diagnosis until the end of life" (1). With a 5-year breast cancer survival rate of 90%, issues of survivorship should be discussed at the start of the treatment (2). Issues such as fertility preservation, risk of cardiac toxicity, neuropathy, and lymphedema should be assessed prior to starting surgery, chemotherapy, and radiation therapy as treatment will leave permanent effects. As the National Comprehensive Cancer Network (NCCN) states, surviving cancer can have a large "impact on health, physical and mental states, health behaviors, professional and personal identity, sexuality, and financial standing" of the individual (3). The Institute of Medicine suggests that there should be standards for survivorship care that address prevention of recurrent and new cancer, surveillance of spread, assessment of late effects, intervention for consequences of cancer and its treatment, coordination of care between primary physician and specialists, and development of survivorship plans to delineate these roles, educate, and communicate with the survivor (3). The American Cancer Society (ACS) and the American Society of Clinical Oncology (ASCO) jointly published guidelines based on the previously noted goals and completed a systematic review of the literature to examine the evidence for the practice of survivorship (4). A panel of experts convened to discuss consensus recommendations when evidence-based literature was not available.

Combining the NCCN, ACS, and ASCO guidelines, this chapter reviews breast cancer survivorship as it relates to:

1. Surveillance for breast cancer recurrence
2. Screening for secondary primary cancers
3. Assessment, management, and interventions of physical and psychosocial long-term and late effects including:
   - Cardiac toxicity
   - Cognitive impairment and fatigue
   - Distress, depression, anxiety, and sleep disorders
   - Lymphedema, musculoskeletal health, and bone health
   - Neuropathy and pain
   - Infertility, premature menopause, and sexual health
   - Body image and health promotion
4. Survivorship care planning and coordination

SURVEILLANCE FOR BREAST CANCER RECURRENCE

Recurrence of breast cancer is a major fear for survivors. All breast cancer patients should be educated on symptoms of local, regional, and distant recurrence and encouraged to seek medical attention at any concern. Palpation of new masses, nipple discharge, change in skin and breast contours, axillary/clavicular/cervical lymphadenopathy, localized bone pain, nausea, weight loss, and headaches should prompt full workup. While there are strong recommendations from ASCO against the use of routine laboratory tests, tumor markers, and systemic imaging in patients treated with curative intent, the importance of routine follow-up and physical exams for signs of recurrence cannot be overstated (5).

> ➤ We recommend breast cancer survivors have a thorough history and physical exam every 3 to 6 months for the first 3 years, every 6 to 12 months for years 4 and 5, and annually after the fifth year (6). While systemic imaging is not recommended in routine breast cancer follow-up, breast-specific imaging remains important for detecting an in-breast recurrence or new primary breast cancer.
>
> ➤ After breast conservation surgery, we recommend a mammogram at 4 to 6 months after completion of radiation and then annually unless specific mammographic findings require earlier follow-up (6).

Routine addition of contrast enhanced breast MRI for screening after diagnosis of breast cancer remains controversial and should be based on the risk of second cancer and concerning features (extremely dense breast tissue or occult breast cancer on initial mammography) that would make mammography alone insufficient.

> ➤ A lifetime risk of breast cancer greater than 20% to 25%, personal or first degree family history of high penetrance deleterious mutation (BRCA mutation/ Li–Fraumeni/Cowden syndrome), and history of chest radiation therapy qualifies a patient for MRI surveillance for breast cancer (7).

While official recommendations remain indeterminate for patients with dense breasts and previous abnormal biopsies of atypical ductal hyperplasia/lobular carcinoma in-situ (ADH/LCIS), the use of MRI can be considered as recent data suggests lifetime risk exceeding 30% for ADH (7,8). A discussion of the increased sensitivity of MRI and the high false positive rates needs to occur prior to the test being performed.

SCREENING FOR SECOND PRIMARY CANCER

The average breast cancer patient should be screened for other cancers (cervical, colorectal, endometrial, and lung) as per ACS guidelines for the general population (4,9).

Routine screening for endometrial cancer with annual gynecologic exams is recommended for postmenopausal patients on selective estrogen-receptor modulators (SERMs) (tamoxifen) (4,10). While in the absence of symptoms routine endometrial imaging or endometrial biopsies are not recommended, new onset bleeding should prompt a complete workup (10).

Enhanced screening for second primaries for patients with hereditary genetic syndromes, such as the **hereditary breast and ovarian cancers, Lynch syndrome, Li–Fraumeni, hereditary diffuse gastric cancer, and Cowden syndrome,** should be guided by recommendations from the NCCN (11). As previously discussed in Chapter 9, a thorough review of family history and referral for genetic counseling and testing is important for patients with concerning family histories. Extended gene panels using next generation testing now identify medium/intermediate penetrance genes as well. The most appropriate management for many of these genes is still unknown (12).

Myelodysplastic syndrome and leukemia are a known rare sequela of chemotherapy and radiation. Alkylating agents (cyclophosphamide) and topoisomerase targeting drugs (anthracyclines) are the most frequently implicated and are used in many adjuvant breast cancer regimens (13).

A review of over 20,000 patients with early-stage breast cancer treated between 1998 and 2007 found a marrow neoplasm cumulative incidence rate of 0.48% and a rate of 0.54 per 1,000 person years for patients treated with surgery/chemotherapy/radiation as compared to 0.16 for those treated with surgery alone. The hazard ratio for all three modalities was 7.6 (95% CIs [1.6, 35.8]; $P = .01$). Among patients who developed acute leukemia, two thirds had complex cytogenetics. While the breast cancer stage, race, and tumor characteristics were not significantly different in those who developed marrow neoplasm versus those without, patients with marrow neoplasms were significantly older (13). While there is no recommendation for routine testing with a complete blood count, incidentally discovered cytopenias or symptoms such as infections/fatigue/bruising/bleeding should prompt workup (4).

ASSESSMENT AND MANAGEMENT OF PHYSICAL AND PSYCHOSOCIAL LONG-TERM AND LATE EFFECTS

Cardiac Toxicity

Anthracyclines, monoclonal antibodies, left breast radiation (especially when the internal mammary lymph nodes are targeted), hormonal therapy with aromatase inhibitors (AIs), and early menopause have been associated with varying degrees of cardiovascular effects and cardiac toxicity (4). Preexisting cardiac disease and risk stratification should be taken into consideration prior to initiating therapies.

> ➤ Medical management of cardiac toxicities involves prompt referral to cardiology when abnormalities are detected and treatment with beta-blockers, angiotensin converting enzyme (ACE) inhibitors, and lipid lowering agents as appropriate.

ASCO and ACS have no specific long-term follow-up recommendations in the follow-up of asymptomatic breast cancer patients treated with adjuvant chemotherapy. They recommend patients receive education of possible cardiac symptoms, smoking cessation, diet, exercise, and monitoring of periodic lipid levels per the U.S. Preventive Services Task Force recommendations (4).

Anthracyclines

Chronic/late-onset anthracycline-induced cardiac toxicity presents within a few months to decades after the last dose of chemotherapy and progresses from an asymptomatic cardiomyopathy to overt heart failure. The cause of the cardiac toxicity is still unclear, but the primary mechanism is likely related to oxidative stress and damage to myocytes (14,15).

A study of older breast cancer patients who received anthracycline-based chemotherapy compared to no chemotherapy demonstrated hazard ratios for cardiomyopathy, CHF, and heart disease of 2.48 (95% CIs [2.10, 2.93]), 1.38 (95% CIs [1.25, 1.52]), and 1.35 (95% CIs [1.26, 1.44]), respectively (16).

The strongest risk factor for the development of cardiac toxicity is the lifetime cumulative dose of anthracycline. The risk of cardiac toxicity increases sharply after 400 to 450 mg/m^2 for doxorubicin although with substantial individual variation (17).

A baseline pretreatment transthoracic echocardiogram (echo) or multigated acquisition (MUGA) scan should be performed prior to administration of anthracycline-based chemotherapy. In the adjuvant setting, concurrent and posttreatment heart function assessments are not usually necessary in the low-risk patient. However, we often check an echo within 1 year of completion of anthracycline in patients with one or more cardiac risk factors (age >65 years, cumulative doxorubicin dose of 300 mg/m^2, underlying cardiovascular disease, and low-normal left ventricular ejection fraction (LVEF) of 50%–54%) (3). Mortality due to anthracycline cardiac toxicity has improved with the use of drugs for heart failure such as ACE inhibitors and beta-blockers.

Dexrazoxane is a chelating agent that has a cardioprotective effect when treating with high-dose anthracyclines (18). However, there is a theoretical risk of decreasing the efficacy of anthracycline treatment with the chelator. Therefore, dexrazoxane is not recommended for breast cancer patients who are undergoing potentially curative/adjuvant treatment with anthracycline-based regimens. For patients with metastatic disease receiving higher cumulative doses of doxorubicin, dexrazoxane should be added after initial doses exceed 300 mg/m^2. Routine assessment of ejection fraction should occur after 250 to 300 mg/m^2 and again between 400 and 450 mg/m^2. Once a dose of 500 mg/m^2 is reached, monitoring of ejection fraction should be completed every 50 mg/m^2. A decline in ejection fraction of less than the lower limit of normal or the clinical development of heart failure are indications for stopping the chemotherapy. Epirubicin is an anthracycline also used in the treatment of breast cancer with the maximum cumulative dose limit at 900 mg/m^2 (18).

HER2 Directed Therapy

As opposed to anthracyclines, the cardiac toxicity of HER2 targeted monoclonal antibodies (trastuzumab and pertuzumab) usually presents as a reversible, dose-independent, asymptomatic decrease in LVEF. It is considered a "Type II" cardiac toxicity as there is a loss of contractility, but no myocyte destruction (19).

Concern regarding trastuzumab's cardiac toxicity was noted early in its history. A black box warning of cardiac toxicity was placed on the drug after the large phase III trial for metastatic breast cancer found an incidence of heart failure of 27% when combined with anthracycline and 13% when combined with paclitaxel, compared to 8% in patients treated without trastuzumab (20). Follow-up clinical studies that excluded patients with preexisting decreased ejection fraction showed significantly less cardiac toxicity.

In the BCIRG006 adjuvant trial, a sustained subclinical loss of mean LVEF (>10% relative decline) was noted in 18.6% of study participants in the anthracycline/docetaxel/trastuzumab arm, 9.4% in the docetaxel/carboplatin/

trastuzumab arm, and 11.2% in the anthracycline/docetaxel arm, while the rate of clinical heart failure was low; 2%, 0.4%, and 0.7%, respectively (21).

A meta-analysis of nearly 12,000 patients receiving trastuzumab showed that the overall incidence of cardiac toxicity resulting in congestive heart failure was 2.5% compared to 0.4% of controls (RR 5.11; $P < .00001$) (22).

Risk factors for trastuzumab-induced cardiac toxicity include anthracycline exposure (concurrent or previous), increased age, hypertension, and obesity (23,24).

As described in Chapters 5 and 6, pertuzumab is a second monoclonal antibody that targets HER2 and is used in combination with trastuzumab in the neoadjuvant and metastatic setting (25). TRYPHAENA was a phase II neoadjuvant study that evaluated the cardiac safety of this medication. The rate of decreased LVEF ranged from 2.6% to 5.6% and symptomatic congestive heart failure from 0% to 2.7% (25). The nonanthracycline regimen of docetaxel/carboplatin/trastuzumab/pertuzumab had the lowest incidence of cardiac dysfunction with the highest pathologic complete response rate (25).

When used in the neoadjuvant setting, the package insert recommends cardiac monitoring every 6 weeks. If a drop in LVEF to <45% or an absolute decrease of 10 points with a LVEF of 45% to 49% is noted the drug is withheld. Reassessment should occur within 3 weeks and the medications can be resumed when the LVEF >49% (26).

In the metastatic setting, trastuzumab, pertuzumab, and ado-trastuzumab emtansine HER2 targeted agents are utilized for treatment. These drugs can cause asymptomatic declines in the LVEF and rare symptomatic heart failure.

In the metastatic setting, cardiac assessment every 3 months is appropriate with a guideline to hold therapy for ado-trastuzumab, if LVEF falls to less than 40% or if 40% to 45% with more than a 10-point decrease from baseline, while for pertuzumab + trastuzumab, to hold treatment if LVEF is below 45% or 45% to 49% and more than a 10-point drop from baseline (27,28).

Lapatinib, an oral, reversible, tyrosine kinase epidermal growth factor receptor (EGFR) (ERBB1) and HER2 inhibitor, is approved for treatment of advanced breast cancer. A pooled analysis of 3,689 patients enrolled in clinical trials with lapatinib showed low levels of cardiac toxicity for lapatinib; cardiac events were usually asymptomatic reversible declines in LVEF with similar rates for patients who were exposed versus not to anthracyclines or trastuzumab in the past (29). See the summary of cardiac monitoring recommendations for HER2 agents in Box 11.1.

Radiation

Older radiotherapy techniques for breast cancer involved significant doses of radiation to the heart. A meta-analysis from the Early Breast Cancer Trialists Collaborative Group (EBCTCG) of 40 trials found that while radiotherapy decreased the annual mortality rate from breast cancer, there was significant increase in the annual mortality rate from other causes (21% increase) that was largely attributable to cardiac and vascular events (30). The spectrum of radiation-related cardiac disease includes myocardial damage and coronary artery disease when mediastinal radiation is used (31). SEER Medicare analyses have demonstrated that the risk of cardiac death is not elevated for women treated since 1990 (32). This improvement could be related to improved techniques or possibly decreased targeting of the internal mammary lymph nodes. While current breast radiotherapy doses to the

Box 11.1 Cardiac Monitoring Recommendations for HER2 Directed Agents

- Pretreatment and serial echo or multigated acquisition (MUGA) study at approximately every 3 month intervals (26).
- Follow cardiac function with the same test and do not switch from MUGA to echo and vice versa in the same patient.
- If the LVEF falls >15 points from baseline or ≥10 points and below the institutional limits of normal, hold HER2 directed therapy for 4 weeks and repeat cardiac imaging.
- If the LVEF returns to normal, HER2 therapy can be reinitiated; otherwise, repeat cardiac imaging in 4 weeks.
- Any symptoms of CHF (increased dyspnea on exertion, edema, weight gain, new murmur) should prompt an immediate evaluation for cardiac toxicity.
- HER2 directed agents are discontinued for the development of clinical heart failure.
- Cardiac toxicity is more frequent and severe when trastuzumab is used in combination with anthracyclines; thus, in practice they are not given concurrently. It is unclear if one potentiates the effects of the other or if each has an independent mechanism (23).

Source: From Ref. (23). Perez EA, Suman VJ, Davidson NE, et al. Cardiac safety analysis of doxorubicin and cyclophosphamide followed by paclitaxel with or without trastuzumab in the North Central Cancer Treatment Group N9831 adjuvant breast cancer trial. *J Clin Oncol.* 2008;26(8):1231–1238.

heart are significantly less, there is no entirely safe dose and the effects of radiation to the heart are dose-dependent (33).

Cognitive Impairment and Fatigue

Seventy-five percent of breast cancer patients report decline of cognitive function during their treatment and 35% report continuing impairment after treatment ends (34–36). The presence of treatable and contributing factors of cognitive impairment such as depression, insomnia, substance abuse, medication effects, and causes of fatigue should be evaluated (3,4). However, often no distinct cause can be identified and the patient is assumed to have cognitive impairment related to treatment.

"Chemo brain" is a lay term given to this phenomenon and it can be a source of fear and anxiety for those patients about to embark on cancer treatment (37). These subtle yet significant effects on cognitive functioning can have a large impact on quality of life (37,38).

Breast cancer patients appear to be particularly susceptible to cognitive deficits for numerous reasons including effects of cancer itself, emotional stress of the diagnosis, and the sequelae of chemotherapy and hormone therapy. Multiple studies have confirmed objective evidence of cognitive decline after chemotherapy (37–39). Analyses using a battery of neuropsychological tests have shown deficits in various cognitive domains including visuospatial ability, executive function, information processing speed, and verbal and visual memory (40,41). Most of these deficits were small to moderate but consistent throughout different studies looking at effects of adjuvant chemotherapy on neurocognitive function. Studies with brain imaging in breast cancer patients who have received chemotherapy show structural changes reflective of treatment effects (42,43). The exact timing and duration of the impairment is still unclear (41). Risk factors for cognitive impairment include older age; cyclophosphamide, methotrexate, and fluorouracil (CMF) regimen; and lower cognitive reserve (44,45).

In addition to cytotoxic agents, breast cancer patients with hormone-receptor-positive breast cancer receive adjuvant hormonal therapy. Tamoxifen has been found to have a negative impact on cognitive function (39). Along the same principles, AIs, which are known to cause estrogen-deprived states, have also been shown to cause mild cognitive impairment when compared to tamoxifen; however, the role of these agents in posttreatment cognitive dysfunction has not been well established (46,47).

As health care providers for breast cancer survivors, understanding the possibility of cognitive dysfunction and its effect on quality of life and function in society is essential.

- The clinical validation that posttreatment cognitive dysfunction is a real entity and reassurance to the patient that the cognitive effects are not progressive and have not been associated with progression to dementia helps ease many patients' concerns.
- Neuropsychological testing, occupational therapy, and speech therapy has been helpful for some patients in developing coping techniques.
- Encouragement of physical activity, meditation, mindfulness stress reduction, limitation of alcohol, and promotion of good sleep hygiene may benefit cancer-associated cognitive dysfunction (3).

Fatigue is very common in cancer patients treated with radiation and chemotherapy, and some patients experience longer lasting symptoms causing disruptions in quality of life and increased distress. The NCCN defines cancer-related fatigue as the "a distressing persistent, subjective sense of physical, emotional, and/or cognitive tiredness or exhaustion related to cancer or cancer treatment that is not proportional to recent activity and interferes with usual functioning." Fatigue can be exacerbated by medications, anemia, nutritional deficiency, thyroid dysfunction, adrenal insufficiency, cardiac or pulmonary dysfunction, pain, deconditioning, depression, and insomnia; these entities should be evaluated based on history (3,4).

DISTRESS, DEPRESSION, ANXIETY, AND SLEEP DISORDERS

Distress is the "multifactorial unpleasant emotional experience of a psychological (ie, cognitive, behavioral, emotional), social, and or spiritual nature that may interfere with the ability to cope effectively with cancer and/or its physical symptoms, and its treatment." Breast cancer patients may be uniquely susceptible to depression, anxiety, and resultant distress due to decreased estrogen levels secondary to hormone therapy and chemotherapy (48). Estrogen has been shown to have anti-depressive effects, and treatment for breast cancer can lead to an estrogen-deprived state (48). It is important to routinely assess breast cancer survivors for distress and mental health disorders and offer appropriate counseling, treatments, and referrals as necessary.

We recommend the use of the distress thermometer, Patient Health Questionnaire-9 or -12, or the General Anxiety Disorder 7 item scale; validated screening tools for distress, depression, and anxiety; these should be implemented regularly. Identification of substance abuse is also important as it can exacerbate any mental illness (49–51). NCCN also recommends screening for panic disorder, posttraumatic stress disorder, and suicidal ideations (3).

In collaboration with their primary care physicians, breast cancer survivors should undergo routine assessments for signs and symptoms of insomnia, depression, anxiety, and distress. For those at higher risk, a more thorough assessment may be needed. To ensure appropriate and timely management, there should be a low threshold to refer these patients to mental health professionals for evaluation and management. Counseling, mindful meditation, hope therapy, and making meaningful interventions have helped many breast cancer survivors (52). Other times, pharmacologic assistance may be needed as well.

Major depressive disorder (MDD) was found to have a prevalence of 22% among breast cancer survivors and only 11.6% in the general cancer population (4). The rate of depression in breast cancer (4.5%–46%) is higher than rates in most other cancer types, behind only oropharyngeal (22%–57%) and pancreatic cancers (33%–50%) (53). In the first year after diagnosis patients are at the highest risk for MDD, especially for younger patients and those who have received chemotherapy (48). These high rates of depression may be due to a multitude of factors including body image issues, physical effects of treatment, loss of sexual function, ongoing fatigue, and perpetual concern about recurrence.

Anxiety rates are also very high in breast cancer patients. One large cohort study found pure anxiety symptoms in 14.7% and mixed anxiety/depression in 10.8% of patients (54). Despite the high rates of depression and anxiety among breast cancer patients, dedicated studies on management of these patients are lacking. Pharmacotherapy and psychotherapy are the mainstay of treatment for mild to moderate depression and anxiety. Studies that included patients with breast cancer have shown selective serotonin reuptake inhibitors (SSRIs), serotonin–norepinephrine reuptake inhibitors (SNRIs), tricyclic antidepressants, and mirtazapine to be effective treatment.

Patients should be counseled on the expected side effects and the multiple weeks it takes for SSRIs and SNRIs to become effective. A review of the side effects may be helpful in treating concomitant problems the patient may face (insomnia, appetite issues, pains, hot flashes). Short-term use of benzodiazepines in cases of anxiety may be necessary but long-term use should be limited.

For those taking tamoxifen, the antidepressive medications duloxetine, sertraline, fluvoxamine, paroxetine, fluoxetine, and bupropion may inhibit metabolism of tamoxifen to its active metabolites via the cytochrome P450 2D6 enzymes, leading to a decrease in therapeutic effect of tamoxifen. In this situation, alternative antidepressants should be considered if possible (55).

Sleep disorders are prominent in cancer patients and may contribute to cognitive impairment, fatigue, and depression. Treating contributing factors such as pain, hot flashes, sleep apnea, and activating medications are important steps in addressing sleep disorders. Review of sleep hygiene, exercise times, caffeine consumption, and meditation techniques may help regulate sleep. Cognitive behavior therapy is also recommended. Pharmacologic agents can be used short term, but most recommend limited exposure.

LYMPHEDEMA, MUSCULOSKELETAL PAIN, AND BONE HEALTH

Musculoskeletal symptoms are commonly reported in patients who are undergoing or have undergone treatment for breast cancer. Twenty-five to sixty percent of breast cancer patients experience chronic pain as a result of their treatments (56). Surgery may cause chest wall pain and difficulties in movement of the upper extremity on the side of surgery.

> ➤ Lymphedema, decrease in shoulder range of motion, and axillary web syndrome (scarring in the axilla) may occur after surgery. Patients should be referred for physical therapy following surgery or if symptoms develop.

According to a meta-analysis of 72 studies, the risk of lymphedema in patients undergoing sentinel lymph node biopsy (6%) is lower than axillary dissection (20%) (57). Postoperative radiation to the axillary and supraclavicular lymph nodes can increase the risk of lymphedema with a significant impact being related to the extent of the axillary dissection (58). Obesity also increases the risk of lymphedema. Significant lymphedema can be difficult to treat and therefore primary prevention and early identification of mild cases prior to progression are very important.

Secondary prevention to minimize limb swelling after the development includes good skin hygiene and prevention of infection, use of sleeves/gloves/elevation, and obtaining ideal body weight.

For patients with significant lymphedema, treatments (in order of increasing intensity for severity) can include increased hours of compression from garments, massage for manual lymphatic drainage, complete decongestive therapy, and pneumatic compression.

MUSCULOSKELETAL PAIN/SYMPTOMS

Bone Pain

Systemic treatments with chemotherapeutics, antiresorptive agents, and granulocyte colony stimulating factors (G-CSF) are associated with bone pain. G-CSF can trigger an inflammatory response and increase histamine levels; antihistamines such as loratadine are thought to antagonize these effects and relieve pain associated with G-CSF (59). The antiresorptive agents zoledronic acid and denosumab have a side-effect profile that includes musculoskeletal pain (60). It is important to alert patients to these acute side effects so that they can be prepared to manage them appropriately. However, given that this pain is short-lived, most patients tolerate these therapies well.

Musculoskeletal Symptoms of Hormonal Therapy

Hormonal therapy has been associated with musculoskeletal effects; given the daily administration, the side effect can be chronic and greatly affect quality of life. Arthralgia is seen in up to 50% of patients treated with AIs, which is the most effective adjuvant treatment of early-stage hormone-receptor-positive breast cancer in postmenopausal women (61,62).

Aromatase inhibitor-induced musculoskeletal symptoms (AIMSS) are generally symmetric pain, stiffness, and soreness affecting joints in the hands, knees, hips, lower back, shoulders, and feet. These joint symptoms are distinct from inflammatory arthritis with negative inflammatory markers (63). The musculoskeletal side effects can have a significant impact on quality of life and lead to nonadherence and premature discontinuation of treatment, jeopardizing the potential therapeutic benefits of AIs (64–66). These symptoms are thought to be secondary to estrogen deprivation (67). No specific risk factors have been identified, but studies have suggested younger patients and those with prior taxane exposure may be more susceptible (68–70). One large study showed that 5% to 25% of patients discontinued AI therapy during the first 2 years and only 32% to 73% finish the recommended 5 years (71). Anecdotal evidence and previous studies show AIMSS to be a major contributor.

Patient education and active management of AIMSS plays a large role in successful treatment with AIs. Patients should be made aware of potential joint symptoms prior to treatment. If these symptoms occur, aggressive management should be pursued to maximize adherence. Management of AIMSS can pose a challenge. Nonpharmacologic modalities such as **exercise and acupuncture** have been shown to have statistically significant reductions in pain and lead to improvements in quality of life (72–74). **The most widely used pharmacologic agents are nonsteroidal anti-inflammatory drugs and acetaminophen, although the effect is modest. Other pharmacologic agents including tramadol, tricyclic antidepressants, and duloxetine may be used at times; we discourage routine use of narcotics for management of AIMSS symptoms** (63,75).

> ➤ If symptoms are interfering with daily activities, we recommend switching to a different AI (although side-effect profiles are similar) or tamoxifen to complete duration of therapy.

Bone Loss

The loss of bone mineral density and the development of osteopenia and osteoporosis are important late effects of chemotherapy, premature ovarian failure, gonadotropin-releasing hormone (GnRH) suppressors, and AIs (4,76,77). All women should be counseled on the importance of bone health and weight bearing exercise and the avoidance of excessive alcohol and smoking; in addition, calcium (1,200 mg/day) and vitamin D (1,000 IU/day) supplementation should be recommended (78).

Women on AIs are at the highest increased risk for bone loss, so screening by dual energy x-ray absorptiometry (DEXA) is recommended at least every 2 years (4). Premenopausal women who experience early menopause from cancer therapies and are willing to consider osteoporosis treatment should also receive testing (78). In women found to have osteoporosis or a high 10-year risk of hip (>3%) or major osteoporotic fracture (>20%) by FRAX score, pharmacologic treatment with bisphosphonates and denosumab should be implemented (78). Evaluation of the risk of osteonecrosis of the jaw and appropriate dental consult should be addressed prior to starting the agents.

Neuropathy

Peripheral neuropathy is one of the common side effects of breast cancer treatment and may have great impact on quality of life (79,80). Chemotherapy-induced peripheral neuropathy (CIPN) is a common side effect of regimens containing platinum, vinca alkaloids, and/or taxanes (81).

While taxanes are an integral part of standard treatment of breast cancer and have been shown to improve survival in early-stage breast cancer, grade 2 to 3 CIPN can be experienced by up to 16% of patients (82–84). In another study, 28.7% of patients were diagnosed with CIPN within the first year after diagnosis (85). CIPN is more commonly seen with paclitaxel than with docetaxel and the degree of neurotoxicity has been associated with cumulative dose of these agents (86–90).

No standardized assessment tool for CIPN exists, and CIPN remains mostly a clinical diagnosis (91). Common clinical features include paresthesia, dysesthesia, shock-like sensation, altered proprioception, and imbalance (92). Several mechanisms have been identified to explain taxane-induced neuropathy. Ultimately, it is likely a combination of axonal damage, damage to peripheral nerves, and myelinopathy (92). Risk factors for developing neuropathy include other comorbid conditions associated with neuropathy such as diabetes and alcohol consumption (86,88).

There are no approved treatments specifically for CIPN. Most of the treatments are aimed at symptom management. The most effective management strategy is to prevent the development by carefully assessing symptoms of neuropathy during chemotherapy treatments and adjusting treatment if needed to try to prevent long-term damage. Duloxetine has been shown to have some benefit in treating CIPN and is recommended by ASCO Clinical Practice Guidelines (82). Other pharmacologic agents that may be effective include gabapentin, tramadol, and tricyclic antidepressants. Nonpharmacologic modes of symptom management including acupuncture, electrical stimulation therapies like spinal cord stimulation, or transcutaneous or percutaneous electrical nerve stimulation may be helpful and are described more in Chapter 10.

Although most effects are reversible, long-term follow-up and continued evaluation for neurotoxicity is an important part of posttreatment health assessments in breast cancer survivors.

INFERTILITY, MENOPAUSAL SYMPTOMS, GYNECOLOGIC AND SEXUAL HEALTH

Infertility

The risk of infertility due to premature ovarian failure from chemotherapy needs to be discussed prior to the initiation of systemic therapy. Infertility can have a large impact on patients' distress and quality of life (93). In many cases, a reproductive endocrinologist can perform egg harvesting and possible in vitro fertilization prior to chemotherapy for implantation at a later date. Alternatively, the Prevention of Early Menopause Study (POEMS) showed that goserelin (a GnRH agonist) administered 1 week prior to chemotherapy resulted in less premature ovarian failure at 2 years and led to higher pregnancy and live births as secondary outcomes (94). Of note, this study was in hormone-receptor-negative patients.

> ➤ Early recognition of the need for counseling and referral to infertility specialists is important to prevent delays in chemotherapy and lead to optimal long-term results for young patients.

Vasomotor Symptoms—Hot Flashes

One of the most common complaints from women who undergo premature menopause from chemotherapy and those who are treated with hormone therapies is the vasomotor symptom of hot flashes.

A hot flash is characterized by sudden onset of feelings of heat which "seem to come from nowhere" and spread upwards through the body, chest, neck, and face. The frequency, duration, and intensity of the hot flash are highly individualized and the syndrome may be associated with sweating, dizziness, heart palpitations, and light-headedness.

In the Anastrozole, Tamoxifen, Alone or in Combination (ATAC) trial, rates of hot flashes were 36% for patients receiving anastrozole and 41% for patients receiving tamoxifen (95). The Tamoxifen Exemestane Adjuvant Multinational (TEAM) trial evaluated menopausal symptoms and again found higher rates of hot flashes in patients taking tamoxifen; they noted hot flashes peaked at 3 months after the start of treatment and were decreasing by 12 months (96).

Clinical recommendations for hot flashes:

1. Nonpharmacologic treatment of hot flashes to include avoidance of triggers (alcohol, hot beverages, smoking, tight clothes), behavioral modifications (meditation, biofeedback), and acupuncture (97).
2. Pharmacologic treatment for patients can include the use of serotonin reuptake inhibitors, SNRIs, gabapentin, and clonidine.
3. Again, it is important to avoid treatment with a strong inhibitor of CYP2D6 (paroxetine, fluoxetine, duloxetine, sertraline) when patients are on tamoxifen as there is reduction in the efficacy of tamoxifen. Venlafaxine (Effexor) is the recommended agent for patients receiving tamoxifen.

Sexual Side Effects

From body image concerns to the physical effects of vaginal dryness and atrophy with estrogen deprivation, the loss of sexual desire, intimacy, and pleasure is common in breast cancer survivors. This can result in high levels of distress and decreases in quality of life. Recommended treatments for atrophic vaginitis and vaginal dryness resulting in dyspareunia include lubricants and moisturizers. When water-based products are insufficient, silicone-based products may provide more relief (4).

For some women with severe cases of dyspareunia, small quantities of vaginal estrogens 2 to 3 times per week need to be considered and typically provide relief of symptoms (98). It is important to remember that vaginal treatment with estrogen preparations (creams or tablets) is associated with a small amount of systemic absorption of estrogen and therefore has to be considered carefully in the context of the risk of recurrence and type of adjuvant treatment (AI).

In one retrospective study of 1,472 breast cancer patients, there was no increase risk of breast cancer recurrence in the 69 patients (4.7%) using vaginal estrogen (through low-dose estradiol tablets or estriol cream) (99). We recommend vaginal estrogen only after moisturizer and lubricants have been unsuccessful. It is important to mention that SERMs (tamoxifen) are less likely to cause vaginal dryness and can be used instead of an AI for adjuvant therapy in hormone-receptor-positive patients.

When intimacy and body image issues are prominent causes of sexual dissatisfaction, psychotherapy and counseling can provide support. A referral to a sexual health specialist can be considered if necessary.

BODY IMAGE CONCERNS AND HEALTHY LIVING

In patients treated for breast cancer there is a daily reminder of the disease through scars, a missing breast, loss of sensation to the breast, and changes in breast shape that accompany treatment. Discussion of the psychological implications and validation of the feeling of normality can help patients deal with their concerns. Patients are often helped with support groups. Prescriptions for wigs, customized breast prosthesis, and bras are helpful for patients.

> ➤ Certain studies have shown that weight gain after breast cancer treatment is associated with increased risk of recurrence and death (100). Encouraging patients to exercise and eat healthy are the key preventative health strategies that should be addressed regularly. Nutritional counseling, physical training, and support groups can all provide support in this long-term endeavor.

SURVIVORSHIP CARE PLANNING

Given the complexity of all these issues, the Commission on Cancer set a goal that comprehensive survivorship care plans be provided to all patients by 2019. These comprehensive plans are written documentation of the diagnosis, treatment, and follow-up plan for cancer survivors. These documents serve as a communication tool between oncologists, patients, and primary care providers. The care plans need to be explained and delivered to patients at the end of their active treatment so that patients are not lost to follow-up. They summarize the plan for management of the multitude of issues that may develop during or after treatment. However, survivorship cannot be addressed in one visit or with one care plan. It should be continuously addressed by all members of the care team and updated as new issues arise and old issues resolve.

The physical, social, and emotional toll of cancer and its treatment can be lifelong. Breast cancer survivors deserve a well thought out plan that addresses all their needs.

➤ MANAGEMENT PEARLS

1. Patients are considered survivors from the moment of diagnosis. Survivorship issues should be addressed in the planning of therapy and take into account comorbidities and the personal concerns of the patient.
2. Patients with early-stage disease should not receive routine systemic imaging (CTs, PET scans, or bone scans). Any concerning sign or symptom should prompt directed imaging.
3. Patients with early-stage disease should follow up with their provider every 3 to 6 months for the first 3 years, every 6 to 12 months in years 4 and 5, and then yearly after 5 years.
4. After breast conservation surgery, we recommend a diagnostic mammogram at 4 to 6 months after completion of radiation and then annually unless specific mammographic findings require earlier follow-up.
5. Neuropathy, hot flashes, joint aches, depression, anxiety, memory impairments, and vaginal dryness are common side effects of breast cancer treatment and should be discussed regularly. There are many treatment options to control symptoms.
6. Studies have shown that weight gain after breast cancer treatment is associated with increased risk of recurrence and death. Encouraging patients to exercise and eat healthy are the key preventative health strategies that should be addressed regularly. Nutritional counseling, physical training, and support groups can all provide support in this long-term endeavor.
7. Patients should receive a survivorship care plan to summarize their treatment and delineate their follow-up within 1 year of diagnosis. This can be shared with their primary physician and help bridge transitions of care.

REFERENCES

1. Definitions—Office of Cancer Survivorship [Internet]. National Cancer Institute. http://cancercontrol.cancer.gov/ocs/statistics/definitions.html. Updated May 30, 2014.
2. SEER Stat Fact Sheets: Female Breast Cancer [Internet]. Bethesda, MD: National Cancer Institute. http://seer.cancer.gov/csr/1975_2013
3. NCCN Clinical Practice Guidelines in Oncology—Survivorship [Internet]. National Comprehensive Cancer Network; https://www.nccn.org/professionals/physician_gls/pdf/survivorship.pdf. Updated 2016.
4. Runowicz CD, Leach CR, Henry NL, et al. American Cancer Society/American Society of Clinical Oncology breast cancer survivorship care guideline. *CA Cancer J Clin.* 2016;66(1):43–73.
5. Schnipper LE, Smith TJ, Raghavan D, et al. American Society of Clinical Oncology identifies five key opportunities to improve care and reduce costs: the top five list for oncology. *J Clin Oncol.* 2012;30(14):1715–1724.
6. Khatcheressian JL, Hurley P, Bantug E, et al. Breast cancer follow-up and management after primary treatment: American Society of Clinical Oncology clinical practice guideline update. *J Clin Oncol.* 2013;31(7):961–965.

7. Saslow D, Boetes C, Burke W, et al. American Cancer Society guidelines for breast screening with MRI as an adjunct to mammography. *CA Cancer J Clin*. 2007;57(2):75–89.

8. Hartmann LC, Sellers TA, Frost MH, et al. Benign breast disease and the risk of breast cancer. *N Engl J Med*. 2005;353(3):229–237.

9. Smith RA, Manassaram-Baptiste D, Brooks D, et al. Cancer screening in the United States, 2015: a review of current American Cancer Society guidelines and current issues in cancer screening. *CA Cancer J Clin*. 2015;65(1):30–54.

10. Runowicz CD. Gynecologic surveillance of women on tamoxifen: first do no harm. *J Clin Oncol*. 2000;18(20):3457–3458.

11. NCCN Clinical Practice Guidelines in Oncology: Genetic/Familial High Risk Assesment: Breast and Ovarian [Internet]. National Comprehensive Cancer Network. https://www.nccn.org/professionals/physician_gls/pdf/genetics_screening.pdf. Updated February 2016.

12. Slavin TP, Niell-Swiller M, Solomon I, et al. Clinical application of multigene panels: challenges of next-generation counseling and cancer risk management. *Front Oncol*. 2015;5:208.

13. Wolff AC, Blackford AL, Visvanathan K, et al. Risk of marrow neoplasms after adjuvant breast cancer therapy: the national comprehensive cancer network experience. *J Clin Oncol*. 2015;33(4):340–348.

14. Franco VI, Henkel JM, Miller TL, Lipshultz SE. Cardiovascular effects in childhood cancer survivors treated with anthracyclines. *Cardiol Res Pract*. 2011;2011:134679.

15. Singal PK, Iliskovic N, Li T, Kumar D. Adriamycin cardiomyopathy: pathophysiology and prevention. *Faseb J*. 1997;11(12):931–936.

16. Doyle JJ, Neugut AI, Jacobson JS, et al. Chemotherapy and cardiotoxicity in older breast cancer patients: a population-based study. *J Clin Oncol*. 2005;23(34):8597–8605.

17. Gianni L, Herman EH, Lipshultz SE, et al. Anthracycline cardiotoxicity: from bench to bedside. *J Clin Oncol*. 2008;26(22):3777–3784.

18. Hensley ML, Hagerty KL, Kewalramani T, et al. American Society of Clinical Oncology 2008 clinical practice guideline update: use of chemotherapy and radiation therapy protectants. *J Clin Oncol*. 2009;27(1):127–145.

19. Ewer MS, Vooletich MT, Durand JB, et al. Reversibility of trastuzumab-related cardiotoxicity: new insights based on clinical course and response to medical treatment. *J Clin Oncol*. 2005;23(31):7820–7826.

20. Slamon DJ, Leyland-Jones B, Shak S, et al. Use of chemotherapy plus a monoclonal antibody against HER2 for metastatic breast cancer that overexpresses HER2. *N Engl J Med*. 2001;344(11):783–792.

21. Slamon D, Eiermann W, Robert N, et al. Adjuvant trastuzumab in HER2-positive breast cancer. *N Engl J Med*. 2011;365(14):1273–1283.

22. Moja L, Tagliabue L, Balduzzi S, et al. Trastuzumab containing regimens for early breast cancer. *Cochrane Database Syst Rev*. 2012;(4):CD006243.

23. Perez EA, Suman VJ, Davidson NE, et al. Cardiac safety analysis of doxorubicin and cyclophosphamide followed by paclitaxel with or without trastuzumab in the North Central Cancer Treatment Group N9831 adjuvant breast cancer trial. *J Clin Oncol*. 2008;26(8):1231–1238.

24. Romond EH, Jeong JH, Rastogi P, et al. Seven-year follow-up assessment of cardiac function in NSABP B-31, a randomized trial comparing doxorubicin and cyclophosphamide followed by paclitaxel (ACP) with ACP plus trastuzumab as adjuvant therapy for patients with node-positive, human epidermal growth factor receptor 2-positive breast cancer. *J Clin Oncol*. 2012;30(31):3792–3799.

25. Schneeweiss A, Chia S, Hickish T, et al. Pertuzumab plus trastuzumab in combination with standard neoadjuvant anthracycline-containing and anthracycline-free chemotherapy regimens in patients with HER2-positive early breast cancer: a randomized phase II cardiac safety study (TRYPHAENA). *Ann Oncol.* 2013;24(9):2278–2284.
26. Herceptin [package insert]. San Franscisco, CA: Genetech. 2016.
27. Kadcyla Highlights of Prescribing [package insert]. San Francisco, CA: Genetech. 2016.
28. Perjeta Prescribing Highlights [package insert]. San Francisco, CA: Genetech. 2016.
29. Perez EA, Koehler M, Byrne J, et al. Cardiac safety of lapatinib: pooled analysis of 3689 patients enrolled in clinical trials. *Mayo Clin Proc.* 2008;83(6):679–686. doi:10.4065/83.6.679
30. Early Breast Cancer Trialists' Collaborative Group. Favourable and unfavourable effects on long-term survival of radiotherapy for early breast cancer: an overview of the randomised trials. *Lancet.* 2000;355(9217):1757–1770.
31. Adams MJ, Lipsitz SR, Colan SD, et al. Cardiovascular status in long-term survivors of Hodgkin's disease treated with chest radiotherapy. *J Clin Oncol.* 2004;22(15):3139–3148.
32. Giordano SH, Kuo YF, Freeman JL, et al. Risk of cardiac death after adjuvant radiotherapy for breast cancer. *J Natl Cancer Inst.* 2005;97(6):419–424.
33. Moslehi J. The cardiovascular perils of cancer survivorship. *N Engl J Med.* 2013;368(1055):e6.
34. Stan D, Loprinzi CL, Ruddy KJ. Breast cancer survivorship issues, *Hematol Oncol Clin North Am.* 2013;77:805–827.
35. Von Ah D, Habermann B, Carpenter JS, Schneider BL. Impact of perceived cognitive impairment in breast cancer survivors. *Eur J Oncol Nurs.* 2013;78:236–241.
36. Janelsins MC, Kohli S, Mohile SG, et al. An update on cancer- and chemotherapy-related cognitive dysfunction: current status. *Semin Oncol.* 2011;38(3):431–438.
37. Wefel JS, Saleeba AK, Buzdar AU, Meyers CA. Acute and late onset cognitive dysfunction associated with chemotherapy in women with breast cancer. *Cancer.* 2010;116(14):3348–3356.
38. Stewart A, Bielajew C, Collins B, et al. A meta-analysis of the neuropsychological effects of adjuvant chemotherapy treatment in women treated for breast cancer. *Clin Neuropsychol.* 2006;20(1):76–89.
39. Jansen CE, Miaskowski C, Dodd M, et al. A metaanalysis of studies of the effects of cancer chemotherapy on various domains of cognitive function. *Cancer.* 2005;104(10):2222–2233.
40. Jim HS, Phillips KM, Chait S, et al. Meta-analysis of cognitive functioning in breast cancer survivors previously treated with standard-dose chemotherapy. *J Clin Oncol.* 2012;30(29):3578–3587.
41. Castellon SA, Ganz PA, Bower JE, et al. Neurocognitive performance in breast cancer survivors exposed to adjuvant chemotherapy and tamoxifen. *J Clin Exp Neuropsychol.* 2004;26(7):955–969.
42. McDonald BC, Saykin AJ. Alterations in brain structure related to breast cancer and its treatment: chemotherapy and other considerations. *Brain Imaging Behav.* 2013;7(4):374–387.
43. Falleti MG, Sanfilippo A, Maruff P, et al. The nature and severity of cognitive impairment associated with adjuvant chemotherapy in women with breast cancer: a meta-analysis of the current literature. *Brain Cogn.* 2005;59(1):60–70.

44. Deprez S, Amant F, Smeets A, et al. Longitudinal assessment of chemotherapy-induced structural changes in cerebral white matter and its correlation with impaired cognitive functioning. *J Clin Oncol.* 2012;30(3):274–281.

45. Ahles TA, Saykin AJ, McDonald BC, et al. Longitudinal assessment of cognitive changes associated with adjuvant treatment for breast cancer: impact of age and cognitive reserve. *J Clin Oncol.* 2010;28(29):4434–4440.

46. Schagen SB, van Dam FS, Muller MJ, et al. Cognitive deficits after postoperative adjuvant chemotherapy for breast carcinoma. *Cancer.* 1999;85(3):640–650.

47. Bender CM, Sereika SM, Brufsky AM, et al. Memory impairments with adjuvant anastrozole versus tamoxifen in women with early-stage breast cancer. *Menopause.* 2007;14(6): 995–998.

48. Fann JR, Thomas-Rich AM, Katon WJ, et al. Major depression after breast cancer: a review of epidemiology and treatment. *Gen Hosp Psychiatry.* 2008;30(2):112–126.

49. Mark T. Hegel, Moore CP, et al. Distress, psychiatric syndromes, and impairment of function in women with newly diagnosed breast cancer. *Cancer,* 2006;107(12):2924–2931.

50. Hinz A, Mehnert A, Kocalevent RD, et al. Assessment of depression severity with the PHQ-9 in cancer patients and in the general population. *BMC Psychiatry.* 2016;16:22. doi:10.1186/s12888-016-0728-6

51. Goldberg DP, Gater R, Sartorius N, et al. The validity of two versions of the GHQ in the WHO study of mental illness in general health care. *Psychol Med,* 1997;27(1):191–197.

52. Casellas-Grau A, Font A, Vives J. Positive psychology interventions in breast cancer. A systematic review. *Psycho-Oncology.* 2014;23(1):9–19.

53. Massie MJ. Prevalence of depression in patients with cancer. NIH State-of-the-Science Conference on Symptom Management in Cancer: Pain, Depression, and Fatigue. 2002; 29. https://consensus.nih.gov/2002/2002CancerpainDepressionFatigueSOS022Program .pdf#page=28

54. Brintzenhofe-Szoc KM, Levin TT, Li Y, et al. Mixed anxiety/depression symptoms in a large cancer cohort: prevalence by cancer type. *Psychosomatics.* 2009;50(4):383–391.

55. Desmarais JE, Looper KJ. Interactions between tamoxifen and antidepressants via cytochrome P450 2D6. *J Clin Psychiatry.* 2009;70(12):1478–1697.

56. Andersen KG, Kehlet H. Persistent pain after breast cancer treatment: a critical review of risk factors and strategies for prevention. *J Pain.* 2011;12(7):725–746.

57. DiSipio T, Rye S, Newman B, Hayes S. Incidence of unilateral arm lymphoedema after breast cancer: a systematic review and meta-analysis. *Lancet Oncol.* 2013;14(6):500–515.

58. Chang DT, Feigenberg SJ, Indelicato DJ, et al. Long-term outcomes in breast cancer patients with ten or more positive axillary nodes treated with combined-modality therapy: the importance of radiation field selection. *Int J Radiat Oncol Biol Phys.* 2007;67(4):1043–1051.

59. Lambertini M, Del Mastro L, Bellodi A, Pronzato P. The five "Ws" for bone pain due to the administration of granulocyte-colony stimulating factors (G-CSFs). *Crit Rev Oncol.* 2014;89(1):112–128.

60. Bock O, Boerst H, Thomasius F, et al. Common musculoskeletal adverse effects of oral treatment with once weekly alendronate and risedronate in patients with osteoporosis and ways for their prevention. *J Musculoskelet Neuronal Interact.* 2007;7(2):144.

61. Burstein HJ, Prestrud AA, Seidenfeld J, et al. American Society of Clinical Oncology clinical practice guideline: update on adjuvant endocrine therapy for women with hormone receptor-positive breast cancer. *J Clin Oncol.* 2010;28(23):3784–3796.

62. Buzdar AU, Coombes RC, Goss PE, Winer EP. Summary of aromatase inhibitor clinical trials in postmenopausal women with early breast cancer. *Cancer*. 2008;112(S3): 700–709.

63. Burstein HJ. Aromatase inhibitor-associated arthralgia syndrome. *Breast*. 2007;16(3): 223–234.

64. Crew KD, Greenlee H, Capodice J, et al. Prevalence of joint symptoms in postmenopausal women taking aromatase inhibitors for early-stage breast cancer. *J Clin Oncol*. 2007;25(25):3877–3883.

65. Garreau JR, DeLaMelena T, Walts D, et al. Side effects of aromatase inhibitors versus tamoxifen: the patients' perspective. *Am J Surg*. 2006;192(4):496–498.

66. Hershman DL, Kushi LH, Shao T, et al. Early discontinuation and nonadherence to adjuvant hormonal therapy in a cohort of 8,769 early-stage breast cancer patients. *J Clin Oncol*. 2010;28(27):4120–4128.

67. Coleman R, Bolten W, Lansdown M, et al. Aromatase inhibitor-induced arthralgia: clinical experience and treatment recommendations. *Cancer Treat Rev*. 2008;34(3): 275–282.

68. Mao JJ, Stricker C, Bruner D, et al. Patterns and risk factors associated with aromatase inhibitor-related arthralgia among breast cancer survivors. *Cancer*. 2009;115(16):3631–3639.

69. Menas P, Merkel D, Hui W, et al. Incidence and management of arthralgias in breast cancer patients treated with aromatase inhibitors in an outpatient oncology clinic. *J Oncol Pharm Pract*. 2012;18(4):387–393.

70. Henry NL, Azzouz F, Desta Z, et al. Predictors of aromatase inhibitor discontinuation as a result of treatment-emergent symptoms in early-stage breast cancer. *J Clin Oncol*. 2012;30(9):936–942.

71. Murphy CC, Bartholomew LK, Carpentier MY, et al. Adherence to adjuvant hormonal therapy among breast cancer survivors in clinical practice: a systematic review. *Breast Cancer Res Treat*. 2012;134(2):459–478.

72. Crew KD, Capodice JL, Greenlee H, et al. Randomized, blinded, sham-controlled trial of acupuncture for the management of aromatase inhibitor-associated joint symptoms in women with early-stage breast cancer. *J Clin Oncol*. 2010;28(7):1154–1160.

73. DeNysschen C, Burton H, Ademuyiwa F, et al. Exercise intervention in breast cancer patients with aromatase inhibitor-associated arthralgia: a pilot study. *Eur J Cancer Care (Engl)*. 2014;23(4):493–501.

74. Irwin ML, Cartmel B, Gross CP, et al. Randomized exercise trial of aromatase inhibitor-induced arthralgia in breast cancer survivors. *J Clin Oncol*. 2015;33(10):1104–1111.

75. Henry NL, Banerjee M, Wicha M, et al. Pilot study of duloxetine for treatment of aromatase inhibitor-associated musculoskeletal symptoms. *Cancer*. 2011;117(24):5469–5475.

76. Ramaswamy B, Shapiro CL. Osteopenia and osteoporosis in women with breast cancer. *Semin Oncol*. 2003;30(6):763–775.

77. Hadji P, Aapro MS, Body JJ, et al. Management of aromatase inhibitor-associated bone loss in postmenopausal women with breast cancer: practical guidance for prevention and treatment. *Ann Oncol*. 2011;22(12):2546–2555.

78. Watts NB, Diab DL. Long-term use of bisphosphonates in osteoporosis. *J Clin Endocrinol Metab*. 2010;95(4):1555–1565.

79. Khasraw M, Posner JB. Neurological complications of systemic cancer. *Lancet Neurol*. 2010;9(12):1214–1227.

80. Eckhoff L, Knoop A, Jensen M, Ewertz M. Persistence of docetaxel-induced neuropathy and impact on quality of life among breast cancer survivors. *Eur J Cancer.* 2015;51(3):292–300.

81. Giglio P, Gilbert MR. Neurologic complications of cancer and its treatment. *Curr Oncol Rep.* 2010;12(1):50–59.

82. Hershman DL, Lacchetti C, Dworkin RH, et al. Prevention and management of chemotherapy-induced peripheral neuropathy in survivors of adult cancers: American Society of Clinical Oncology clinical practice guideline. *J Clin Oncol.* 2014;32(18): 1941–1967.

83. De Iuliis F, Taglieri L, Salerno G, et al. Taxane induced neuropathy in patients affected by breast cancer: Literature review. *Crit Rev Oncol.* 2015;96(1):34–45.

84. Wood AJ, Shapiro CL, Recht A. Side effects of adjuvant treatment of breast cancer. *N Engl J Med.* 2001;344(26):1997–2008.

85. Hershman DL, Weimer LH, Wang A, et al. Association between patient reported outcomes and quantitative sensory tests for measuring long-term neurotoxicity in breast cancer survivors treated with adjuvant paclitaxel chemotherapy. *Breast Cancer Res Treat.* 2011;125(3):767–774.

86. Rivera E, Cianfrocca M. Overview of neuropathy associated with taxanes for the treatment of metastatic breast cancer. *Cancer Chemother Pharmacol.* 2015;75(4):659–670.

87. Jung BF, Herrmann D, Griggs J, et al. Neuropathic pain associated with non-surgical treatment of breast cancer. *Pain.* 2005;118(1–2):10–14.

88. Lee JJ, Swain SM. Peripheral neuropathy induced by microtubule-stabilizing agents. *J Clin Oncol.* 2006;24(10):1633–1642.

89. Freilich RJ, Balmaceda C, Seidman AD, et al. Motor neuropathy due to docetaxel and paclitaxel. *Neurology.* 1996;47(1):115–118.

90. Grisold W, Cavaletti G, Windebank AJ. Peripheral neuropathies from chemotherapeutics and targeted agents: diagnosis, treatment, and prevention. *Neuro Oncol.* 2012;14(suppl 4):iv45–iv54.

91. Pereira S, Fontes F, Sonin T, et al. Chemotherapy-induced peripheral neuropathy after neoadjuvant or adjuvant treatment of breast cancer: a prospective cohort study. *Support Care Cancer.* 2015:1–11.

92. Stubblefield MD, Burstein HJ, Burton AW, et al. NCCN task force report: management of neuropathy in cancer. *J Natl Compr Canc Netw.* 2009;7(suppl 5):S1–S26.

93. Trivers KF, Fink AK, Partridge AH, et al. Estimates of young breast cancer survivors at risk for infertility in the U.S. *Oncologist.* 2014;19(8):814–822.

94. Moore HC, Unger JM, Phillips K, et al. Goserelin for ovarian protection during breast-cancer adjuvant chemotherapy. *N Engl J Med.* 2015;372(10):923–932.

95. Howell A, Cuzick J, Baum M, et al. Results of the ATAC (Arimidex, Tamoxifen, Alone or in Combination) trial after completion of 5 years' adjuvant treatment for breast cancer. *Lancet.* 2005;365(9453):60–62.

96. Jones SE, Cantrell J, Vukelja S, et al. Comparison of menopausal symptoms during the first year of adjuvant therapy with either exemestane or tamoxifen in early breast cancer: report of a Tamoxifen Exemestane Adjuvant Multicenter trial substudy. *J Clin Oncol.* 2007;25(30):4765–4771.

97. Bakkum-Gamez JN, Laughlin SK, Jensen JR, et al. Challenges in the gynecologic care of premenopausal women with breast cancer. *Mayo Clin Proc.* 2011;86(3):229–240.

98. Biglia N, Peano E, Sgandurra P, et al. Low-dose vaginal estrogens or vaginal moisturizer in breast cancer survivors with urogenital atrophy: a preliminary study. *Gynecol Endocrinol.* 2010;26(6):404–412.

99. Dew J, Wren B, Eden J. A cohort study of topical vaginal estrogen therapy in women previously treated for breast cancer. *Climacteric.* 2003;6(1):45–52.

100. Kroenke CH, Chen WY, Rosner B, Holmes MD. Weight, weight gain, and survival after breast cancer diagnosis. *J Clin Oncol.* 2005;23(7):1370–1378.

Index

abemaciclib, 184–185
accelerated partial breast irradiation
    (APBI), 62
acupuncture, 275
  AIMSS management, 270
  fatigue, 272
  lymphedema management, 271–272
  neuropathic pain, 272
  vasomotor symptoms control, 270–271
ADAPT trial, 142
Adjuvant Lapatinib and/or Trastuzumab
    Treatment Options (ALTTO),
    135–136
Adjuvant Paclitaxel Trastuzumab (APT)
    trial, 135
alcohol intake, breast cancer risk, 267
Alliance 012202 trial, 151
AMAROS trial, 93–94
American Cancer Society (ACS), 286
American College of Surgeons Oncology
    Group (ACOSOG) Z0011 trial, 93,
    101
American College of Surgeons Oncology
    Group (ACOSOG) Z1071 study, 149
American Society of Clinical Oncology
    (ASCO), 286
anastrozole, 29, 31, 34, 63, 65–66, 113, 146,
    179–180
anthracyclines, 134, 288–289
antiresorptive agents, 294
anxiety, 293
APHINITY trial, 135
Arimidex, Tamoxifen, Alone or in
    Combination (ATAC) trial, 111, 297
aromatase inhibitor-induced
    musculoskeletal symptoms
    (AIMSS), 270, 295
aromatase inhibitors (AI), 29
  early-stage invasive breast cancer
    comparisons, 113
    sequential therapy, 111–113
    vs. tamoxifen, 111
  metastatic breast cancer
    postmenopausal women, 178–181

premenopausal women, 183–184
arthralgia, 294
atypical ductal hyperplasia (ADH)
  core biopsy, 22
  cribriforming cellular proliferation, 22
  monotonous cellular proliferation, 22
  risk of future malignancy, 23
  surgical excision, 23
  treatment, 23
atypical lobular hyperplasia (ALH)
  histology, 23
  risk of future malignancy, 24
  surgical excision, 24
  treatment, 24
autologous/implant combined
    reconstruction, 240
autologous reconstruction
  advantages, 238–239
  disadvantages, 239–240
  donor sites, 238
  selection, 238

Baker Capsular Contracture Scale, 236
basal-like invasive carcinoma, 86
BCIRG 001 trial, 129
BCIRG 005 trial, 129
BIG 1-98 trial, 111
BOLERO-2 trial, 180
bone loss, 295
bone metastases, 200–202, 209
bone pain, 294
brain metastases
  graded prognostic assessment, 206, 207
  heterogeneity, 206
  radiation, 207–208
  risk factors, 206
  surgery, 207
BRCA gene mutations
  carriers, 252
  genetics, 251–252
  invasive ductal adenocarcinoma, 252
  lifetime risk, 252, 254
  ovarian cancer risks, 253

breast conserving surgery (BCS)
  contraindications, 90
  ductal carcinoma in situ, 52–53
  eligibility for, 90
  margins, 89
  vs. mastectomy, 90
  vs. MRM, 95
  radiation
    deep inspiratory breath-hold, 96–97
    GammaPod, 100–101
    intensity-modulated radiation therapy,
      98
    internal mammary node radiation,
      102–104
    large node negative breast cancer, 104
    lumpectomy cavity boost irradiation,
      99–100
    node-positive cancer, 101–102
    partial breast irradiation, 100
    postmastectomy radiation, 102–105
    whole breast irradiation, 98–99
  without radiation, 95–96
breast imaging
  biopsy, 12–13
  BI-RADS, 2–3
  breast pain, 11
  CEM, 2
  concordant lesions, 14
  diagnostic exam, 1
  discordant lesions, 14–15
  high-risk lesions, 15
  implant abnormalities, 12
  mammography (*see* mammography)
  MRI (*see* magnetic resonance imaging)
  needle localizations, 12–14
  nipple discharge, 11–12
  nuclear medicine modalities, 2
  palpable breast lump, 10–11
  screening mammography, 1
  ultrasound (*see* ultrasound)
breast imaging reporting and data system
    (BI-RADS)
  assessment categories, 3
  principles, 2
  recommendation, 3
breast reconstruction
  autologous/implant combined
    reconstruction, 240
  autologous reconstruction, 238–240
  external prosthesis, 231
  implant-based reconstruction, 232–238
  oncoplasty, 240–247
  types of, 231
British Columbia trial, 104
buparlisib, 184

Cancer and Leukemia Group B (CALGB)
    9343 trial, 96
Cancer and Leukemia Group B (CALGB)
    9344 study, 129
Cancer and Leukemia Group B (CALGB)
    9741 trial, 129–130
capsular contracture, 235–236
cardiotoxicity
  anthracyclines, 288–289
  HER2 directed therapy, 289–290
  radiotherapy, 290–291
chemo brain, 291
chemoprevention
  aromatase inhibitors, 29
  risk reduction, 28
  SERMs, 28–29
chemotherapy. *See also* neoadjuvant
    chemotherapy
  CMF and AC, 126
  Her2 blockade, 196–199
  HER2-positive disease, 130–136
  MammaPrint trials, 124–125
  Oncotype Dx trials, 123–124
  phyllodes tumors, 43, 46
  pregnancy-associated breast cancer,
    225–227
  maintenance, 189
  regimens, 125–130
  single agent, 186–189
  single agent vs. combination, 286
  taxane schedule, 130
  triple negative breast cancer, 136–137
  triplets and dose dense, 129–130
  tumor genomic multigene assays, 121–123
chemotherapy-induced peripheral
    neuropathy (CIPN), 296
cognitive impairment, 291–292
Collaborative Trials in Neoadjuvant Breast
    Cancer (CTNeoBC), 139
complementary and integrative medicine
    (CIM)
  acupuncture, 270–272, 275
  diet, 265–267
  exercise and physical activity, 267–268
  mind–body therapies, 268–269
  online resources, 276
  population-based study, 264
  prevalence, 264

supplements and botanical products, 273–274
  touch therapy, 272–273
complete decongestive therapy (CDT), 271
computed tomography (CT), 16
CONFIRM trial, 179
contrast enhanced mammography (CEM), 2
Cowden syndrome, 255
cribriform carcinoma, 83
cribriform ductal carcinoma in situ, 51
cyclin-dependent kinase inhibitor, 181, 184
cyclophosphamide, methotrexate, and 5-fluorouracil (CMF), 126

Danish 82b trial, 103–104
deep inferior epigastric perforator (DIEP) flap reconstruction, 241, 247
denusomab, 294
depression, 292–293
dexrazoxane, 289
dietary guidance, cancer survivors, 265–267, 275
digital breast tomosynthesis (DBT), 4–5, 6
distress, 292
docetaxel and cyclophosphamide (TC), 129
dual energy x-ray absorptiometry (DEXA), 295
ductal carcinoma in situ (DCIS)
  accelerated partial breast irradiation, 62
  breast conservation, 55–59
  chemoprevention, 63–66
  clinical presentation, 49, 50
  diagnostic evaluation, 49
  endocrine therapy, 62–63
  epidemiology, 49
  grading, 50–52
  high-grade, 51, 52
  hormone receptor expression, 52
  hypofractionation, 61
  intermediate, 51
  low-grade, 51
  lymph node evaluation, 55
  margins, 53–54
  mastectomy, 54–55
  microcalcifications, 50
  Paget disease of the nipple, 51
  pathology, 50
  pleomorphic morphology, 50
  radiotherapy, 59
  risk factors, 49
  surgical management, 52–53
  systemic therapy, 62–63
  unusual variants, 52

Early Breast Cancer Trialists Collaborative Group (EBCTCG), 55, 57, 95, 104, 109, 113, 290
early-stage invasive breast cancer
  breast conserving surgery (*see* breast conserving surgery)
  breast lesion immunophenotype, 88
  characteristics, 73
  clinical staging, 76–78
  cribriform carcinoma, 83
  epidemiology, 73
  extramammary malignancies, 88
  histologic grading system, 84–85
  initial laboratory tests, 75
  invasive ductal carcinoma, 81
  invasive lobular carcinoma, 82–83
  local/regional staging, 75
  mastectomy, 90–91
  medullary carcinoma, 83
  metaplastic carcinoma, 84
  micropapillary carcinoma, 83
  modifiable risk factors, 74–75
  mucinous carcinoma, 83, 84
  multidisciplinary evaluation, 75
  multigene tests, 88
  neoadjuvant chemotherapy (*see* neoadjuvant chemotherapy)
  neoadjuvant hormonal therapy (*see* neoadjuvant hormonal therapy)
  nonmodifiable risk factors, 74
  pathologic staging, 76, 78–81
  pretreatment workup, 75
  prognostic markers, 85–88
  psychosocial assessment, 76
  radical mastectomy, 89
  sentinel lymph node biopsy, 92–94
  symptoms and signs, 73
  systemic adjuvant therapy (*see* systemic adjuvant therapy)
  systemic imaging, 75–76
  TNM classification, 76–80
  tubular carcinoma, 83
Eastern Cooperative Oncology Group (ECOG), 130
eLecTRA trial, 195
electroacupuncture (EA), 270
EMILIA study, 197

ENCORE 301 trial, 185
endocrine therapy, 62–63
  duration, 177
  indications, 176–177
  positivity and response, 177
entinostat, 185
epirubicin, 289
estrogen receptor (ER) positivity, 85, 86
  early-stage invasive breast cancer, 137, 141
  metastatic breast cancer
    aromatase inhibitor, 178–181, 183–184
    cyclin-dependent kinase inhibitor,
      184–185
    estrogen therapy, 182
    HDAC inhibitor, 185
    ovarian suppression/ablation, 182–183
    PI3K inhibitors, 184
    progestins, 181–182
    selective estrogen receptor modulators,
      178, 183
European Organisation for Research and
    Treatment of Cancer (EORTC)
    10853 trial, 54
European Organisation for Research and
    Treatment of Cancer (EORTC)
    22881-10882 trial, 99
European Organisation for Research and
    Treatment of Cancer (EORTC)
    22922 trial, 101
everolimus, 180
exemestane, 29, 180
ExteNET trial, 136
external radiation therapy (XRT), 53–54

F-18 fluoro-deoxyglucose positron emission
    tomography (F-18 FDG PET), 17
FACT trial, 180
FALCON trial, 180
fat grafting, 246
fatigue, 272, 292
Femara versus Anastrozole Clinical
    Evaluation (FACE) trial, 113
FIRST trial, 179
flat epithelial atypia (FEA)
  columnar cell change, 26
  histology, 26
  lifetime malignancy risk, 27
  surgical excision, 26
  treatment, 26
full field digital mammography (FFDM),
    4–6
fulvestrant, 179–180

GammaPod, 100–101
genetic counseling
  cancer predisposition, 257
  family history, 256–257
  genetic risk evaluation, 256
  informed consent, 256
Genetic Information Nondiscrimination
    Act (GINA), 259
genetic testing, 257–259
GeparQuinto, 141
graded prognostic assessment, 206, 207
granulocyte colony stimulating factor
    (G-CSF), 226–227, 294
grayscale ultrasound, 2, 9
Grupo Español de Investigación del Cáncer
    de Mama (GEICAM) trial, 143

Herceptin Adjuvant (HERA) trial, 131
hereditary breast cancer syndromes
  BRCA1 and *BRCA2*, 251–254
  Cowden syndrome, 255
  genetic counseling, 256–257
  genetic testing, 257–259
  hereditary diffuse gastric cancer
      syndrome, 254–255
  insurance protection, 259
  Li–Fraumeni syndrome, 255–256
hereditary diffuse gastric cancer syndrome
    (HDGC), 254–255
high-risk breast disease
  atypical ductal hyperplasia, 22–23
  atypical lobular hyperplasia, 23–24
  chemoprevention, 28–29
  flat epithelial atypia, 26–27
  lobular carcinoma in situ, 24–26
  prevention trials, 29–35
  prophylactic mastectomy, 35
  surveillance, 35
histone deacetylase (HDAC) inhibitor, 185
HORIZON trial, 181
hormonal therapy. *See also* neoadjuvant
    hormonal therapy
  aromatase inhibitors, 110–113
  CDK inhibitor, 184–185
  endocrine therapy, 106, 109, 176–178
  HDAC inhibitor, 185
  HER2 therapy, 195
  musculoskeletal symptoms, 294–295
  ovarian ablation and suppression,
      113–114
  PI3K inhibitor, 184
  postmenopausal women

aromatase inhibitor, 178–181
    estrogen therapy, 182
    progestins, 181–182
    SERMs, 178
  pregnancy-associated breast cancer, 227
  premenopausal women
    aromatase inhibitors, 183–184
    cyclin-dependent kinase inhibitor, 184
    ovarian suppression/ablation, 182–183
    SERMs, 183
  recommendations, 115–121
  sequential lines, 177–178
  tamoxifen therapy, 109–110
hot flash, 297
human epidermal growth factor receptor 2
    (HER2) positivity
  early-stage invasive breast cancer
    ado-trastuzumab emtansine, 138
    chemotherapy regimens, 134–135
    lapatinib, 135–136
    neoadjuvant chemotherapy, 141,
      144–145
    neratinib, 136
    pertuzumab, 135
  immunohistochemistry, 87
  invasive BC, 86–87
  metastatic breast cancer
    BOLERO-1 study, 199–200
    and chemotherapy, 195–199
    fluorescence in situ hybridization, 87
    and hormone therapy, 195
    overexpression, 190
    trastuzumab and pertuzumab, 199
    triple-positive ER/PR/HER2+ MBC,
      190, 195
  testing guidelines, 87
hypofractionation, 61

implant-based reconstruction
  acellular dermal matrix sling, 234
  advantages, 235
  breast implants, 233–234
  capsular contracture, 235–236
  direct-to-implant reconstruction, 237–238
  disadvantages, 235
  implant rupture, 237
  infection, 235
  mastectomy flap ischemia, 236
  selection, 232–233
  seroma, 236–237
  surveillance, 237
  tissue expanders, 233

  visible rippling/wrinkling, 237
infertility, 296–297
intensity-modulated radiation therapy
    (IMRT), 98
Intergroup Exemestane Study (IES), 112
internal mammary node radiation,
    102–104
International Breast Cancer Intervention
    Study I (IBIS-I), 30
  design, 29
  hazard ratio, 29
  risk reduction, 29, 32
  side effects, 32
International Breast Cancer Intervention
    Study II (IBIS-II), 31, 34
International Breast Cancer Study Group
    (IBCSG)-24-01 trial, 93
intraductal papilloma (IP)
  histology, 27
  lifetime malignancy risk, 28
  surgical excision, 27
  treatment, 28
intrauterine growth retardation (IUGR),
    224
invasive ductal carcinoma (IDC), 81
invasive lobular carcinoma (ILC), 82–83

Ki-67 proliferative index, 88

LANDSCAPE study, 197
lapatinib, 135–136, 141, 197–198, 290
lapatinib and trastuzumab combination
    therapy, 141
Li–Fraumeni syndrome, 255–256
lobular carcinoma in situ (LCIS)
  histology, 24
  lifetime malignancy risk, 26
  pleomorphic, 25
  small monotonous dyscohesive cells, 25
  surgical excision, 24–25
  treatment, 25
lumpectomy cavity boost irradiation,
    99–100
lymphedema, 271–272, 294

magnetic resonance imaging (MRI)
  biopsy, 13
  contraindications, 7
  gadolinium-based agents, 7
  patient surveillance, 17

magnetic resonance imaging (MRI) (*cont.*)
  recommendations, 7, 8
  sensitivity and specificity, 7, 17
  staging evaluation, 15, 16
  technique, 7
  technology, 7
major depressive disorder, 293
MammaPrint trials
  EORTC 10041 and BIG 3-04, 125
  MINDACT, 125
  RASTER study, 124
  Symphony trial, 125
  TransBig trial, 124–125
Mammary Prevention 3 (MAP3) trial, 31, 34
mammography, 1
  breast composition, 5–6
  digital breast tomosynthesis, 6
  mortality reduction, 4
  patient surveillance, 17
  staging evaluation, 15
  2D mammography, 4–6
  uncertainty, 44
MARIANNE trial, 197
massage, 275
mastectomy
  ductal carcinoma in situ, 54–55
  local–regional relapse risk factors,
    149–151
  modified radical, 91
  nipple-sparing, 91
  simple, 90
  skin-sparing, 91
mastectomy flap ischemia, 236
medroxyprogesterone acetate, 181–182
medullary carcinoma, 83
megestrol acetate, 181–182
metastatic breast cancer (MBC)
  antiresorptive therapy, 200–202
  bone metastases, 209
  brain metastases, 206–208
  chemotherapy, 186–194
  choice of therapy, 175
  5-year survival, 174
  follow-up, 175
  genomic tumor tissue testing, 175
  HER2 positivity, 190, 195–200
  history and physical exam, 174–175
  hormone therapy, 176–185
  imaging, 175
  laboratory examination, 175
  local–regional therapy, 204
  oligometastatic disease, 202–206

  spinal cord compression, 209
  therapy response and duration, 176
  tissue diagnosis, 174
  triple-positive ER/PR/HER2+, 190, 195
MIcroarray for 0–3 Node+ Disease
    may Avoid Chemotherapy Trial
    (MINDACT), 125
microarRAy-prognoSTics-in-breast-cancER
    (RASTER) study, 124
micropapillary ductal carcinoma in situ, 51
mind–body therapies, 268–269, 275
mindfulness-based stress reduction
    (MBSR), 269
mucinous carcinoma, 83, 84
Multiple Outcomes of Raloxifene
    Evaluation (MORE), 30, 33
musculoskeletal pain/symptoms, 294–296

National Cancer Institute (NCI), 286
National Comprehensive Cancer Network
    (NCCN), 1, 255, 286
National Surgical Adjuvant Breast and
    Bowel Project (NSABP) B-06 trial,
    95
National Surgical Adjuvant Breast and Bowel
    Project (NSABP) B-17 trial, 53
National Surgical Adjuvant Breast and
    Bowel Project (NSABP) B-20 trial,
    123
National Surgical Adjuvant Breast and
    Bowel Project (NSABP) B-21 trial,
    95–96
National Surgical Adjuvant Breast and Bowel
    Project (NSABP) B-32 trial, 93
National Surgical Adjuvant Breast and Bowel
    Project (NSABP) B-33 trial, 112
National Surgical Adjuvant Breast and
    Bowel Project, Prevention-1
    (NSABP P-1), 30, 32
needle biopsy, 13, 14
neoadjuvant chemotherapy (NACT)
  benefits, 138
  clinical trials for radiation after, 151
  CTNeoBC, 140
  I-SPY 1 trial, 139
  locally advanced breast cancer, 138
  NEOSPHERE, 142
  proliferative index, 138
  receptor status
    HER2-negative neoadjuvant regimens,
      143

HER2-positive neoadjuvant regimens,
144–145
HR+ HER2– BC, 140
TNBC, 140–141
NeOAdjuvant Herceptin (NOAH) study,
141
neoadjuvant hormonal therapy (NAHT)
ACOSOG Z1031, 146
assessment of response, 146–147
duration, 146
GEICAM trial, 143
IMPACT trial, 146
vs. NACT, 143
patient selection, 146
PEPI score, 147
PROACT trial, 146
P024 trial, 146
Neoadjuvant Study of Pertuzumab +
Herceptin in an Early Regimen
Evaluation (NEOSPHERE), 142
neoadjuvant therapy (NST)
ACOSOG Z1031 trial, 147
axillary lymph nodes, 148
clinically positive lymph nodes prior to,
148–149
inflammatory breast cancer, 148
NSABP B-18 trial, 147
radiation, 149
neratinib, 136
neuropathy, 296
nipple discharge, 11
nipple-sparing mastectomy (NSM), 245,
246
ductal carcinoma in situ, 55
implant reconstruction, 91
nodal status, 81

oncoplastic reconstruction
delayed immediate reconstruction, 243
delayed reconstruction, 243
fat grafting, 246
fat necrosis, 241
immediate reconstruction, 243
lumpectomy, 242
nipple reconstruction, 244–246
radiation therapy, 243–244
unilateral reconstruction, 246, 247
volume-removal procedures, 240–242
volume-replacement techniques, 242
Oncotype Dx trials, 123–124
organic foods, breast cancer risk, 266
ovarian ablation and suppression, 113–114,
182–183

PALOMA-2 trial, 181
partial breast irradiation, 100
Patient Protection and Affordable Care Act
(PPACA), 259
PATRICIA trial, 198
pertuzumab, 135, 142
pertuzumab-induced cardiac toxicity,
290
phyllodes tumors (PTs)
benign, 40
borderline, 41
chemotherapy, 43, 46
clinical presentation, 39
diagnosis, 41
epidemiology, 39
vs. fibroadenomas, 39
leaf-like architecture, 40–41
malignant, 40, 41
pathologic classification, 39–40
pathology, 39
prognosis, 42
radiation therapy, 42–45
wide local excision, 41–42
physical activity recommendations,
267–268, 275
PI3K inhibitors, 184
pleomorphic lobular carcinoma, 82
positron emission tomography–computed
tomography (PET–CT), 15–16
postmastectomy radiation (PMRT),
102–104
power Doppler, 9
pregnancy-associated breast cancer
(PABCa)
breast examination, 223
chemotherapy, 225–227
epidemiology, 223–224
fetal risks, 224–225
hormonal therapy, 227
incidence, 223
risk factors, 223
surgery, 227–228
Preoperative Endocrine Prognostic Index
(PEPI score), 147
PRIME II study, 96
progesterone receptor (PR), 85
progestins, 181–182
prophylactic mastectomy, 35
Protocol for Herceptin as Adjuvant therapy
with Reduced Exposure (PHARE)
trial, 131, 134
proton radiotherapy, 103
P024 trial, 146

qigong, 269

radiotherapy
    cardiotoxicity, 290–291
    deep inspiratory breath-hold, 96–97
    ductal carcinoma in situ (DCIS), 59
    GammaPod, 100–101
    intensity-modulated radiation therapy, 98
    internal mammary node radiation,
        102–104
    large node negative breast cancer, 104
    lumpectomy cavity boost irradiation,
        99–100
    node-positive cancer, 101–102
    oncoplastic reconstruction, 243–244
    partial breast irradiation, 100
    phyllodes tumors, 42–45
    postmastectomy radiation, 102–105
    whole breast irradiation, 98–99
raloxifene, 28
Royal Marsden Trial, 30, 32–33

SEER Medicare analyses, 290
selective estrogen receptor modulators
        (SERMs), 28–29
    postmenopausal women, 178
    premenopausal women, 183
SENTINA trial, 149
sentinel lymph node biopsy (SLNB)
    axillary lymph node dissection, 92
    clinically negative axillary lymph nodes,
        93–94
    clinically positive axillary lymph nodes,
        94
    ductal carcinoma in situ, 55
    patient eligibility, 92
    pregnancy-associated breast cancer,
        227–228
    technique, 92
SERM Clinical Trials Meta-Analysis, 34–35
skin-sparing mastectomy (SSM), 54–55, 91,
        245, 246
sleep disorders, 293–294
SoFEA trial, 180
soy isoflavones, breast cancer risk, 267
spinal cord compression, 209
stereotactic biopsy, 12–13
Study of Tamoxifen and Raloxifene (STAR)
        P-2, 31, 33–34
sugar, breast cancer risk, 266–267
Suppression of Ovarian Function Trial
        (SOFT), 113

survivorship
    anxiety, 293
    cancer recurrence, 286–287
    cardiotoxicity, 288–291
    care planning, 298
    cognitive impairment, 291–292
    depression, 292–293
    distress, 292
    fatigue, 292
    infertility, 296–297
    lymphedema, 294
    musculoskeletal pain/symptoms,
        294–296
    second primary cancer screening,
        287–288
    sexual side effects, 297–298
    sleep disorders, 293–294
    vasomotor symptoms, 297
SWOG 0226 trial, 180
SWOG 8814 trial, 123
SWOG S0221 trial, 130
Symphony trial, 125
systemic adjuvant therapy
    BC mortality rates, 106
    chemotherapy
        CMF and AC, 126
        HER2-positive disease, 130–135
        MammaPrint trials, 124–125
        Oncotype Dx trials, 123–124
        regimens, 126–128
        side effects, 114
        taxane, 129, 130
        triple negative breast cancer, 136–137
        triplets and dose dense, 129–130
        tumor genomic multigene assays,
            121–123
    clinicopathologic factors, 107–108
    guidelines, 106
    hormonal therapy
        aromatase inhibitors, 110–113
        endocrine therapy, 106, 109
        ovarian ablation and suppression,
            113–114
        recommendations, 115–121
        tamoxifen therapy, 109–110
    tumor genomic factors, 107–108

tai chi, 269
Tamoxifen and Exemestane Trial (TEXT),
        113
Tamoxifen Exemestane Adjuvant
        Multinational (TEAM), 112, 297

tamoxifen therapy, 28
  ATLAS trial, 110
  ductal carcinoma in situ, 63
  EBCTCG trial, 109
  with everolimus, 180
  NSABP B-14 trial, 109–110
  postmenopausal women, 178
  pregnancy-associated breast cancer, 227
  premenopausal women, 183
  recurrence rate, 109
  side effects, 110
TAMRAD trial, 180
TAnDEM trial, 195
target of rapamycin (mTOR) inhibitor, 180
temsirolimus, 181
TH3RESA study, 196
tissue expanders, 233
toremifene, 178
total skin-sparing mastectomies (TSSMs), 246
traditional Chinese medicine (TCM), 269
transarterial chemoembolization (TACE), 205–206
TransBig trial, 124–125
trastuzumab-induced cardiac toxicity, 289–290
Trastuzumab+Pertuzumab in Neoadjuvant HER2-Positive Breast Cancer (TRYEPHENA), 142, 290
Trial Assigning Individualized Options in Treatment (TAILORx), 123

tubular carcinoma, 83
2D mammography, 4–6
Tykerb Evaluation After Chemotherapy (TEACH), 135

UK/ANZ DCIS trial, 64–65
UK Standardization of Breast Radiotherapy (START) A and START B trials, 98–99
ultrasound
  biopsy, 12
  color Doppler, 9
  elastography, 9
  grayscale, 2, 9
  guidelines, 10
  and mammography, 9–10
  patient surveillance, 17
  power Doppler, 9
  technique, 9
usual ductal hyperplasia (UDH), 22

Van Nuys Predictive Index, 57
volume-replacement techniques, 240–242

whole breast irradiation, 98–99

yoga, 269

zoledronic acid, 294